THE WONDERFUL WORLD OF JAMES HERRIOT

THE WONDERFUL WORLD OF

JAMES HERRIOT

Introduction by
Jim Wight and Rosie Page

EDITED BY EMMA MARRIOTT

MACMILLAN

First published 2022 by Macmillan
an imprint of Pan Macmillan
The Smithson, 6 Briset Street, London EC1M 5NR
EU representative: Macmillan Publishers Ireland Ltd, 1st Floor,
The Liffey Trust Centre, 117–126 Sheriff Street Upper,
Dublin 1, D01 YC43
Associated companies throughout the world
www.panmacmillan.com

ISBN 978-1-0350-0853-7

1 3 5 7 9 8 6 4 2

A CIP catalogue record for this book is available from the British Library.

Internal illustrations by Claire Harrup

Typeset in Sabon LT Std by Palimpsest Book Production Ltd, Falkirk, Stirlingshire
Printed and bound by CPI Group (UK) Ltd, Croydon, CR0 4YY

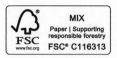

Visit **www.panmacmillan.com** to read more about all our books
and to buy them. You will also find features, author interviews and
news of any author events, and you can sign up for e-newsletters
so that you're always first to hear about our new releases.

To Mum and Dad – the best parents

Contents

INTRODUCTION

by Jim Wight and Rosie Page

Our father, James Alfred Wight, practised as a veterinary surgeon in Yorkshire for almost fifty years. He tended to the animals of his Thirsk practice around the clock, and later chronicled his experiences of veterinary practice, writing under the pen name of James Herriot. The love he had for his profession, along with the countryside around him and the people who lived there, fuelled his imagination and resulted in eight books, all of which sold in their millions around the world.

Literary success, however, didn't come to Alf Wight until he was in his fifties, as it was only then that he could set aside his evenings for writing. To us, he was simply a devoted father and a busy veterinary surgeon who spent long days and many nights driving around the hills of Yorkshire visiting his animal patients. As children, we often joined him on his farm visits, jumping into the car, always with a dog or two in the back, the cold, sweet-scented air of North Yorkshire all around. We didn't come just to watch, though, we were there to help – to open and close gates, run back and forth to the car to fetch syringes or penicillin, knowing exactly which packets to reach for before we could even read. Dad relished spending time with us, and we loved seeing him at work, so much so that we both ended up as medics with local practices – Jim as a veterinary surgeon working with Dad and Rosie as a GP in Thirsk.

From an early age, we both learned invaluable lessons about animals, not least that sows can be fearsome creatures, as thirteen-year-old Jim discovered when he was trapped in a sty and one came roaring towards him, only to have Dad holler: 'You have got to get in and out quickly! It's no good being frightened of the bloody things!' The odd escaped cow presented a similar risk, proving that animals are nothing if not unpredictable – mishaps that would later feature in Dad's books! But we loved it all and for a small child nothing can match the thrill of holding a new-born lamb or discovering a litter of kittens in some straw or puppies in a basket. Just as Dad spent hours driving around the hills of North Yorkshire, so did we, first as passengers in a variety of aged cars – often having to jump out of our Austin A70 so Dad could coax it up the notoriously steep Sutton Bank – and then as teenagers, both of us learning to drive as we bumped along farm tracks, taking Dad on his rounds.

Our father first arrived in the North Yorkshire town of Thirsk – fictionalized as Darrowby in his books – in 1940, and he lived and worked in the area for the rest of his life. He never lost his soft Glaswegian accent, however, having spent the previous twenty-three years in the Scottish city, at its schools and then at the Glasgow Veterinary College where he trained. Suddenly immersed in a rural world, he witnessed a community on the cusp of change, when rural vets spent much of their days out and about on small family farms, tending to cows in cobbled byres, birthing sheep in open fields or chasing piglets, reared for the Yorkshire delicacy of fatty bacon, around in rickety tin sheds. Working all hours, he met an array of unforgettable characters, principal of whom was his long-time practice partner Donald Sinclair, immortalized in the books as Siegfried Farnon.

While his job demanded much of his time, and was physically exhausting, our father had for many years dreamed of writing and putting his experiences down on paper: the Yorkshire he had grown to love, the quirky people he had met, the array of animals he treated and the vast changes he had seen in veterinary practice. He had always been a voracious reader; his school diaries and letters as a young man are full of the kind of colourful and humorous descriptions that he would utilize to such great effect in his later books.

It took a long twenty years, however, for him to turn his dream of writing a book into reality. At first, he wrote short stories on various topics, treating his writing largely as a hobby, tapping away at his typewriter in the evenings. After some gentle prodding from our mother, he decided, in 1965, to focus on writing a full-length book about a world he knew: veterinary practice. Over the next eighteen months, still working full-time and often at night, he crafted a novel based on his experiences. Entitling it *The Art and Science*, he sent it off to the publisher Collins. Ultimately Collins turned it down for publication but he received an encouraging reply from one of their readers, Juliana Wadham, who gave him a crucial piece of advice. As his stories were clearly based on his own life and real events, why not write it in the first person as a semi-autobiographical work?

Dad took to the idea enthusiastically and he immediately set about reworking his book into an account of his first year in veterinary practice. By the summer of 1968, it was finished, with a new title of *If Only They Could Talk*, as suggested by a local dairy farmer and friend of Dad's, Arthur Dand. Surprisingly, Collins turned the book down again, much to

Juliana Wadham's disappointment. Their loss, however, would turn into another publisher's gain, when Michael Joseph accepted the book for publication. The only change they required was that he alter his pen name from James Walsh, who was a real person on the veterinary register. Dad kept 'James' but came up with the alternative 'Herriot', inspired by the Birmingham City and future Scotland goal-keeper Jim Herriot. He considered himself first and foremost a veterinary surgeon, which is why he went to some lengths to preserve his anonymity as an author, not only changing his name but setting the story in the Yorkshire Dales, thirty miles from Thirsk, and in 1937 rather than 1940 when he really arrived.

If Only They Could Talk introduced Darrowby, the Yorkshire Dales, James's erratic partner Siegfried and his younger brother Tristan, and many of the extraordinary individuals that would populate the James Herriot books. Descriptions are vivid, characters and dialogue brilliantly drawn, the language light and accessible, with stories that are by turns hilarious and incredibly touching. Most of the tales in the book are based on real events and are reproduced just as they happened. Like James Herriot, Alf fell asleep under an acacia tree in the garden of the practice while waiting for his interview; he too treated an indulged Pekinese dog with 'flop-bott'; Siegfried's arguments with his brother were just as explosive and the dialogue true to the word; and Tristan really did prang his brother's beloved Rover – and the list goes on. Some of the incidents and events may have been combined but the vast majority were based on real cases and many of them, such as the first calving story in the book – Dad face down on a cold floor, his arm deep in a straining cow for seemingly hours, without being offered so much as a cup of tea afterwards – we remember Dad telling us, much to our and his amusement.

Introduction

The first James Herriot book was published in the UK in April 1970. While our father was thrilled, he was also nervous about how some people would react to being portrayed in the book, not wanting to upset friends or clients. He often changed their names and occasionally their gender in a bid to disguise their real identity, while some characters combined the traits of several individuals. Sometimes this worked but his descriptions and characters were often so well drawn that people couldn't help but recognize themselves or others in the books. Generally, people were flattered to be included; some were even annoyed if they weren't, as was the case with Mr Smedley, a little old man who came into the practice one day waving his stick and shouting: 'Why haven't you put me in your books, Mr Wight?'

Sales for the first book were steady but not meteoric in the first few months after publication. We were both in our twenties by this time. Jim, having graduated in veterinary science from the University of Glasgow, had been working with our father at the Thirsk practice for three years, while Rosie, who had studied medicine at Cambridge, had just begun her first job as a junior doctor at the Raigmore Hospital in Inverness. At that point, no one at the hospital had heard of the name James Herriot. Rosie once lent a copy of *If Only They Could Talk* to the hospital librarian, Malize McBride, who was married to Hamish, one of the doctors there. Rosie remembers Hamish coming into breakfast the following morning and cursing her to the heights because his wife had read the book right through the night, waking him up intermittently by laughing so much – the story of James dressed up in the ridiculous rubber suit when cleansing a cow had reduced her to tears of laughter. Hamish, however, got his own back when he read the book the following night and kept her awake with his chuckling!

This of course all boded well for Dad's book. We knew it was good and immensely entertaining but we had no idea then just how much people would grow to love his stories and what the future held in store. Dad was simply happy to have fulfilled his dream of having a book published. At the time, we'd sit in the kitchen and joke with Dad, saying, OK, now you've had a book published, why not do a film? We'd roar with laughter about who might play him and I think we agreed that the smooth-voiced Leslie Phillips could be perfect for Siegfried. To us, this was just a bit of fun and a million miles away from our day-to-day lives – little did we know this would all play out in reality.

Towards the end of 1970 *If Only They Could Talk* was reprinted and the publishers asked Dad whether he'd consider writing a follow-up. Having enjoyed writing the first book so much, he'd already begun working on a second manuscript, entitled *It Shouldn't Happen to a Vet,* which was duly delivered and published in January 1972. As with the first book, the *London Evening Standard* serialized it, boosting sales, and Michael Joseph committed to a bigger print run. This book covered Dad's second year in practice and included the array of personalities and the charming humour that worked so well in the first book, although it introduced a new character: our mother, Joan Danbury, renamed as Helen Alderson. While our mother was happiest out of the spotlight, she was perfectly content to feature in the book. She wasn't a farmer's daughter as Helen is, but so much else about their first few months together is true: the chaotic first dates, their small wedding in Thirsk and a working honeymoon testing cattle for tuberculin amid the grassy, meadow-sweet hills of the Dales.

A third book, *Let Sleeping Vets Lie*, was published in April 1973 and flew off the shelves, rapidly rising to the top of the bestseller lists. *Vet in Harness* followed in 1974 and by the time *Vets Might Fly* was published in 1976 Michael Joseph were printing in the region of 60,000 hardback copies, as they did for *Vet in a Spin* in 1977. Now James Herriot was a household name and paperback sales of the books were spectacular; by 1979 each of the first six books had sold more than a million copies – an achievement only then matched by Ian Fleming, the author of the James Bond series.

Having worked long hours throughout his life, just about keeping his head above water, the financial rewards of Dad's success were welcome, principally because he no longer had to worry about money – although it never motivated him. He continued to run the Thirsk practice with Jim, who as a qualified veterinary surgeon had joined in 1967; we were all leading busy lives and Dad's books were just one of many issues we discussed as a family. If he was reading the newspaper, he might mention that one of his books was at the top of the bestseller list, but before anyone had time to respond he'd have moved on to why Sunderland FC hadn't beaten Wolverhampton the previous Saturday. He and his day-to-day life remained largely unaltered by his success.

By 1980 there were few households that didn't have at least one copy of the James Herriot books on their shelves; the readership spanned all ages and backgrounds and prompted a surge in applications to study veterinary science. The love for Dad's books was not just limited to the UK: they also sold well in Europe, Canada, Australia and Japan, and were hugely popular in the United States. There, the first two books were combined into one omnibus edition, entitled *All Creatures Great and Small* and published in November 1972. The book rocketed into the bestseller list and by the end of 1973 paperback sales in the US had reached a million copies. The subsequent four books were also combined into two volumes and sales were equally as impressive, catapulting our father to worldwide fame. While Dad was naturally excited that so many people enjoyed his stories, he was not comfortable with the media attention that was suddenly focused on him. He turned down countless television interviews and public appearances and even kept his face off the books as much as possible. In 1973 he was persuaded to tour the US twice, flying from city to city for book signings and television appearances. It made for a wonderful experience, but he was always pleased to be back in Yorkshire, and by the time he returned from his second tour in the autumn of 1973 he was so drained, and in fact ill with bronchitis, that he vowed never to do another tour: 'I love America and its people but I'm not going back, just yet . . .' and he never did return.

Jim was also pleased to have Dad back home, largely because the Thirsk practice was so busy. While Dad was working on his books, Jim shared many of the night call-outs with the practice assistants so that Dad could concentrate on daytime shifts and his writing, but Dad always prioritized his work as a veterinary surgeon. By then, throngs of tourists from across the globe had begun turning up at 23 Kirkgate, with queues snaking down the street on the two afternoons our father set aside to sign books and speak to visitors. While Jim may have grumbled a little at the distraction, Dad felt he owed as much to his fans, especially those who had travelled from as far away as the US to come and see him. As the queue grew, he also decided to set up a collection for a stray-dog sanctuary, the Jerry Green Foundation Trust, which under the leadership of Sister Ann Lilley (Sister Rose in the books) features in *The Lord God Made Them All*.

While visitors to the practice were principally there to see the real James Herriot, and were often overcome with excitement to meet him – which always bemused Dad – they were also delighted if Donald Sinclair (better known to them as Siegfried) made an appearance. This of course tickled us as, since we had grown up in and around the practice, Donald and his younger brother Brian (on whom Tristan was based) were like family. They were a constant presence in our lives, Donald was Jim's godfather and we always referred to him and his wife as 'Uncle Donald and Auntie Audrey'.

Because Jim worked alongside our father and Donald, he had a taste of rural veterinary practice as it had been for Dad. As a result, quite a few stories from the first six books were experienced by Jim and related to Dad afterwards. Dad was continually on the lookout for fresh stories and he asked Jim and others at the Thirsk practice to remember anything interesting that happened to them on their rounds. He would jot the details down in notebooks, his writing virtually indecipherable to anyone else, distilling them into simple headings to which he'd repeatedly refer as he wrote.

By 1975 the idea we once laughed about – seeing Dad's book on the big screen – turned into reality when the first movie of *All Great Creatures Great and Small*, originally made for a US audience, was released in cinemas in the UK. With Simon Ward playing Dad and Anthony Hopkins starring as Siegfried, Dad was thrilled, if not a little astonished to see his little stories set in Yorkshire in movie theatres. Another film, *It Shouldn't Happen to a Vet*, followed in 1976, this time with John Alderton as James Herriot and Colin Blakely as Siegfried. Two years later the BBC aired the first television series of *All Creatures Great and Small*. Shot in the Yorkshire Dales, it went on to become a huge hit, adored by fans of all ages and regularly attracting 15 million viewers each week. Broadcast from 1978 to 1990, the seven series featured the virtually unknown

Christopher Timothy as Dad, the much-esteemed Robert Hardy as Siegfried, the future Doctor Who, Peter Davison, as Tristan, and Carol Drinkwater and then Lynda Bellingham played Helen. Once again, visitors poured into the Yorkshire Dales and Thirsk, both from the UK and across the world, and that area of North Yorkshire was soon labelled as 'Herriot Country'. As various small businesses popped up bearing the Herriot name, it gradually dawned upon us that people were latching on to Dad's success, that his books were drawing people in from far and wide. Dad simply took it in his stride and paid little attention to that kind of thing, although he was amused by one brochure he saw: 'Come to our hotel, deep in the Yorkshire Dales, home of James Herriot, the world's most famous vet . . . No pets.'

While most around Thirsk knew that Alf Wight was the man behind James Herriot, many of his fans were unaware that Herriot wasn't the author's real name, although his fame had grown to such an extent that a letter sent in the 1970s to 'James Herriot, Vet, England' still somehow made its way to the practice, albeit with various possible locations scratched out and a jokey note from our postman reading: 'It shouldn't happen to a postman . . .' Awards and honours also began to flood in for Dad, including an OBE in February 1979 followed by an invitation to join Her Majesty the Queen for lunch later in the year, where he learned that the Queen, a renowned animal lover, was a fan of his books and known to 'laugh out loud' when reading them. In 1982 he received the Fellowship of the Royal College of Veterinary Surgeons, of which he was particularly proud and in 1984 he won the Yorkshire Salver in recognition of his services to Yorkshire. In 1991 he was also offered the honorary position of Life President of the Sunderland Football Club. Having been a keen football and club supporter all his life, he regarded this honour as particularly pleasing but preferred not to sit in the directors' box, instead continuing to sit among the crowd in the terraces where he could soak up the atmosphere.

Dad continued to work full-time right up to 1980 when he was almost sixty-five years old. Unlike other bestselling authors, he chose not to move abroad, which meant that the bulk of his earnings went into Her Majesty's coffers in the form of tax. He was never a greedy man and maintained, 'I love living in Yorkshire among my friends and family', and that was that. While he was immensely proud of his literary achievements, he always knew what made him happiest and was unaltered by the success he achieved, writing in 1980: 'In my early days as a young vet with a family I had either to work round the clock or starve but it was during those hard days when I spent every waking hour dashing about the countryside usually with my children in the car that happiness seemed to steal up behind me and tap me on the shoulder.'

The seventh James Herriot book, *The Lord God Made Them All*, was published in 1981 and went on to become a major bestseller both in the UK and US. That year, Dad decided to put down his pen and focus on his life in North Yorkshire, keen to spend more time with the family, his grandchildren in whom he always delighted, and the dogs who were his constant companions throughout his life. Five years later, he was persuaded to write some new material for the television series of *All Creatures Great and Small*, which led eventually to the publication of his final book *Every Living Thing* in 1992. The long-awaited return of James Herriot proved to be another hit.

Despite his huge success as a writer, Dad was, however, happiest when he was at home in Yorkshire and considered himself fortunate to have hit upon a profession he loved, always maintaining that he was 'ninety-nine per cent vet and one per cent author'. As much as he loved writing and being a published author he preferred to be treated simply as the local vet, recognizing that many of his clients had little time for books. As he put it, 'The farmers round here couldn't care less about my book-writing activities. If one of them has a cow with its calf bed hanging out, he doesn't want to see Charles Dickens rolling up!' The reality was, however, that many of the local farmers read his books and enjoyed them, and they were quietly proud to have James Herriot as their vet but they were not the type to gush about his achievements, which suited Dad very well. Whereas American fans were vocal in their adulation, the Yorkshire community around him were more reserved, although they derived pleasure in having a bestselling author in their midst. Throughout the twenty years that Rosie worked as a GP in Thirsk, it was a rare day that anyone referred to her being the daughter of a famous author – as far as the local community was concerned, Alf Wight and his family were just one of them.

Dad always felt fortunate to have met so many interesting people through his work and they in turn enriched his life. His stories are full of the characters he met – the farmers who have long since gone, as well as Donald and Brian Sinclair, who are pivotal to the books. The pair could be frustrating and chaotic, but both were skilled veterinary surgeons, very funny and always good company, and many stories in Dad's books revolved around them. Dad remained good friends with them throughout his life, and both were just as characterful in later years.

Growing up with Dad and working in the same community to which he dedicated his life means we know well the people and places on which all the classic James Herriot books are based. This book contains some of our favourite stories from the series – many of which we still laugh about, and we still see several of the families and former clients of Dad and Jim as we walk around Thirsk today. Creating this book has rekindled precious memories, of the small farms that once dotted the landscape, the wonderful animals, and of a bygone world, all of which Dad brought alive with such skill and tenderness that we wish we'd told him more often just how glorious a writer he was.

Chapter 1

JAMES HERRIOT

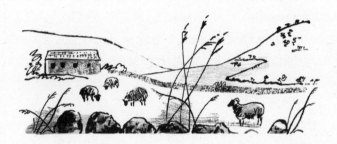

Farnon guided me to a seat, ordered two beers and turned to face me. 'Well, you can have this job if you want it. Four quid a week and full board. OK?'

The suddenness struck me silent. I was in. And four pounds a week! I remembered the pathetic entries in the *Record*. 'Veterinary surgeon, fully experienced, will work for keep.'

The BVMA had had to put pressure on the editor to stop him printing these cries from the heart. It hadn't looked so good to see members of the profession offering their services free. Four pounds a week was affluence.

'Thank you,' I said, trying hard not to look triumphant. 'I accept.'

'Good.' Farnon took a hasty gulp at his beer. 'Let me tell you about the practice. I bought it a year ago from an old man of eighty. Still practising, mind you, a real tough old character. But he'd got past getting up in the middle of the night, which isn't surprising. And, of course, in lots of other ways he had let things slide — hanging on to all the old ideas. Some of those ancient instruments in the surgery were his. One way and another, there was hardly any practice left and I'm trying to work it up again now. There's very little profit in it so far, but if we stick in for a few years, I'm confident we'll have a good business. The farmers are pleased to see a younger man taking over and they welcome new treatments and operations. But I'm having to educate them out of the three and sixpenny consulting fee the old chap used to charge and it's been a hard slog. These Dalesmen are wonderful people and you'll like them, but they don't like parting with their brass unless you can prove they are getting something in return.'

James Herriot is delighted to accept the position of assistant to veterinary surgeon Siegfried Farnon MRCVS, owner of a practice in the Yorkshire market town of Darrowby. Earlier that day, on a sunny June morning in 1937, the newly qualified vet had made his first trip to the Yorkshire Dales. Arriving at Skeldale House for his interview, Siegfried had shown James around the practice before taking the wheel of his battered Hillman for a whirlwind tour of the local farms. They are now enjoying a drink at a village pub, where Siegfried gives James a quick rundown of the job and the challenges of veterinary work in the Dales.

James jumps at the chance of a job, not only because he's taken an instant liking to the erratic but charming Siegfried and to the breathtaking scenery of Yorkshire, but also because he knows he's lucky to be offered a position. As the real James Herriot, James Alfred Wight, put it, 'the depression of the thirties was still lying over our profession like a dark blanket and jobs were desperately scarce. For every vacant appointment advertised in the *Veterinary Record*, there were eighty applicants and for those who did manage to find a post, the remuneration was often pitiful.' On top of this, the draught horse, once the mainstay of veterinary work, was rapidly disappearing in the towns and rural areas, so the young vet was entering a challenging world.

Later in *It Shouldn't Happen to a Vet* James muses on how he came to Yorkshire and what led him to become a veterinary surgeon. He envisaged a very different life to the one he has, his workplace now the fells and dales of Yorkshire, dressed 'in shirt sleeves and Wellingtons, smelling vaguely of cows'.

> I could remember the very moment. I was thirteen and I was reading an article about careers for boys in the *Meccano Magazine* and as I read, I felt a surging conviction that this was for me. And yet what was it based upon? Only that I liked dogs and cats and didn't care much for the idea of an office life; it seemed a frail basis on which to build a career. I knew nothing about agriculture or about farm animals and though, during the years in college, I learned about these things I could see only one future for myself; I was going to be a small animal surgeon. This lasted right up to the time I qualified – a kind of vision of treating people's pets in my own animal hospital where everything would be not just modern but revolutionary. The fully equipped operating theatre, laboratory and X-ray room; they had all stayed crystal clear in my mind until I had graduated MRCVS.

An article in the *Meccano Magazine* had similarly caught the eye of Alf Wight when he was a pupil of Hillhead High School in Glasgow. He was a keen subscriber of the magazine and often read the 'What Shall I Be?' series, which included a feature on veterinary science as a career. That glimmer of interest was then sparked further when the principal of Glasgow Veterinary

College, Dr A. W. Whitehouse, gave a talk at his school and invited any of those interested to visit the college. Alf followed up the invitation, talked further to the principal, and decided there and then that veterinary practice was the profession for him.

It was an unusual choice for a thirteen-year-old boy who had grown up in the city streets of Glasgow and knew nothing about horses or agricultural life. He was born in Sunderland on 3 October 1916 but his family had moved to Glasgow when he was just three weeks old, setting up their first home in a ground-floor apartment in the respectable working-class area of Yoker. His father, Jim Wight, worked in the shipyards on the River Clyde and his mother, Hannah Wight (née Bell), eventually set up a successful dressmaking business, which would keep the family afloat when Jim was later made redundant. Both were musical – his father an accomplished organist and pianist in local cinemas and theatres, and Hannah a gifted singer; Alf himself would inherit his parents' love for music.

While the teenage Alf knew little of country life, he had at the age of twelve acquired an Irish setter puppy, named Don, and there had always been cats in the family home. Don, however, was the main object of Alf's affection and together they would walk for hours in the city streets and parks, as well as in the Kilpatrick Hills and countryside surrounding Glasgow. The bond that existed between Alf and Don sparked a love for animals that Alf carried throughout his life and profession.

Alf determined upon getting the necessary grades to enter veterinary college, and he was always a diligent student, excelling particularly in English and Latin, less so in maths, with a great love for sport and music. He enjoyed his time at school, made friends easily and kept diaries, in which he poked fun at some of his teachers. With an already impish sense of humour and descriptive flair, he once wrote of his Latin master, 'Buckie was in a terrible mood today. Roaring and bellowing at us like a rogue elephant.' He also had a great enthusiasm for a number of pastimes, and loved to read, devouring the classics as well as the works of the great comic writer P. G. Wodehouse. His school career and indeed his life almost came to end when he caught the virulent disease of diphtheria in 1932, causing severe sore throat and headaches, along with painful abscesses all over his body. He recovered and emerged with a new lease of life, determined to embark upon a fitness regime he had read about, involving exercises and cold baths, which he followed religiously for several years. Whenever Alf set upon a new venture or pastime, he always applied himself with determination and enthusiasm and he liked to keep busy. Despite his illness, he left school on 29 June 1933 with the necessary grades to join Glasgow Veterinary College in September of that year, having obtained three Highers (Higher Education Leaving Certificates) in English, Latin and French. While modern veterinary students are expected to have a solid grounding in the sciences, the requirements for students in the 1930s were not so stringent.

When Alf first visited Glasgow Veterinary College as a schoolboy, he remembered Dr Whitehouse telling him that as a veterinary surgeon he would never grow rich but have a life of endless interest and variety. These words proved to be more true than Alf could ever have imagined and capture the spirit of the James Herriot books. The diverse nature of his work is certainly borne out across the series, most notably in *If Only They Could Talk* when James attends to the birth of piglets in a cold farmyard byre. Just hours before, he had attended a glittering party of another client, Mrs Pumphrey, owner of spoiled Pekinese Tricki Woo, where, dressed in black tie, he drank champagne and danced the night away. As he gets into bed that night, the music of the ballroom still in his head, the phone rings and it's Atkinson of Beck Cottage: 'I 'ave a sow 'ere what can't get pigged. She's been on all night. Will you come?'

'Let's have it, then.' I trained the feeble beam on my patient. 'Just a young pig, isn't she?'

'Aye, nobbut a gilt. Fust litter.'

The pig strained again, shuddered and lay still.

'Something stuck there, I reckon,' I said. 'Will you bring me a bucket of hot water, some soap and a towel, please?'

'Haven't got no 'ot water. Fire's out.'

'OK, bring me whatever you've got.'

The farmer clattered away down the byre taking the light with him and, with the darkness, the music came back again. It was a Strauss waltz and I was dancing with Lady Frenswick; she was young and very fair and she laughed as I swung her round. I could see her white shoulders and the diamonds winking at her throat and the wheeling mirrors.

Mr Atkinson came shuffling back and dumped a bucket of water on the floor. I dipped a finger in the water; it was ice cold. And the bucket had seen many hard years – I would have to watch my arms on that jagged rim.

Quickly stripping off my jacket and shirt, I sucked in my breath as a villainous draught blew through a crack on to my back.

'Soap, please,' I said through clenched teeth.

'In t'bucket.'

I plunged an arm into the water, shivered, and felt my way round till I found a roundish object about the size of a golf ball. I pulled it out and examined it; it was hard and smooth and speckled like a pebble from the seashore and, optimistically, I began to rub it between my hands and up my arms, waiting for the lather to form. But the soap was impervious; it yielded nothing.

I discarded the idea of asking for another piece in case this would be construed as another complaint. Instead, I borrowed the light and trekked down the byre into the yard, the mud sucking at my Wellingtons, goose pimples rearing on my chest. I searched around in the car boot, listening to my teeth chattering, till I came on a jar of antiseptic lubricating cream.

Back in the pen, I smeared the cream on my arm, knelt behind the pig and gently inserted my hand into the vagina. I moved my hand forward and as wrist and elbow disappeared inside the pig I was forced to roll over on my side. The stones were cold and wet but I forgot my discomfort when my fingers touched something; it was a tiny tail. Almost a transverse presentation, a biggish piglet stuck like a cork in a bottle.

Using one finger, I worked the hind legs back until I was able to grasp them and draw the piglet out. 'This is the one that's been causing the trouble. He's dead, I'm afraid — been squashed in there too long. But there could be some live ones still inside. I'll have another feel.'

I greased my arm and got down again. Just inside the os uteri, almost at arm's length, I found another piglet and I was feeling at the face when a set of minute but very sharp teeth sank into my finger.

I yelped and looked up at the farmer from my stony bed. 'This one's alive, anyway. I'll soon have him out.'

But the piglet had other ideas. He showed no desire to leave his warm haven and every time I got hold of his slippery little foot between my fingers he jerked it away. After a minute or two of this game I felt a cramping in my arm. I relaxed and lay back, my head resting on the cobbles, my arm still inside the pig. I closed my eyes and immediately I was back in the ball-room, in the warmth and the brilliant light. I was holding out my immense glass while François poured from the magnum; then I was dancing, close to the orchestra this time, and the leader, beating time with one hand, turned round and smiled into my face; smiled and bowed as though he had been looking for me all his life.

I smiled back but the bandleader's face dissolved and there was only Mr Atkinson looking down at me expressionlessly, his unshaven jaw and shaggy eyebrows thrown into sinister relief by the light striking up from the bicycle lamp.

I shook myself and raised my cheek from the floor. This wouldn't do. Falling asleep on the job; either I was very tired or there was still some champagne in me. I reached again and grasped the foot firmly between two fingers and this time, despite his struggles, the piglet was hauled out into the world. Once arrived, he seemed to accept the situation and tottered round philosophically to his mother's udder.

'She's not helping at all,' I said. 'Been on so long that she's exhausted. I'm going to give her an injection.'

Another numbing expedition through the mud to the car, a shot of pituitrin into the gilt's thigh and within minutes the action began with powerful contractions of the uterus. There was no obstruction now and soon a wriggling pink piglet was deposited in the straw; then quite quickly another and another.

'Coming off the assembly line now, all right,' I said. Mr Atkinson grunted.

Eight piglets had been born and the light from the lamp had almost given out when a dark mass of afterbirth welled from the gilt's vulva.

I rubbed my cold arms. 'Well, I should say that's the lot now.' I felt suddenly chilled; I couldn't say how long I had been standing there looking at the wonder that never grew stale: the little pigs struggling onto their legs and making their way unguided to the long double row of teats; the mother with her first family easing herself over to expose as much as possible of her udder to the hungry mouths.

Better get dressed quickly. I had another try at the marble-like soap but it defeated me as easily as the first time. I wondered how long it had been in the family. Down my right side my cheek and ribs were caked with dirt and mucus. I did my best to scrape some off with my fingernails, then I swilled myself down with the cold water from the bucket.

'Have you a towel there?' I gasped.

Mr Atkinson wordlessly handed me a sack. Its edges were stiff with old manure and it smelt musty from the meal it had long since contained. I took it and began to rub my chest and as the sour grains of the meal powdered my skin, the last bubbles of champagne left me, drifted up through the gaps in the tiles and burst sadly in the darkness beyond.

I dragged my shirt over my gritty back, feeling a sense of coming back to my own world. I buttoned my coat, picked up the syringe and the bottle of pituitrin and climbed out of the pen. I had a last look before I left. The bicycle lamp was shedding its final faint glow and I had to lean over the gate to see the row of little pigs sucking busily, utterly absorbed. The gilt carefully shifted her position and grunted. It was a grunt of deep content.

Yes, I was back and it was all right. I drove through the mud and up the hill where I had to get out to open a gate and the wind, with the cold, clean smell of the frosty grass in it, caught at my face. I stood for a while looking across the dark fields, thinking of the night which was ending now. My mind went back to my schooldays and an old gentleman talking to the class about careers. He had said: 'If you decide to become a veterinary surgeon you will never grow rich but you will have a life of endless interest and variety.'

I laughed aloud in the darkness and as I got into the car I was still chuckling. That old chap certainly wasn't kidding. Variety. That was it — variety.

On entering Glasgow Veterinary College, Alf had envisaged a career of looking after small animals, principally dogs. It soon became clear, however, that the college had other ideas.

And I knew exactly what kind of a dog doctor I would be. During the summer holidays between leaving school and going to the College, I carried a vision with me. I could see myself quite clearly, standing masked and gowned in a gleaming operating theatre. I was surrounded by nurses and on the table lay a dog which I was restoring to health by brilliant surgery. Or sometimes I was in a white coat under the spotless walls of a consulting room, ministering to a series of dogs, large, small, tail-wagging, woebegone, but all enchanting and all in need of my services. It was a heavenly prospect.

However, when I rolled up to the College with the new students to start the autumn term, I found that the authorities had no intention of encouraging me in my ambition. They had other plans for me. They were going to make me into a horse doctor.

Veterinary education had stood still despite the fundamental changes which were taking place and all our studies were geared to the horse. The order of priorities, as set out, was quite clear. Horse, ox, sheep, pig, dog. It was a little jingle, repeated over and over and pumped into us as we read our text books. Sisson's great tome, *The Anatomy of the Domestic Animals*, provided exhaustive descriptions of the bones, muscles, digestive system, etc. of the horse, then perhaps about a fifth of the space to the ox and so on down sheep, pig, to the poor dog pushed in at the end.

Glasgow Veterinary College was run on a shoestring when Alf was there, the government having withdrawn its financial support after it was decreed that Scotland only needed one veterinary college. Much of the tuition was undertaken by retired practitioners and centred on the horse-focused curriculum of a bygone age, but the students saw a lot of practice and in their final year they spent most of their days with local vets out in the real world. As a result, Alf gained some valuable practical experience working for the eminent Donald Campbell who had a practice just south of Glasgow in Rutherglen and Bill Weipers (later Sir William Weipers) who ran a small animal surgery in the West End of Glasgow where Alf could indulge his passion for dogs and cats.

In his final two years, during the vacations, Alf also worked further afield, in Dumfries in south-west Scotland at the veterinary practice of Tom Fleming, where he treated large farm animals. He also saw practice in Sunderland, with J. J. McDowall, and stayed with family who still lived in the city of his birth. Following an operation for an anal fistula – a condition that would trouble him for some years – he sat his final exams in July and then December 1939 and qualified as a fully-fledged MRCVS (Member of the Royal College of Veterinary Surgeons).

In the books, James heads straight to Yorkshire after graduation whereas Alf went back to the practice of J. J. McDowall in Sunderland. Although he was there only six months, it was an eventful period, during which he worked hard, day and night, for very little money and often ran surgeries alone. He saw a variety of animals, including dogs, cats and farm animals, and helped at the South Shields Racing Stadium, where McDowall was veterinary surgeon in attendance. Alf drove a tiny and unreliable Ford car, a precursor to the rusty little Austin he would later drive in the Dales. He also picked up some invaluable tips from McDowall, known to him as Mac. Having been surprised not to receive any thanks after he'd just produced two calves from a farmer's cow in fifteen minutes, he was told by Mac never to make a job look too easy. 'Remember this, Fred. It's not *what* you do, it's the way that you do it!' – advice that Alf would later drum into his own assistants in later years. It was a dictum that both Alf and Donald, and their fictional alter egos James and Siegfried, would follow, always mindful that, when treating animals, you invariably have their owners looking on; how you behave around them is critical to your success in the profession. Donald in fact had a set of golden rules he always expounded, which included: be courteous and respectful to farmers; give everything a name and never admit you don't know what's wrong; and never leave a farm without injecting something, even if it's a shot of vitamins, just do something!

While working with McDowall, Alf also learned a great deal about the various types of people he would come across in practice, both the clients and his fellow veterinary colleagues. He liked his boss Mac and they became very good friends, but the elder vet had an explosive temper and a liking for alcohol – not an uncommon trait among veterinary surgeons in those days. Angus Grier, a character who appears in the first two James Herriot books, shares some of the foibles of McDowall, although Grier is a far more disagreeable man. If anything, Grier is more of a composite character, formed out of the horror stories Alf would occasionally hear from student friends who were treated as the lowest form of life when working as assistants in practice.

In *If Only They Could Talk*, Siegfried advises James to take a Border terrier in need of an operation to Angus Grier, who had previously treated the dog. An ill-tempered Aberdonian vet, Grier is based in Brawton, the fictional name used for the Yorkshire spa town of Harrogate.

As I came into the operating room I saw that Siegfried had a patient on the table. He was thoughtfully stroking the head of an elderly and rather woebegone Border terrier.

'James,' he said, 'I want you to take this little dog through to Grier.'

'Grier?'

'Vet at Brawton. He was treating the case before the owner moved into our district. I've seen it a couple of times — stones in the bladder. It needs an immediate operation and I think I'd better let Grier do it. He's a touchy devil and I don't want to stand on his toes.'

'Oh, I think I've heard of him,' I said.

'Probably you have. A cantankerous Aberdonian. Since he practises in a fashionable town he gets quite a few students and he gives them hell. That sort of thing gets around.' He lifted the terrier from the table and handed him to me. 'The sooner you get through there the better. You can see the op and bring the dog back here afterwards. But watch yourself — don't rub Grier the wrong way or he'll take it out on you somehow.'

At my first sight of Angus Grier I thought immediately of whisky. He was about fifty and something had to be responsible for the fleshy, mottled cheeks, the swimmy eyes and the pattern of purple veins which chased each other over his prominent nose. He wore a permanently insulted expression.

He didn't waste any charm on me; a nod and a grunt and he grabbed the dog from my arms. Then he stabbed a finger at a slight, fairish youth in a white coat. 'That's Clinton — final-year student. Do ye no' think there's some pansy-lookin' buggers coming into this profession?'

Grier proceeds to operate on the dog, while niggling constantly at his student. Afterwards, Grier suggests James join him on a visit while they wait for the dog to wake from his anaesthetic. In the car, Angus launches into a long monologue cataloguing the many wrongs he's suffered 'at the hands of wicked clients and predatory colleagues'. He then inflicts on poor James the very humiliation he's been railing against.

We drew up in a particularly dirty farmyard and Grier turned to me. 'I've got a cow tae cleanse here.'

'Right,' I said, 'fine.' I settled down in my seat and took out my pipe. Grier paused, halfway out of the car. 'Are you no' coming to give me a hand?'

I couldn't understand him. 'Cleansing' of cows is simply the removal of retained afterbirth and is a one-man job.

'Well, there isn't much I can do, is there?' I said. 'And my Wellingtons and coat are back in my car. I didn't realize it was a farm visit — I'd probably get messed up for nothing.'

I knew immediately that I'd said the wrong thing. The toad-skin jowls flushed darker and he gave me a malevolent glance before turning away; but halfway across the yard he stopped and stood for a few moments in thought before coming back to the car. 'I've just remembered. I've got something here you can put on. You might as well come in with me — you'll be able to pass me a pessary when I want one.'

It sounded nutty to me, but I got out of the car and went

round to the back. Grier was fishing out a large wooden box from his boot.

'Here, ye can put this on. It's a calving outfit I got a bit ago. I haven't used it much because I found it a mite heavy, but it'll keep ye grand and clean.'

I looked in the box and saw a suit of thick, black, shining rubber. I lifted out the jacket; it bristled with zip-fasteners and press studs and felt as heavy as lead. The trousers were even more weighty, with many clips and fasteners. The whole thing was a most imposing creation, obviously designed by somebody who had never seen a cow calved and having the disadvantage that anybody wearing it would be pretty well immobilized.

I studied Grier's face for a moment but the watery eyes told me nothing. I began to take off my jacket — it was crazy but I didn't want to offend the man.

And, in truth, Grier seemed anxious to get me into the suit because he was holding it up in a helpful manner. It was a two-man operation. First the gleaming trousers were pulled on and zipped up fore and aft, then it was the turn of the jacket, a wonderful piece of work, fitting tightly around the waist and possessing short sleeves about six inches long with powerful elastic gripping my biceps.

Before I could get it on I had to roll my shirtsleeves to the shoulder, then Grier, heaving and straining, worked me into it. I could hear the zips squeaking into place, the final one being at the back of my neck to close a high, stiff collar which held my head in an attitude of supplication, my chin pointing at the sky.

Grier's heart really seemed to be in his work and, for the final touch, he produced a black rubber skull cap. I shrank away from the thing and began to mouth such objections as the collar would allow, but Grier insisted. 'Stand still a wee minute longer. We might as well do the job right.'

When he had finished he stood back admiringly. I must have been a grotesque sight, sheathed from head to foot in gleaming black, my arms, bare to the shoulders, sticking out almost at right angles. Grier appeared well satisfied. 'Well, come on, it's time we got on wi' the job.' He turned and hurried towards the byre; I plodded ponderously after him like an automaton.

Our arrival in the byre caused a sensation. There were present the farmer, two cowmen and a little girl. The men's cheerful greeting froze on their lips as the menacing figure paced slowly, deliberately in. The little girl burst into tears and ran outside.

'Cleansing' is a dirty, smelly job for the operator and a bore for the onlooker who may have to stand around for twenty minutes without being able to see anything. But this was one time the spectators were not bored. Grier was working away inside the cow and mumbling about the weather, but the men weren't listening; they never took their eyes away from me as I stood rigid, like a suit of armour against the wall. They studied each part of the outfit in turn, wonderingly. I knew what they were thinking. Just what was going to happen when this formidable unknown finally went into action? Anybody dressed like that must have some tremendous task ahead of him.

The intense pressure of the collar against my larynx kept me entirely out of any conversation and this must have added to my air of mystery. I began to sweat inside the suit.

The little girl had plucked up courage and brought her brothers and sisters to look at me. I could see the row of little heads peeping round the door and, screwing my head round painfully, I tried to give them a reassuring smile; but the heads disappeared and I heard their feet clattering across the yard.

I couldn't say how long I stood there, but Grier at last finished his job and called out, 'All right, I'm ready for you now.' The atmosphere became suddenly electric. The men straightened up and stared at me with slightly open mouths. This was the moment they had been waiting for.

I pushed myself away from the wall and did a right turn with some difficulty before heading for the tin of pessaries. It was only a few yards away but it seemed a long way as I approached it like a robot, head in the air, arms extended stiffly on either side. When I arrived at the tin I met a fresh difficulty; I could not bend. After a few contortions I got my hand into the tin, then had to take the paper off the pessary with one hand; a new purgatory. The men watched in fascinated silence.

Having removed the paper, I did a careful about-turn and paced back along the byre with measured tread. When I came level with the cow I extended my arm stiffly to Grier who took the pessary and inserted it in the uterus.

I then took up my old position against the wall while my colleague cleaned himself down. I glanced down my nose at the men; their expressions had changed to open disbelief. Surely the mystery man's assignment was tougher than that — he couldn't be wearing that outfit just to hand over a pessary. But when Grier started the complicated business of snapping open the studs and sliding the zips they realized the show was over; and fast on the feeling of let-down came amusement.

As I tried to rub some life back into my swollen arms which had been strangulated by the elastic sleeves, I was surrounded by grinning faces. They could hardly wait, I imagined, to get round to the local that night to tell the tale. Pulling together the shreds of my dignity, I put on my jacket and got into the car. Grier stayed to say a few words to the men, but he wasn't holding their attention; it was all on me, huddling in the seat. They couldn't believe I was true.

Back at the surgery the Border terrier was coming out of the anaesthetic. He raised his head and tried bravely to wag his tail when he saw me. I wrapped him in a blanket, gathered him up and was preparing to leave when I saw Grier through the partly open door of a small storeroom. He had the wooden box on a table and he was lifting out the rubber suit, but there was something peculiar about the way he was doing it; the man seemed to be afflicted by a kind of rigor — his body shook and jerked, the mottled face was strangely contorted and a half-stifled wailing issued from his lips.

I stared in amazement. I would have said it was impossible, yet it was happening right in front of me. There was not a shadow of a doubt about it — Angus Grier was laughing.

While working in Sunderland, Alf continued to scour the *Veterinary Record* for advertised job vacancies. Sunderland had been hit badly by the Depression and the long-term prospects of the job were not guaranteed, nor did Alf relish the prospect of working alongside Mac on a permanent basis. Of the few advertisements he saw, one was based in Thirsk, the job described as 'Mainly agricultural work in a Yorkshire market town'. He wrote for an interview, received a reply, and set off for Thirsk on that fateful morning in June 1940.

In the books, James arrives at the Yorkshire practice in 1937, whereas in reality, Alf made his way to Thirsk three years later, when the country was in the grip of the Second World War. The owner of the practice, Donald Sinclair, on whom Siegfried Farnon was based, was joining the RAF and in need of someone to look after the practice in his absence. Just a few days after Alf accepted the job, Donald left for the RAF, as did the practice assistant Eric Parker four weeks later.

As a result, Alf was left to run the practice single-handedly in an area he knew little about. Long days were spent visiting farms, where he would treat animals with an array of concoctions – Universal Cattle Medicine being the most favoured – in the days when modern drugs had yet to transform veterinary practice. The work itself was tough, as was navigating around the peculiar ways of Dales farmers and the impenetrable Yorkshire dialect. Alf's dreams of becoming a small animal vet in a city practice soon melted away, as he described in *James Herriot's Dog Stories.*

> I spent my time in shirtsleeves and Wellingtons, trudging through mud and muck, wrestling with huge beasts, being kicked, knocked down and trodden on. As a city boy, thrown headlong into the kind of remote rural community I had only read about in books, I was like a poor swimmer trying to keep afloat in the deep end. I was acutely aware that I had no agricultural background and that I had to establish myself among farmers who had spent a lifetime with livestock and often had a jaundiced attitude to what they called 'book learnin''. Life was very full.

Alf, grew to love his work and the community in which he worked, many of whom led tough lives but were honest, plain-speaking and often generous with their hospitality. Money, however was often in short supply and the practice finances were on something of a knife-edge when Alf joined. To supplement their income, he undertook tuberculin testing for the Ministry of Agriculture. The 1930s saw the development of a test for the bacterial disease, bovine tuberculosis (TB), which is dangerous to cattle and to people who drink infected milk. The goal was to eradicate TB entirely and the work, which paid as much as £20 to £30 a day, meant Alf and Donald could afford to employ assistants.

As he rattled about in his little Austin 7 and a variety of aged cars, Alf grew to love the hills and moorland of North Yorkshire, and after a hard day's work he and his fellow bachelors, Donald and Brian, would share a pint or two in the local pub or attend the odd village dance. He soon met his future wife Joan Danbury, immortalized in the books as Helen, the two marrying at St Mary's Church in Thirsk on 5 November 1941. At around the time he met Joan, Alf had signed up to join the RAF, keen to do his bit against the onslaught of Nazi Germany which in March 1941 had bombed his home city of Glasgow, badly damaging his parents' home near the River Clyde in the process. He wasn't called up until the following year and by the time he left for training on 16 November 1942, Joan was pregnant with their first child. The day Alf left was an incredibly sad one for the couple and the next few months would prove challenging for the young vet.

Alf was sent first to Regent's Park in London where he was examined and inoculated and drilled ready for assignment to a training wing. The medical examinations at Regent's Park involved dentist check-ups, where Alf had a tooth pulled out, an unfortunate experience that he related in *Vets Might Fly*. While he yearned to be back with Joan in Thirsk, he was nonetheless determined to do well in the RAF and the extract demonstrates how Alf utilized every life experience, however awkward or painful, as entertaining content for his books. In *Vets Might Fly*, James explains how his fear of dentists dates back to being trapped in a dental chair as a child, the great bulk of Hector McDarroch, a caber-tossing Highlands Games competitor, looming over him with a terrifying drilling machine. Nowadays he prefers much smaller frailer-looking types, such as his Darrowby dentist Mr Grover, so that 'if it came to a stand-up fight I would have a good chance of victory and

escape'. As a consequence, the unknown RAF dentist, nick-
named 'the Butcher', fills James with utter dread, and for very
good reason.

I still don't enjoy going to the dentist but I have to admit that
the modern men are wonderful. I hardly see mine when I go.
Just a brief glimpse of a white coat then all is done from behind.
Fingers come round, things go in and out of my mouth but
even when I venture to open my eyes I see nothing.

Hector McDarroch, on the other hand, seemed to take a
pleasure in showing off his grisly implements, filling the
long-needled syringe right in front of my eyes and squirting
the cocaine ceilingwards a few times before he started on me.
And worse, before an extraction he used to clank about in a
tin box, producing a series of hideous forceps and examining
them, whistling softly, till he found the right one.

So with all this in mind, as I sat in a long queue of airmen
for the preliminary examination, I was thankful I had been to
Mr Grover for a complete check-up. A dentist stood by a chair
at the end of the long room and he examined the young men
in blue one by one before calling out his findings to an orderly
at a desk.

I derived considerable entertainment from watching the
expressions on the lads' faces when the call went out. 'Three
fillings, two extractions!' 'Eight fillings!' Most of them looked
stunned, some thunderstruck, others almost tearful. Now and
again one would try to expostulate with the man in white but
it was no good; nobody was listening. At times I could have
laughed out loud. Mind you, I felt a bit mean at being amused,
but after all they had only themselves to blame. If only they
had shown my foresight they would have had nothing to
worry about.

When my name was called I strolled across, humming a little tune, and dropped nonchalantly into the chair. It didn't take the man long. He poked his way swiftly along my teeth then rapped out, 'Five fillings and one extraction!'

I sat bolt upright and stared at him in amazement.

James tries to argue otherwise but is promptly told to report back the following morning for the extraction. He awaits the appointment with growing apprehension, desperately trying to comfort himself with the assurance that the procedure wouldn't hurt.

I was nurturing this comforting thought when I turned into a large assembly room with numbered doors leading from it. About thirty airmen sat around wearing a variety of expressions from sickly smiles to tough bravado. A chilling smell of antiseptic hung on the air. I chose a chair and settled down to wait. I had been in the armed forces long enough to know that you waited a long time for everything and I saw no reason why a dental appointment should be any different.

As I sat down the man on my left gave me a brief nod. He was fat, and greasy black hair fell over his pimpled brow. Though engrossed in picking his teeth with a match he gave me a long appraising stare before addressing me in rich cockney.

'What room you goin' in, mate?'

I looked at my card. 'Room Four.'

'Blimey, mate, you've 'ad it!' He removed his matchstick and grinned wolfishly.

'Had it . . .? What do you mean?'

'Well, haven't you 'eard? That's the Butcher in there.'

'The . . . the . . . Butcher?' I quavered.

'Yeh, that's what they call the dental officer in there.' He gave an expansive smile. 'He's a right killer, that bloke, I'll tell yer.'

I swallowed. 'Butcher . . .? Killer . . .? Oh come on. They'll all be the same, I'm sure.'

'Don't you believe it, mate. There's good an' there's bad, and that bloke's pure murder. It shouldn't be allowed.'

'How do you know, anyway?'

He waved an airy hand. 'Oh I've been 'ere a few times and I've heard some bleedin' awful screams comin' out of that room. Spoken to some of the chaps afterwards, too. They all call 'im the Butcher.'

I rubbed my hands on the rough blue of my trousers. 'Oh you hear these tales. I'm sure they're exaggerated.'

'Well, you'll find out, mate.' He resumed his tooth-picking. 'But don't say I didn't tell you.'

James waits for almost an hour – his heart thumping as he watches other men leaving Room Four looking shattered, one person reeling as he holds his mouth with both hands. He eventually gets called in to meet the Butcher, who is described as 'about six feet two with rugby-forward shoulders bulging beneath his white coat'. After a hearty laugh, he motions James to the chair, fills a syringe and after a few playful spurts in the air, he puts the needle in. A minute or two later, he then seizes some forceps and starts to grapple with the tooth, until a large crack indicates that the tooth has broken off leaving the root still in James's gum.

He must have been gouging for half an hour when an idea seemed to strike him. Pushing all the forceps to one side he almost ran from the room and reappeared shortly with a tray on which reposed a long chisel and a metal mallet.

At a sign from him the WAAF wound the chair back till I was completely horizontal. Seemingly familiar with the routine, she cradled my head in her arms in a practised manner and stood waiting.

This couldn't be true, I thought, as the man inserted the chisel into my mouth and poised the mallet; but all doubts were erased as the metal rod thudded against the remnants of my tooth and my head in turn shot back into the little WAAF's bosom. And that was how it went on. I lost count of time as the Butcher banged away and the girl hung on grimly to my jerking skull.

The thought uppermost in my mind was that I had always wondered how young horses felt when I knocked wolf teeth out of them. Now I knew.

When it finally stopped I opened my eyes, and though by this time I was prepared for anything I still felt slightly surprised to see the Butcher threading a needle with a length of suture silk. He was sweating and looking just a little desperate as he bent over me yet again.

'Just a couple of stitches,' he muttered hoarsely, and I closed my eyes again.

When I left the chair I felt very strange indeed. The assault on my cranium had made me dizzy and the sensation of the long ends of the stitches tickling my tongue was distinctly odd. I'm sure that when I came out of the room I was staggering, and instinctively I pawed at my mouth.

Minus a tooth, Alf was then posted from Regent's Park to Scarborough on the Yorkshire coast for initial training, arriving there on 19 December 1942. The endless marching and drill meant he soon lost the extra few pounds he'd put on during his first year of marriage. Happy to be back in Yorkshire, he enjoyed his time in Scarborough, where he was billeted in the Grand Hotel and easily passed his exams ready for flight training. While in Scarborough, he also went absent without leave several times to visit Joan – an act of rebellion, wholly out of character for a man who was very much a rule-follower. Alf's visit on 13 February 1943, on the day his son Jim was born, was his third unsanctioned trip away.

On 20 May that year Alf was sent to Winkfield aerodrome near Windsor, where he excelled in flight training and was one of only four men out of fifty to fly solo in a Tiger Moth, the RAF training aircraft, after just two weeks. He was then posted to Salford, Manchester, where he suffered considerable discomfort from an anal fistula again, which required two operations at an RAF hospital in Hereford, which left him in considerable pain and, in the eyes of the RAF, an invalid.

Knowing that his career with the air force was at an end, he was sent to Heaton Park in Manchester where he was assigned to stores, and he eventually left the RAF on 10 November 1943. Some of the stories of his time in the RAF were retold in the James Herriot books, many of them humorous, but in reality it was a difficult period for Alf and he yearned to return to his growing family and to the job he loved.

In *The Lord God Made Them All*, James has returned to the Dales after a year with the RAF. He is pleased to be back at work but there is no gentle easing in for the young vet. The practice is busier than ever and he is soon bumping along the winding country lanes and farm tracks to a never-ending list of patients.

When the gate fell on top of me I knew I was really back home.

My mind drifted effortlessly over my spell in the RAF to the last time I had visited the Ripleys. It was to 'nip some calves' as Mr Ripley said over the phone, or more correctly to emasculate them by means of the Burdizzo bloodless castrator, and when the message came in I realized that a large part of my morning had gone.

It was always something of a safari to visit Anson Hall, because the old house lay at the end of a ridged and rutted track which twisted across the fields through no fewer than seven gates.

Gates are one of the curses of a country vet's life and in the Yorkshire Dales, before the coming of cattle grids, we suffered more than most. We were resigned to opening two or three on many of the farms, but seven was a bit much. And at the Ripleys it wasn't just the number but the character.

The first one which led off the narrow road was reasonably normal — an ancient thing of rusty iron — and as I unlatched it it did at least swing round groaning on its hinges. It was the only one which swung; the others were of wood and of the type known in the Dales as 'shoulder gates'. I could see how they got their name as I hoisted each one up, balanced the top spar on my shoulder and dragged it round. These had no hinges but were tied at one end with binder twine top and bottom.

Even with an ordinary gate there is a fair amount of work involved. You have to stop the car, get out, open the gate, drive through, stop the car again, dismount and close the thing behind you. But the road to Anson Hall was hard labour. The gates deteriorated progressively as I approached the farm and I was puffing with my efforts as I bumped and rattled my way up to number seven.

This was the last and the most formidable — a malignant entity with a personality of its own. Over decades it had been patched and repaired with so many old timbers that probably none of the original structure remained. But it was dangerous.

I got out of the car and advanced a few steps. We were old

foes, this gate and I, and we faced each other for some moments in silence. We had fought several brisk rounds in the past and there was no doubt the gate was ahead on points.

The difficulty was that, apart from its wobbly, loosely nailed eccentricity, it had only one string hinge, halfway down. This enabled it to pivot on its frail axis with deadly effect.

With the utmost care I approached the right-hand side and began to unfasten the binder twine. The string, I noticed bitterly, was, like all the others, neatly tied in a bow, and as it fell clear I grabbed hastily at the top spar. But I was too late. Like a live thing the bottom rail swung in and rapped me cruelly on the shins, and as I tried to correct the balance the top bashed my chest.

It was the same as all the other times. As I hauled it round an inch at a time, the gate buffeted me high and low. I was no match for it.

Another thing which didn't help was that I could see Mr Ripley watching me benevolently from the farmhouse doorway. While I wrestled the gate open, contented puffs rose from the farmer's pipe and he did not stir from his position until I had hobbled over the last stretch of grass and stood before him.

'Now then, Mr Herriot, you've come to nip me a few calves?' A smile of unaffected friendship creased the stubbled cheeks. Mr Ripley shaved once a week — on market day — considering, with some logic, that since only his wife and his cattle saw him on the other six days there was no point in scraping away at his face every morning with a razor.

I bent and massaged my bruised ankles. 'Mr Ripley, that gate! It's a menace! Do you remember that last time I was here you promised me faithfully you'd have it mended? In fact you said you'd get a new one — it's about time, isn't it?'

While work resumes at a busy pace for James, not everything is as it was before. The small farmers, the bread and butter of the Darrowby practice, are soon to be a disappearing breed and a simple injection now has more of an effect than many of the age-old remedies they once poured down the throats of animals.

> There were signs, too, that the small farmer was on the way out. These men, some with only six cows, a few pigs and poultry, still made up most of our practice and were the truly rich characters, but they were beginning to wonder if they could make a living on this scale and one or two had sold out to the bigger men. In our practice now, in the eighties, there are virtually no small farmers left. I can think of only a handful. Old men doggedly doing the things they have always done for the sole reason that they have always done it. They are the last remnants of the men I cherished, living by the ancient values, speaking the old Yorkshire dialect which television and radio have almost extinguished.
>
> I took a last long breath and got into my car. The uncomfortable feeling of change was still with me, but I looked through the window at the great fells thrusting their bald summits into the clouds, tier upon tier of them, timeless, indestructible, towering over the glories beneath, and I felt better immediately. The Dales had not changed at all.

A daughter, Rosie, arrived on 9 May 1947 and the years Alf spent with his young children were some of the happiest in his life. Despite his heavy workload, seven days a week, he always made time for Jim and Rosie, taking them on his rounds or on trips to the hills around Thirsk. The family enjoyed the occasional holiday in the coastal town of

Llandudno in North Wales as well as Runswick Bay and Robin Hood's Bay on the Yorkshire coast. Alf also played the piano and violin and took great pleasure in music. In 1949, he saved up and bought himself a radiogram so that he could listen to his favourite classical composers, from Mozart to Brahms, delighting also in the tenor Beniamino Gigli and jazz musician Duke Ellington, among many others. As a small child Rosie also loved to listen to music on the radiogram and to sing nursery rhymes or Bing Crosby tunes to her father as they drove around the farms on his rounds. Rosie and Jim inherited their father's love of classical music, but Alf wasn't so keen on some of the emerging rock and roll they played, describing their Elvis or Beatles records as being 'like the fiends of hell beating at the door'. Alf was a passionate cricket fan and a life-long football supporter, following Sunderland and Middlesbrough, attending matches whenever he could. The two sports were often the topic of conversation with his clients.

By 1949 he was in full partnership with Donald Sinclair, who by now was married and living with his wife in a country house nearby. Unusually Alf was offered a salaried partnership with Donald when he first joined the practice, receiving five-eighths of the profits while Donald was away in the RAF, and then a salary of four guineas a week on his return, along with a share in the profits from tuberculin testing. From 1946 onwards, Donald agreed to Alf having an equal share of the profits and then in 1949 a full partnership, which resulted in Alf earning more than Donald, largely because he continued to work full-time whereas Donald put in fewer hours. Alf and the family continued to live at 23 Kirkgate until 1953, when he bought a plot of land on Topcliffe Road, then on the periphery of Thirsk, on which he built a new house where the family of four lived for the next twenty-five years. Alf and Donald, however, continued to run the practice in Thirsk for more than thirty years.

∾

While the 1950s was a happy decade for Alf, the first two years of the 1960s marked a difficult period for him. In April 1960 his father died suddenly from a heart attack, the shock of which caused Alf's emotions to spiral into severe depression. He had had a close relationship with his father – and it was some regret to him that his father never witnessed his later literary success – but there were other traits that perhaps made him susceptible to a nervous breakdown. He was a worrier but tended to bottle up his concerns in the pretence that all was well. He fretted about the education of his children, the future of the Thirsk practice, on which his finances depended entirely, and any issues that cropped up with his assistants. He had always felt a sense of responsibility towards his parents and had a close but uneasy relationship with his mother. In the summer of 1960, when he seemed to be suffering the most, his mind haunted by paranoid thoughts and occasional memory lapses, he was advised to have electroconvulsive therapy. As we'll see in chapter ten, it has also been suggested that the strange symptoms he had previously suffered as a result of close contact with disease-infected cattle, as related in *Every Living Thing*, may have contributed to his nervous breakdown.

Alf battled on, always choosing to hide any inner demons, and continued to work full-time, which was probably the best therapy for him as a busy schedule occupied his mind and the landscape of Yorkshire always soothed him. Throughout it all, he was always a caring father and son, continued to write to his mother weekly, and took pleasure from gardening and playing tennis with his wife. In June 1961 Alf and Joan went to Majorca, on their very first trip abroad, on the insistence of Alf's old college friend Eddie Straiton, who offered him his holiday home and to cover his work at the practice. The trip aided Alf's recovery, as did a walking holiday later that summer, roaming the fells and valleys of the Dales and staying in youth hostels with his two children and a friend of Rosie's.

As he started to feel better, Alf was determined to live life to the full and this included seeing more of the world, visiting Russia and Turkey in 1961 and 1962 as an official Ministry of Agriculture veterinarian, a position that, as related in his books, former assistant John Crooks facilitated. Alf was a qualified vet, with experience working as a veterinary tuberculin inspector, so he had the relevant qualifications for the job. He included some of his diary entries from that time in *The Lord God Made Them All*, first explaining why he had made the decision to go to Russia, despite the less than enthusiastic response from some of his clients.

I should like to jump forward in time to 1961 in order to interpolate some extracts from the journal I kept of my Russian adventure.

John was behind it. Although he no longer worked for us he came back often as a friend and had been describing some of his experiences in exporting animals from Hull. He often sailed with these animals as veterinary attendant, but it was the Russian thing which caught my imagination.

'That must have been very interesting,' I said.

John smiled. 'Oh yes, fascinating. I've been out there several times now and it's the real Russia with the lid off, not a tour of the show places they want you to see. You get a glimpse of the country through the eyes of a seaman and you meet the ordinary Russians, the commercial people, the workers.'

'Sounds great!'

'And you get paid for it, too,' John went on. 'That makes it even better.'

I sighed. 'You're a lucky beggar. And these jobs come up pretty regularly?'

'Yes, they do.' He looked at me closely and I suppose my expression must have been wistful. 'Would you like to have a go sometime?'

'Do you mean it?'

'Of course,' he said. 'Just say the word and you can sail on the next one. That'll be some time around the end of October.'

I thumped my fist into my palm. 'Book me in, John. It's really kind of you. Country vetting is fine but sometimes I feel I'm sliding into a rut. A trip to Russia is just what I need.'

'Well, that's grand.' John stood up and prepared to leave. 'I'll let you know the details later but I believe you'll be sailing with a cargo of valuable sheep — breeding animals. The insurance company is bound to insist on veterinary supervision.'

For weeks I went around in a fever of anticipation but there were many people who didn't share my enthusiasm.

One cowman cocked an eye at me. 'Ah wouldn't go there for a bloody big clock,' he said. 'One wrong word and you'll find yourself in t'nick for a long long time.'

He had a definite point. East—West relations were at one of their lowest ebbs at that time and I grew used to my clients making it clear that Russia was one place they would avoid. In fact when I told Colonel Smallwood about it while I was tuberculin testing his cattle a few days before I left, he raised his eyebrows and gave me a cold stare.

'Nice to have known you,' he murmured.

Alf never again let his emotions get the better of him and his recovery from the nervous breakdown also coincided with more earnest attempts at writing, initially as a hobby. He wrote a collection of stories about farmers and his veterinary friends before then trying his hand at writing short stories on other topics, from football to human relationships. Writing served as an emotional outlet for feelings and thoughts that he probably found difficult to express in day-to-day life. The James Herriot that he portrayed in his later books is essentially James Alfred Wight – the deep affection he had for the community and landscape around him, for his family, for his dogs, they are all in the pages of the books, and the man and author are indistinguishable.

Alf stopped working full-time at the Thirsk practice in 1980 but did not retire fully until the end of 1989. His near-fifty years of veterinary practice had, as he had been told as a schoolboy, certainly been full of endless interest and variety, and it was a profession he had always loved. While the elder practitioners he had worked with could be difficult, they had passed on invaluable advice, preparing him for the innumerable challenges that lay ahead – and the advice Siegfried gives James after his very first case in *If Only They Could Talk* does just that. James has had to put a horse down and deal with an ill-tempered client in the form of Mr Soames; Siegfried assures him that humiliation, ridicule and difficult clients are all par for the course in veterinary work.

'It's a funny profession, you know. It offers unparalleled opportunities for making a chump of yourself.'

'But I expect a lot depends on your ability.'

'To a certain extent. It helps to be good at the job, of course, but even if you're a positive genius humiliation and ridicule are lurking just round the corner. I once got an eminent horse specialist along here to do a rig operation and the horse stopped breathing halfway through. The sight of that man dancing frantically on his patient's ribs taught me a great truth — that I was going to look just as big a fool at fairly regular intervals throughout my career.'

I laughed. 'Then I might as well resign myself to it right at the beginning.'

'That's the idea. Animals are unpredictable things, so our whole life is unpredictable. It's a long tale of little triumphs and disasters and you've got to really like it to stick it. Tonight it was Soames, but another night it'll be something else. One thing, you never get bored. Here, have some more whisky.'

I drank the whisky and then some more and we talked. It seemed no time at all before the dark bulk of the acacia tree began to emerge from the grey light beyond the French window, a blackbird tried a few tentative pipes and Farnon was regretfully shaking the last drops from the bottle into his glass.

He yawned, jerked the knot out of his black tie and looked at his watch 'Well, five o'clock. Who would have thought it? But I'm glad we had a drink together — only right to celebrate your first case. It was a right one, wasn't it?'

Chapter 2

THE YORKSHIRE DALES
and DARROWBY

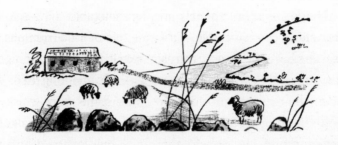

The driver crashed his gears again as he went into another steep bend. We had been climbing steadily now for the last fifteen miles or so, moving closer to the distant blue swell of the Pennines. I had never been in Yorkshire before but the name had always raised a picture of a county as stodgy and unromantic as its pudding; I was prepared for solid worth, dullness and a total lack of charm. But as the bus groaned its way higher I began to wonder. The formless heights were resolving into high, grassy hills and wide valleys. In the valley bottoms, rivers twisted among the trees and solid grey stone farmhouses lay among islands of cultivated land which pushed bright green promontories up the hillsides into the dark tide of heather which lapped from the summits.

A young James Herriot is making his way towards Darrowby in the Yorkshire Dales. Sitting on a rickety little bus, he takes in his first views of North Yorkshire, which instantly dispel his expectations of a dreary landscape. He is enthralled by the

wild beauty of the fells, the grassy hills and windswept moor-
lands, which couldn't be more different to the grey industrial
landscape of his home city of Glasgow.

The James Herriot stories are set in the Yorkshire Dales,
which lie astride the Pennines in North Yorkshire, where sheep
and cattle graze in rich green valleys or up on heather-strewn
moors, separated by countless miles of ancient drystone walls.
The location is about thirty miles to the west of Thirsk, which
is situated in the Hambleton district of North Yorkshire, close
to the North York Moors. This too was the domain of the small
hill farmer and Alf took great pleasure in driving through the
beautiful landscape and villages, coaxing his little car up and
around the Hambleton Hills. Around the flat plain of Thirsk
there is more arable farming than in the valleys and hills of the
Dales, but cattle and sheep are farmed in both areas.

Alf was very familiar with the Dales. The Thirsk practice
covered a large area and, as we've seen, he and Donald
frequently travelled to the Dales to undertake tuberculin
testing of cattle, having been offered the work by Leyburn-
based veterinary surgeon Frank Bingham (recreated as Ewan
Ross in the books). Not only did the government-paid work
provide Donald and Alf with much-needed income but it also
gave Alf an introduction to the majestic beauty of the Dales,
which captivated him for the rest of his life. 'The first thing
that enthralled me about Yorkshire', he wrote, 'was its wild
beauty, the feeling of remoteness and solitude, which keeps
one's sense of wonder alive.'

In *It Shouldn't Happen to a Vet*, the year is 1938 and James
has been in Darrowby for twelve months. Looking at the view
from a high Yorkshire moor, he muses upon how he has changed
and how fortunate he is to be driving across the fells and hills
of the Dales every day.

How on earth, then, did I come to be sitting on a high Yorkshire moor in shirtsleeves and Wellingtons, smelling vaguely of cows?

The change in my outlook had come quite quickly – in fact almost immediately after my arrival in Darrowby. The job had been a godsend in those days of high unemployment, but only, I had thought, a stepping-stone to my real ambition. But everything had switched round, almost in a flash.

Maybe it was something to do with the incredible sweetness of the air which still took me by surprise when I stepped out into the old wild garden at Skeldale House every morning. Or perhaps the daily piquancy of life in the graceful old house with my gifted but mercurial boss, Siegfried, and his reluctant student brother, Tristan. Or it could be that it was just the realization that treating cows and pigs and sheep and horses had a fascin-ation I had never even suspected; and this brought with it a new concept of myself as a tiny wheel in the great machine of British agriculture. There was a kind of solid satisfaction in that.

Probably it was because I hadn't dreamed there was a place like the Dales. I hadn't thought it possible that I could spend all my days in a high, clean-blown land where the scent of grass or trees was never far away; and where even in the driving rain of winter I could sniff the air and find the freshness of growing things hidden somewhere in the cold clasp of the wind.

Anyway, it had all changed for me and my work consisted now of driving from farm to farm across the roof of England with a growing conviction that I was a privileged person.

The sense of gratitude and wonder that James feels working in the Dales, especially when he takes in its wondrous views, never diminishes over the years. In *The Lord God Made Them All*, an old schoolfriend Andrew Bruce drops into the practice and James takes him out on a call to a local farm. Andrew works in a bank and is happy with his lot, until he's introduced to the splendour of the Dales and all of a sudden office life is not quite so appealing.

It was a golden afternoon in October and beyond the stone walls the fell-sides, ablaze with their mantle of dead bracken, rose serenely into a deep, unbroken blue. We passed under a long canopy of tinted leaves thrown over us by the roadside trees then followed a stretch of white-pebbled river before turning along a narrow track which led up the hillside.

Andrew was silent as we climbed into the stark, airy solitude which is the soul of the Dales, but as the track levelled out on the summit he put a hand on my arm.

'Just stop a minute, Jim, will you?' he said.

I pulled up and wound down the window. For a few moments he looked out over the miles of heathery moorland and the rounded summits of the great hills slumbering in the sunshine, then he spoke quietly as though to himself.

'So this is where you work?'

'Yes, this is it, Andy.'

He took a long breath, then another as if greedy for more.

'You know,' he said. 'I've heard a lot about air like wine, but this is the first time I've realized what it means.'

I nodded. I always felt I could never get enough of that air; sharp and cool and tinged only with the grass scent which lingers in the high country.

'Well, you're a lucky beggar, Jim,' Andrew said with a touch of weariness. 'You spend your life driving around in country like this and I'm stuck in a damned office.'

'I thought you liked your job.'

He ran a hand through his hair. 'Oh yes, I suppose playing around with figures is what I'm best at but, oh hell, I have to do it all inside. In fact,' he said, becoming a little worked up, 'when I start to think about it I live and have my being in a bloody, centrally heated box with no windows and electric light blasting down all day, and I share what passes for air with a whole crowd of other people.' He slumped back in his seat. 'Makes me wish I hadn't come out with you.'

'I'm sorry, Andy.'

He laughed ruefully. 'Oh, I didn't really mean that, but honestly, this is idyllic.'

Andrew Bruce was in reality based on Alf's schoolfriend Monty Gilbert who used to join Alf as he walked around the hills of Glasgow when they were both at school. Monty worked and lived in Glasgow and was similarly enchanted by the scenery in Yorkshire when he came to visit. He also left a lasting impression with Alf's children, Jim and Rosie, principally because he had the unusual skill of being able to walk on his hands, making for an unusual sight in the corridor of 23 Kirkgate.

Once the summer months pass, it's not long before the cold north winds pick up, bringing with them snowfall, particularly in the hills. The 1930s and 1940s saw plenty of snow across Yorkshire, sometimes arriving as early as November. While a blanket of snow made for magical views, wintry conditions made life extremely difficult for rural vets like James Herriot. The thin wheels of their cars spun on the ice, blizzards were all too common and snowdrifts blocked the roads. 'To a young Glaswegian like myself,' wrote Alf Wight, 'it was almost unbelievable. Yorkshire, I decided, was the snowiest place I had ever known.'

The treacherous conditions meant Alf often had to abandon his car and walk to remote farms, snowstorms sometimes blinding the path ahead. In *It Shouldn't Happen to a Vet* snowfall comes early in November and yet James and Siegfried must do all they can to make it out to their clients. The following story was in fact experienced by Alf's son Jim, who related it to his father afterwards, but it illustrates the considerable challenges rural vets faced in the winter. Jim had to abandon his car and walk to Tom Cornforth's farm at the top of Hambleton Hills, wading through snow that was waist deep. When he arrived in a howling blizzard, with visibility only two or three yards, he was frankly relieved to have made it.

This was my second winter in Darrowby so I didn't feel the same sense of shock when it started to be really rough in November. When they were getting a drizzle of rain down there on the plain the high country was covered in a few hours by a white blanket which filled in the roads, smoothed out familiar landmarks, transformed our world into something strange and new. This was what they meant on the radio when they talked about 'snow on high ground'.

When the snow started in earnest it had a strangling effect on the whole district. Traffic crawled laboriously between the mounds thrown up by the snowploughs. Herne Fell hung over Darrowby like a great gleaming whale and in the town the people dug paths to their gates and cleared the drifts from their front doors. They did it without fuss, with the calm of long use and in the knowledge that they would probably have to do it again tomorrow.

Every new fall struck a fresh blow at the vets. We managed to get to most of our cases but we lost a lot of sweat in the process. Sometimes we were lucky and were able to bump along in the wake of a council plough but more often we drove as far as we could and walked the rest of the way.

After a night of continuous snow, the practice receives a call from Mr Clayton who has a beast 'with a touch o' cold'. When James enquires what the road to his farm is like, he gives the typically airy response of a hardened Dales farmer: 'Road? Road? Road's right enough. Just tek a bit o' care and you'll get here without any trouble.' In fact, after driving over ten miles, James's fingers throbbing painfully with the cold, the road into Mr Clayton's valley is blocked solid, the snowploughs having not even attempted to clear it. James is forced to hitch on his rucksack and hike the rest of the way.

The flat moorland on the fell top was a white immensity rolling away to the horizon with the sky pressing down like a dark blanket. I could see the farm down there in its hollow and it, too, looked different; small, remote, like a charcoal drawing against the hills bulking smooth and white beyond. A pine wood made a dark smudge on the slopes but the scene had been wiped clean of most of its familiar features.

I could see the road only in places – the walls were covered over most of their length, but the farm was visible all the way. I had gone about half a mile towards it when a sudden gust of wind blew up the surface snow into a cloud of fine particles. Just for a few seconds I found myself completely alone. The farm, the surrounding moor, everything disappeared and I had an eerie sense of isolation till the veil cleared.

It was hard going in the deep snow and in the drifts I sank over the tops of my Wellingtons. I kept at it, head down, to within a few hundred yards of the stone buildings. I was just thinking that it had all been pretty easy, really, when I looked up and saw a waving curtain of a million black dots bearing down on me. I quickened my steps and just before the blizzard hit me I marked the position of the farm. But after ten minutes' stumbling and slithering I realized I had missed the place. I was heading for a shape that didn't exist; it was etched only in my mind.

I stood for a few moments feeling again the chilling sense of isolation. I was convinced I had gone too far to the left and after a few gasping breaths, struck off to the right. It wasn't long before I knew I had gone in the wrong direction again. I began to fall into deep holes, up to the armpits in the snow, reminding me that the ground was not really flat on these high moors but pitted by countless peat hags.

As I struggled on I told myself that the whole thing was ridiculous. I couldn't be far from the warm fireside at Pike House — this wasn't the North Pole. But my mind went back to the great empty stretch of moor beyond the farm and I had to stifle a feeling of panic.

The numbing cold seemed to erase all sense of time. Soon I had no idea of how long I had been falling into the holes and crawling out. I did know that each time it was getting harder work dragging myself out. And it was becoming more and more tempting to sit down and rest, even sleep; there was something hypnotic in the way the big, soft flakes brushed noiselessly across my skin and mounted thickly on my closed eyes.

I was trying to shut out the conviction that if I fell down many more times I wouldn't get up when a dark shape hovered suddenly ahead. Then my outflung arms touched something hard and rough. Unbelievingly I felt my way over the square stone blocks till I came to a corner. Beyond that was a square of light — it was the kitchen window of the farm.

After James thumps on the door of the farm, Mr Clayton appears and takes him over to the calf house where there are four long-haired little bullocks, along with a fifth one with a purulent discharge coming from its nose – the patient. The freezing blizzard conditions are of no concern to Mr Clayton.

As my numb fingers fumbled in a pocket for my thermometer a great gust of wind buffeted the door, setting the latch clicking softly and sending a faint powdering of snow into the dark interior.

Mr Clayton turned and rubbed the pane of the single small window with his sleeve. Picking his teeth with his thumbnail he peered out at the howling blizzard.

'Aye,' he said, and belched pleasurably. 'It's a plain sort o' day.'

In *The Lord God Made Them All* James resorts to using skis to get to some of the more remote farms. The winter of 1946–7 was particularly brutal across the UK, and much of the country was swathed in a blanket of snow and ice. In the Dales, sub-zero temperatures persisted well into mid-March as James remembers.

That was in 1947, the year of the great snow. I have never known snow like that before or since and the odd thing was that it took such a long time to get started. Nothing happened in November and we had a green Christmas, but then it began to get colder and colder. All through January a north-east wind blew, apparently straight from the Arctic, and usually after a few days of this sort of unbearable blast, snow would come and make things a bit warmer. But not in 1947.

Each day we thought it couldn't get any colder, but it did, and then, borne on the wind, very fine flakes began to appear over the last few days of the month. They were so small you could hardly see them but they were the forerunners of the real thing. At the beginning of February big, fat flakes started a steady relentless descent on our countryside and we knew, after all that build-up, that we were for it.

Eventually, even in North Yorkshire, the snow recedes and normal life resumes. Throughout the year, a typical routine for Alf was to take a quick break between farm visits, stopping the car somewhere remote and picturesque to take whichever dog companions he had with him for a walk. With not a soul around, he could unwind properly and take in the scenery around him – a short respite from what are often busy days for a rural vet.

I drove gingerly down through the wood and before starting up the track on the other side I stopped the car and got out with Sam leaping eagerly after me.

This was a little lost valley in the hills, a green cleft cut off from the wild country above. One of the bonuses in a country vet's life is that he sees these hidden places. Apart from old Arnold nobody ever came down here, not even the postman who left the infrequent mail in a box at the top of the track and nobody saw the blazing scarlets and golds of the autumn trees nor heard the busy clucking and murmuring of the beck among its clean-washed stones.

I walked along the water's edge watching the little fish darting and flitting in the cool depths. In the spring these banks were bright with primroses and in May a great sea of bluebells flowed among the trees but today, though the sky was an untroubled blue, the clean air was touched with the sweetness of the dying year.

I climbed a little way up the hillside and sat down among the bracken now fast turning to bronze. Sam, as was his way, flopped by my side and I ran a hand over the silky hair of his ears. The far side of the valley rose steeply to where, above the gleaming ridge of limestone cliffs, I could just see the sunlit rim of the moor.

In such hidden spots, time often feels like it stands still. When it came to rural life in Yorkshire, Alfred Wight also witnessed something of a vanishing world. When he arrived in 1940, the hills and moors around Thirsk and in the Dales were still full of small farms, some with a herd of sheep, a few cows and perhaps the odd pig or horse. Over the subsequent decades, many of these small farms struggled to makes ends meet and were sold. Isolated farms and smallholdings, many of them without even a road or track leading to them, gradually vanished, as did the presence of the draught horse. In the wake of the tractor, the great Shire or Clydesdale horses no longer pulled the ploughs or provided the heavy labour on farms, although many farmers kept them on. Nonetheless, in just a few years, Alf would see the numbers of horses in the region plummet.

While modern life is gradually making itself felt in the Dales, there is still the odd household which has been entirely untouched by modernity. The Bramleys – made up of three brothers and a sister – who feature in *It Shouldn't Happen to a Vet* are a prime example of one such family. There is no road to their farmhouse, which doesn't bother them as they rarely venture into the outside world. Miss Bramley only visits Darrowby on the odd market day and the middle brother Herbert last came into town in 1929 to have a tooth out. James is one of the few people to venture to their farm, when he calls in to treat their vast collection of much-loved cats.

After twenty minutes of slithering in and out of the unseen puddles and opening a series of broken, string-tied gates, I reached the farmyard and crossed over to the back door. I was about to knock when I stopped with my hand poised. I found I was looking through the kitchen window and in the interior, dimly lit by an oil lamp, the Bramleys were sitting in a row.

They weren't grouped round the fire but were jammed tightly on a long, high-backed wooden settle which stood against the far wall. The strange thing was the almost exact similarity of their attitudes; all four had their arms folded, chins resting on their chests, feet stretched out in front of them. The men had removed their heavy boots and were stocking-footed, but Miss Bramley wore an old pair of carpet slippers.

I stared, fascinated by the curious immobility of the group. They were not asleep, not talking or reading or listening to the radio — in fact they didn't have one — they were just sitting.

I had never seen people just sitting before and I stood there for some minutes to see if they would make a move or do anything at all, but nothing happened. It occurred to me that this was probably a typical evening; they worked hard all day, had their meal; then they just sat till bedtime.

James and Siegfried also witness the last days of the small dairy farm, each typically made up of ten or so cows, all of them named and kept in a cobbled byre or sent out to graze in the fields. The bigger, more industrial dairy farms which are replacing them are more productive in terms of milk yield but, as James laments, they are far less welcoming. In the late 1930s, farmers were still hand-milking their cows, many of them the red or brown shorthorn breed which once predominated in the Yorkshire Dales before the advent of the black and white Friesians. In *Let Sleeping Vets Lie*, James calls in on the small dairy farmer Mr Pickersgill who just about makes a living from his smallholding and whose cows are suffering from mastitis.

I had happened in at the little byre late one afternoon when Mr Pickersgill and his daughter Olive were milking their ten cows. I had watched the two at work as they crouched under the row of roan and red backs and one thing was immediately obvious; while Olive drew the milk by almost imperceptible movements of her fingers and with a motionless wrist, her father hauled away at the teats as though he was trying to ring in the new year.

James deduces that Mr Pickersgill's heavy-handed milking method is the cause of the problem and he now has the tricky task of telling the experienced farmer that he must try a more gentle technique.

It wouldn't be easy because Mr Pickersgill was an impressive man. I don't suppose he had a spare penny in the world but even as he sat there in the kitchen in his tattered, collarless flannel shirt and braces he looked, as always, like an industrial tycoon. You could imagine that massive head with its fleshy cheeks, noble brow and serene eyes looking out from the financial pages of *The Times*. Put him in a bowler and striped trousers and you'd have the perfect chairman of the board.

I was very chary of affronting such natural dignity and anyway, Mr Pickersgill was fundamentally a fine stocksman. His few cows, like all the animals of that fast-dying breed of small farmer, were fat and sleek and clean. You had to look after your beasts when they were your only source of income

61

and somehow Mr Pickersgill had brought up a family by milk production eked out by selling a few pigs and the eggs from his wife's fifty hens.

It is Darrowby of course where James and Siegfried live and work, a fictional town that Alf Wight largely based on Thirsk, although it also contains, as Alf wrote, 'something of Richmond, Leyburn, Middleham and a fair chunk of my imagination'. On first arriving, in *If Only They Could Talk*, James is immediately taken with the small market town.

> Darrowby didn't get much space in the guide books but when it was mentioned it was described as a grey little town on the river Darrow with a cobbled market place and little of interest except its two ancient bridges. But when you looked at it, its setting was beautiful on the pebbly river where the houses clustered thickly and straggled unevenly along the lower slopes of Herne Fell. Everywhere in Darrowby, in the streets, through the windows of the houses you could see the fell rearing its calm, green bulk more than two thousand feet above the huddled roofs.
>
> There was a clarity in the air, a sense of space and airiness that made me feel I had shed something on the plain, twenty miles behind. The confinement of the city, the grime, the smoke – already they seemed to be falling away from me.

Darrowby is a bustling place, with at least one weekly market, and plenty of shops, inns and various facilities for those living in the town and its environs. Dr Allison – a character based on Alf Wight's family doctor Harry Addison – is just a few doors down from the Skeldale House practice and there's at least one bank, a dentist, along with Howarth's the chemist, Pickersgill's the ironmonger and the Darrowby Plaza, the location for James and Helen's disastrous date at the cinema. Houses vary in size and age and there are still Dickensian-like yards and tiny streets in the old part of the town, accessed through an arch and narrow passage where the likes of old Mr Dean and his Labrador Bob live.

Like many towns across the UK, Darrowby also has an abundance of public houses and inns – Thirsk had at least nineteen when Alf worked there. Farmers would head to the pubs, especially on market day, and many villages had at least one ale house or inn, where locals could swap stories and unwind in front of a fire after a day's hard labour. In the post-war years, pubs in Yorkshire, as opposed to the large hotel-like inns, typically had no bars, only a stone-flagged kitchen-like room where the largely male regulars would sit at oak tables or on high-back wooden benches in front of a fire burning in a range. They were often quiet places, with the landlords supplementing their usually meagre incomes with a smallholding of a few animals.

Pubs were often judged on their fires, the food and, most importantly, their beer, and local breweries – Tetley's of Leeds, Cameron's of Hartlepool and Tadcaster rivals Samuel Smith and John Smith – competed for customer loyalty. Alf, Donald and Brian, like their fictional counterparts, enjoyed relaxing in a local pub, where they could enjoy a good beer, a roaring fire and pleasant company. During or after rounds, they were also useful places to escape to, where, half-starved and frozen from wrestling farm animals out in the fields, they could warm up and fill their bellies with home-cooked meals prepared on the range. During Alf's courting days, a drink at a pub often preceded a trip to a local dance or the cinema. On returning from the RAF in 1943 he briefly lived with his wife Joan and her family in the village of Sowerby. Their house was conveniently located next door to the Crown and Anchor pub, which is still trading, and Alf shared many pints with his father-in-law and other friends there.

Brian was a great frequenter of the local pubs, just as Tristan is in the books. Like many Yorkshiremen, Tristan considers himself something of a beer connoisseur, and he'll often carouse long after James and Siegfried have turned in. In *The Lord God Made Them All*, James and Helen have just had their daughter Rosie and Tristan is keen to celebrate at a local pub. He mentally goes through all the options, including the pub they frequent most often, the Drovers' Arms, which was based on the Golden Fleece in Thirsk. It's clear Tristan, who has a sharp mind and bags of charm, has an encyclopedic knowledge when it comes to the pubs of Darrowby and beer drinking.

'We've got to wet this baby's head, Jim,' he said seriously.

I was ready for anything. 'Of course, of course, when are you coming over?'

'I'll be there at seven,' he replied crisply, and I knew he would be.

Tristan was concerned about the venue of the celebration. There were four of us in the sitting room at Skeldale House – Siegfried, Tristan, Alex Taylor and myself. Alex was my oldest friend – we started school together in Glasgow at the age of four – and when he came out of the army after five years in the Western Desert and Italy he came to spend a few weeks with Helen and me in Darrowby. It wasn't long before he had fallen under the spell of the country life and now he was learning farming and estate agency with a view to starting a new career. It was good that he should be with me tonight.

Tristan's fingers drummed on the arm of his chair as he thought aloud. His expression was fixed and grave, his eyes vacant.

'We'd normally go to the Drovers' but they've got that big party on tonight, so that's no good,' he muttered. 'We want a bit of peace and quiet. Let's see now, there's the George and Dragon — Tetley's beer, splendid stuff, but I've known them a bit careless with their pipes and I've had the odd sour mouthful. And of course we have the Cross Keys. They pull a lovely pint of Cameron's and the draught Guinness is excellent. And we mustn't forget the Hare and Pheasant — their bitter can rise to great heights although the mild is ordinary.' He paused for a moment. 'We might do worse than the Lord Nelson — very reliable ale — and of course there's always . . .'

'Just a minute, Triss,' I broke in. 'I went round to Nurse Brown's this evening to see Helen, and Cliff asked if he could come with us. Don't you think it would be rather nice to go to his pub since the baby was born in his house?'

Tristan narrowed his eyes. 'Which pub is that?'

'The Black Horse.'

'Ay yes, ye-es.' Tristan looked at me thoughtfully and put his fingertips together. 'Russell and Rangham's. A good little brewery, that. I've had some first-rate pints in the Black Horse, though I've noticed a slight loss of nuttiness under very warm conditions.' He looked anxiously out of the window. 'It's been hot today. Perhaps we'd . . .'

'Oh for heaven's sake!' Siegfried leaped to his feet. 'You sound like an analytical chemist. It's only beer you're talking about, after all.'

Tristan looked at him in shocked silence but Siegfried turned to me briskly. 'I think that's a pleasant idea of yours, James. Let's go with Cliff to the Black Horse. It's a quiet little place.'

And, indeed, as we dropped to the chairs in the bar parlour I felt we had chosen the ideal spot. The evening sunshine sent long golden shafts over the pitted oak tables and the high-backed settles where a few farm men sat with their glasses. There was nothing smart about this little inn, but the furniture, which hadn't been changed for a hundred years, gave it an air of tranquillity. It was just right.

The local inns provide not just beer and company but also a communal space for auctions, games, such as dominoes or darts, or meetings. In *The Lord God Made Them All*, one pub regular even offers haircuts at his local, the Hare and Pheasant – a character based on the Thirsk barber John Wallace. Even at his own premises, as Jim Wight remembers, he'd frequently disappear in the middle of a haircut, only to return twenty minutes later to inform you that he'd just eaten the best ham sandwich ever.

Josh Anderson was one of the local barbers. He liked his job, but he also liked his beer. In fact he was devoted to it, even to the extent of taking his scissors and clippers to the pub with him every night. For the price of a pint he would give anybody a quick trim in the gents' lavatory.

Habitués of the Hare and Pheasant were never surprised to find one of the customers sitting impassively on the toilet seat with Josh snip-snipping round his head. With beer at sixpence a pint it was good value, but Josh's clients knew they were taking a chance. If the barber's intake had been moderate they would escape relatively unscathed because the standard of hair-styling in the Darrowby district was not very fastidious, but if he had imbibed beyond a certain point terrible things could happen.

Josh had not as yet been known to cut off anybody's ear, but if you strolled around the town on Sundays and Mondays you were liable to come across some very strange coiffures.

In *Every Living Thing* James is saddened to see the Lord Nelson, a typical Yorkshire pub of Darrowby, refurbished, its traditional features swept away. The new pubs are more profitable, noisier and attract a younger crowd, but they drive some (but not all) of the local clientele away.

Bob Stockdale was the sole survivor of the cataclysm which had struck the Lord Nelson inn. In dirty Wellington boots and flat cap, he sat there on a high stool at the end of the bar counter, seemingly oblivious of the endless torrent of piped music and the babel of voices from the jostling pack of smart young people.

I fought my way to the bar, collected a pint of bitter and, as I stood surveying the scene from a space against the wall, my thoughts drifted sadly back to the old days. A year ago the Lord Nelson was a typical Yorkshire country pub and I remembered an evening when I dropped in there with a friend from Glasgow, the city of my youth. There was just one big room then, rather like a large kitchen, with a log fire burning in a black cooking range at one end and a dozen farm men sitting on high-backed oak settles, their pints resting on tables of pitted wood. Those settles were a draught-proof refuge from the cold winds which whistled along the streets of the village outside and over the high pastures where those men spent their days.

The conversation never rose above a gentle murmur over which the ticking of a wall clock and the click of dominoes added to the atmosphere of rest and quiet.

'Gosh, it's peaceful in here,' my friend said. Wonderingly, he watched the proprietor, in shirt and braces, proceed unhurriedly down to the cellar and emerge with a long enamel jug from which he replenished the glasses, regulating the flow expertly to achieve the required head of froth.

'A bit different from West Nile Street,' I said.

He grinned. 'It certainly is. In fact, it's unbelievable. How does a place like this pay? Only a few chaps here, and they aren't drinking much.'

'I think it hardly pays at all. Maybe a few pounds a week, but the owner has a smallholding — there are cows, calves and pigs just through that wall — and he looks on this as a pleasant sideline.'

My friend took a pull at his glass, stretched out his legs and half closed his eyes. 'Anyway, I like it. You can relax here. It's lovely.'

It was indeed lovely and most of the pubs around Darrowby were still attractive, but as I looked at the modernized Lord Nelson I wondered how long they would stay that way.

When the new owner took over he didn't waste any time in starting his revolution. He wasn't a farmer, he was an experienced landlord and he could see rich possibilities in the old inn in the pretty village of Welsby tucked among the fells. The kitchen range disappeared and was replaced by a smart bar counter with a background of mirrors and gleaming bottles; the antique settles and tables were swept away, and horse brasses, hunting horns and sporting prints appeared on the walls. The end wall was knocked down and people ate in an elegant dining room where once I calved the cows and tended the pigs.

Two things happened almost at once; droves of young people swarmed out to Welsby in their cars from the big Yorkshire towns, and the old clientele melted away. I never knew where those farm men went, probably to pubs in the neighbouring villages – just Bob Stockdale stayed. I couldn't understand why, but he was a quiet man, a bit of a loner, and maybe he felt that he had sat in that room several nights a week for years and, despite all the changes, he didn't want to leave it. Anyway, whenever I called in, he was there, perched on the same stool, with his old bitch, Meg, tucked underneath.

Dancing was also a common form of entertainment and, in the days of James Herriot, most of the villages and rural communities held dances on Saturday nights in simple wooden-built structures, the village institutes. (Most now have been pulled down and replaced by brick structures.) Locals would gather to whirl around to music and help themselves to the great quantities of food on offer while musicians played the tunes of the day. They were full of life and Alf and Joan often attended. In *If Only They Could Talk* Tristan and James take two nurses, Connie and Brenda, to a dance in the village of Poulton. Tristan suggests they first have a drink at a pub – 'We'll just have a little toothful to get us in the mood.' The landlord plies them with draught Magnet beer, poured from a tall white enamelled jug, and before they know it, they've consumed pints of the stuff, before they decide to head to the dance.

After the brightness of the inn the darkness pressed on us like a blanket and we groped our way up the steep street till we could see the institute standing on its grassy mound. Faint rays of light escaped through the chinks in the curtained windows and we could hear the music and a rhythmic thudding.

A cheerful young farmer took our money at the door and when we went into the hall we were swallowed up in a tight mass of dancers. The place was packed solidly with young men in stiff-looking dark suits and girls in bright dresses, all sweating happily as they swayed and wheeled to the music.

On the low platform at one end, four musicians were playing their hearts out – piano, accordion, violin and drums. At the other end, several comfortable, middle-aged women stood behind a long table on trestles, presiding over the thick sandwiches of ham and brawn, homemade pies, jugs of milk and trifles generously laid with cream.

All round the walls more lads were standing, eyeing the unattached girls. I recognized a young client. 'What do you call this dance?' I yelled above the din.

'The Eva Three Step,' came back the reply.

This was new to me but I launched out confidently with Connie. There was a lot of twirling and stamping and when the men brought their heavy boots down on the boards the hall shook and the noise was deafening. I loved it – I was right on the peak and I whirled Connie effortlessly among the throng. I was dimly aware of bumping people with my shoulders but, try as I might, I couldn't feel my feet touching the floor. The floating sensation was delicious. I decided that I had never been so happy in my life.

After half a dozen dances I felt ravenous and floated with Connie towards the food table. We each ate an enormous wedge of ham and egg pie which was so exquisite that we had the same again. Then we had some trifle and plunged again into the crush. It was about halfway through a St Bernard's Waltz that I began to feel my feet on the boards again – quite heavy and dragging somewhat. Connie felt heavy too. She seemed to be slumped in my arms.

She looked up. Her face was very white. 'Jus' feeling a bit queer – 'scuse me.' She broke away and began to tack erratically towards the ladies' room. A few minutes later she came out and her face was no longer white. It was green. She staggered over to me. 'Could do with some fresh air. Take me outside.'

As a young man in his twenties, James makes the most of his new home and he certainly feels he has landed on his feet when it comes to Darrowby and the Yorkshire Dales. Such was the case with Alf, who soon became part of the community, describing Thirsk as a 'happy town', with 'an abundance of good shops with smiling people behind the counters and some splendid inns with welcoming landlords'.

Chapter 3

SIEGFRIED FARNON *and* SKELDALE HOUSE

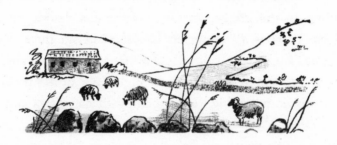

'Mr Farnon is expecting me. He wrote asking me to come today.'

'Mr Herriot?' she said thoughtfully. 'Surgery is from six to seven o'clock. If you wanted to bring a dog in, that would be your best time.'

'No, no,' I said, hanging on to my smile. 'I'm applying for the position of assistant. Mr Farnon said to come in time for tea.'

'Assistant? Well, now, that's nice.' The lines in her face softened a little. 'I'm Mrs Hall. I keep house for Mr Farnon. He's a bachelor, you know. He never said anything to me about you, but never mind, come in and have a cup of tea. It shouldn't be long before he's back.'

Mrs Hall, housekeeper of Skeldale House, is used to answering the front door. On the iron railings outside, a brass plate bears the name of Mr S. Farnon MRCVS, Veterinary Surgeon, and those ringing the bell are usually clients keen for Mr Farnon to see to their animals. This time it's a young man smiling nervously at the door, name of James Herriot, who has come for an interview with her employer.

From Darrowby's main square, the young vet has walked along the quiet street of Trengate until he reached Skeldale House, the only house to have ivy climbing untidily over its bricks. It has a fine, white-painted doorway and graceful, wide windows on the ground floor. The paint is flaking here and there but there is a 'changeless elegance' about the old house and James immediately likes the look of it. Mrs Hall ushers James in and for the first time, he enters the house which will become his home and workplace, where a new life awaits him.

I followed her between whitewashed walls, my feet clattering on the tiles. We turned right at the end into another passage and I was beginning to wonder just how far back the house extended when I was shown into a sunlit room.

It had been built in the grand manner, high-ceilinged and airy with a massive fireplace flanked by arched alcoves. One end was taken up by a French window which gave on a long, high-walled garden. I could see unkempt lawns, a rockery and many fruit trees. A great bank of peonies blazed in the hot sunshine and at the far end, rooks cawed in the branches of a group of tall elms. Above and beyond were the green hills with their climbing walls.

Ordinary-looking furniture stood around on a very worn carpet. Hunting prints hung on the walls and books were scattered everywhere, some on shelves in the alcoves but others piled on the floor in the corners. A pewter pint pot occupied a prominent place at one end of the mantelpiece. It was an interesting pot. Cheques and banknotes had been stuffed into it till they bulged out of the top and overflowed onto the hearth beneath. I was studying this with astonishment when Mrs Hall came in with a tea tray.

'I suppose Mr Farnon is out on a case,' I said.

'No, he's gone through to Brawton to visit his mother. I can't really say when he'll be back.' She left me with my tea.

While James waits for Siegfried, the doorbell constantly rings, each time causing the five dogs of the house to hurl themselves towards the door, leaping and yelping. With no sign of Mrs Hall, James answers the door and greets first Mr Bert Sharpe who has a cow 'wot wants borin' out', then Mr Mulligan, whose dog is 'womitin' bad', and finally a mysterious red-haired girl, Diana Brompton, who comes in to wait for Siegfried. James awkwardly attempts polite conversation with her, until she eventually marches out of the room, clearly annoyed with waiting. James then decides to wander out into the walled garden, flops down onto the knee-deep grass and rests his head against an acacia tree. As the sun beats down on him and a gentle breeze stirs the wisteria covering the back of the house, he half closes his eyes and dozes, conjuring images in his mind of Siegfried – a man with a curiously Germanic-sounding name . . .

And I opened my eyes. Somebody was saying 'Hello', but it wasn't Herr Farrenen. A tall, thin man was leaning against the wall, his hands in his pockets. Something seemed to be amusing him. As I struggled to my feet, he heaved himself away from the wall and held out his hand. 'Sorry you've had to wait. I'm Siegfried Farnon.'

He was just about the most English-looking man I had ever seen. Long, humorous, strong-jawed face. Small, clipped moustache, untidy, sandy hair. He was wearing an old tweed jacket and shapeless flannel trousers. The collar of his check shirt was frayed and the tie carelessly knotted. He looked as though he didn't spend much time in front of a mirror.

Siegfried proceeds to show him around the well-stocked practice dispensary and then to take him for a spin in his battered Hillman to visit Bert Sharpe's cow and some other farms in the area. Siegfried's unorthodox driving – which veers between hurtling along tiny country roads at seventy miles per hour or idling along with his elbows on the wheel, only to slam on his brakes to point out some pedigree shorthorn cows – matches his erratic, unpredictable nature. His boundless energy, however, comes with considerable charm, and once James begins to work alongside Siegfried, it's soon clear how well respected and liked he is by those who live in the Dales.

Donald Vaughan Sinclair, on whom Siegfried was based, also forgot that Alf Wight was coming for an interview in June 1940. Born in 1911, Donald was older than Alf by some five years. A graduate of the Royal School of Veterinary Studies in Edinburgh, he had bought the Thirsk practice at 23 Kirkgate in 1939. Mrs Weatherill was the practice housekeeper, and she too wasn't surprised that Donald was out when Alf arrived as her employer was also forgetful or at least easily distracted as he charged about from place to place. Like Siegfried, Donald had a small, clipped moustache and the tweedy, slightly dishevelled appearance of an English gentleman, but he was attractive with it and something of a charmer when it came to the ladies.

He warmed to Alf instantly and offered him the position. In reality, Donald left for the RAF almost immediately and it was some months before Alf worked with him closely but because *If Only They Could Talk* is set in 1937, Siegfried remains in Darrowby and James soon gets a sense of the confusion and disarray that invariably accompanies day-to-day life with the more senior vet.

Siegfried Farnon charged round the practice with fierce energy from dawn till dark and I often wondered what drove him on. It wasn't money because he treated it with scant respect. When the bills were paid, the cash went into the pint pot on the mantelpiece and he grabbed handfuls when he wanted it. I never saw him take out a wallet, but his pockets bulged with loose silver and balled-up notes. When he pulled out a thermometer they flew around him in a cloud.

After a week or two of headlong rush he would disappear; maybe for the evening, maybe overnight and often without saying where he was going. Mrs Hall would serve a meal for two, but when she saw I was eating alone she would remove the food without comment.

He dashed off the list of calls each morning with such speed that I was quite often sent hurrying off to the wrong farm or to do the wrong thing. When I told him later of my embarrassment he would laugh heartily.

There was one time when he got involved himself. I had just taken a call from a Mr Heaton of Bronsett about doing a PM on a dead sheep.

'I'd like you to come with me, James,' Siegfried said. 'Things are quiet this morning and I believe they teach you blokes a pretty hot post-mortem procedure. I want to see you in action.'

We drove into the village of Bronsett and Siegfried swung the car left into a gated lane.

'Where are you going?' I said. 'Heaton's is at the other end of the village.'

'But you said Seaton's.'

'No, I assure you . . .'

'Look, James, I was right by you when you were talking to the man. I distinctly heard you say the name.'

I opened my mouth to argue further but the car was hurtling down the lane and Siegfried's jaw was jutting. I decided to let him find out for himself.

We arrived outside the farmhouse with a screaming of brakes. Siegfried had left his seat and was rummaging in the boot before the car had stopped shuddering. 'Hell!' he shouted. 'No post-mortem knife. Never mind, I'll borrow something from the house.' He slammed down the lid and bustled over to the door.

The farmer's wife answered and Siegfried beamed on her. 'Good morning to you, Mrs Seaton, have you a carving knife?'

The good lady raised her eyebrows. 'What was that you said?'

'A carving knife, Mrs Seaton, a carving knife, and a good sharp one, please.'

'You want a carving knife?'

'Yes, that's right, a carving knife!' Siegfried cried, his scanty store of patience beginning to run out. 'And I wonder if you'd mind hurrying. I haven't much time.'

The bewildered woman withdrew to the kitchen and I could hear whispering and muttering. Children's heads peeped out at intervals to get a quick look at Siegfried stamping irritably on the step. After some delay, one of the daughters advanced timidly, holding out a long, dangerous-looking knife.

Siegfried snatched it from her hand and ran his thumb up and down the edge. 'This is no damn good!' he shouted in exasperation. 'Don't you understand I want something really sharp? Fetch me a steel.'

The girl fled back into the kitchen and there was a low

77

rumble of voices. It was some minutes before another young girl was pushed round the door. She inched her way up to Siegfried, gave him the steel at arm's length and dashed back to safety.

Siegfried prided himself on his skill at sharpening a knife. It was something he enjoyed doing. As he stropped the knife on the steel, he warmed to his work and finally burst into song. There was no sound from the kitchen, only the ring of steel on steel backed by the tuneless singing; there were silent intervals when he carefully tested the edge, then the noise would start again.

When he had completed the job to his satisfaction he peered inside the door. 'Where is your husband?' he called.

There was no reply so he strode into the kitchen, waving the gleaming blade in front of him. I followed him and saw Mrs Seaton and her daughters cowering in the far corner, staring at Siegfried with large, frightened eyes.

He made a sweeping gesture at them with the knife. 'Well, come on, I can get started now!'

'Started what?' the mother whispered, holding her family close to her.

'I want to PM this sheep. You have a dead sheep, haven't you?'

Explanations and apologies followed.

Later, Siegfried remonstrated gravely with me for sending him to the wrong farm.

'You'll have to be a bit more careful in future, James,' he said seriously. 'Creates a very bad impression, that sort of thing.'

While Siegfried fails to acknowledge his own shortcomings, such as forgetting appointments or driving to the wrong farm, he is not shy in doling out advice and pointing out James's flaws, only then to prove he is just as guilty of them. In *If Only They Could Talk* Siegfried advises James not to get so worked up over a case. Shortly after, a client sends Siegfried into such a violent rage that he's lucky to escape with his life.

Sometimes he would give me advice on how to live. As when he found me hunched over the phone which I had just crashed down; I was staring at the wall, swearing softly to myself.

Siegfried smiled whimsically. 'Now what is it, James?'

'I've just had a torrid ten minutes with Rolston. You remember that outbreak of calf pneumonia? Well, I spent hours with those calves, poured expensive drugs into them. There wasn't a single death. And now he's complaining about this bill. Not a word of thanks. Hell, there's no justice.'

Siegfried walked over and put his arm round my shoulders. He was wearing his patient look again. 'My dear chap,' he cooed. 'Just look at you. Red in the face, all tensed up. You mustn't let yourself get upset like this; you must try to relax. Why do you think professional men are cracking up all over the country with coronaries and ulcers? Just because they allow themselves to get all steamed up over piffling little things like you are doing now. Yes, yes, I know these things are annoying, but you've got to take them in your stride. Keep calm, James, calm. It just isn't worth it − I mean, it will all be the same in a hundred years.'

He delivered the sermon with a serene smile, patting my shoulder reassuringly like a psychiatrist soothing a violent patient.

I was writing a label on a jar of red blister a few days later when Siegfried catapulted into the room. He must have kicked the door open because it flew back viciously against the rubber stop and rebounded almost into his face. He rushed over to the desk where I was sitting and began to pound on it with the flat of his hand. His eyes glared wildly from a flushed face.

'I've just come from that bloody swine Holt!' he shouted.

'Ned Holt, you mean?'

'Yes, that's who I mean, damn him!'

I was surprised. Mr Holt was a little man who worked on the roads for the county council. He kept four cows as a side-line and had never been known to pay a veterinary bill, but he was a cheerful character and Siegfried had rendered his unpaid services over the years without objection.

'One of your favourites, isn't he?' I said.

'Was, by God, was,' Siegfried snarled. 'I've been treating Muriel for him. You know, the big red cow second from the far end of his byre. She's had recurrent tympany — coming in from the field every night badly blown — and I'd tried about everything. Nothing did any good. Then it struck me that it might be actinobacillosis of the reticulum. I shot some sodium iodine into the vein and when I saw her today the difference was incredible — she was standing there, chewing her cud, right as rain. I was just patting myself on the back for a smart piece of diagnosis, and do you know what Holt said? He said he knew she'd be better today because last night he gave her half a pound of Epsom salts in a bran mash. That was what had cured her.'

Siegfried took some empty cartons and bottles from his pockets and hurled them savagely into the wastepaper basket. He began to shout again.

'Do you know, for the past fortnight I've puzzled and worried and damn nearly dreamed about that cow. Now I've found the cause of the trouble, applied the most modern treatment and the animal has recovered. And what happens? Does the owner express his grateful thanks for my skill? Does he hell — the entire credit goes to the half-pound of Epsom salts. What I did was a pure waste of time.'

He dealt the desk another sickening blow.

'But I frightened him, James,' he said, his eyes staring. 'By God, I frightened him. When he made that crack about the salts, I yelled out, "You bugger!" and made a grab for him. I think I would have strangled him, but he shot into the house and stayed there. I didn't see him again.'

Siegfried threw himself into a chair and began to churn his hair about. 'Epsom salts!' he groaned. 'Oh God, it makes you despair.'

I thought of telling him to relax and pointing out that it would all be the same in a hundred years, but my employer still had an empty serum bottle dangling from one hand. I discarded the idea.

Siegfried is quick to lose his temper but it's his younger brother Tristan who brings out the worst in him. Tristan is studying at the Edinburgh Veterinary College and returns to Skeldale House during his vacations. Siegfried boils with frustration over Tristan's indolence and failure to pass his exams and James is witness to countless arguments between the pair, which usually result in Siegfried ranting at his brother and throwing him out of the house.

The relationship between Donald and his younger brother Brian, the real-life persona of Tristan, was equally combative, just as relations often are between siblings, but the two had such outlandish personalities that their squabbles sometimes took on epic proportions. Like Tristan, Brian Sinclair was a student of veterinary science and by the time he returned to the practice during the Christmas vacation of 1940 Donald had already been discharged from the RAF – at nearly thirty, he'd lied about his age, and lacked the reflexes required for air instruction. Once the RAF discovered his true age, they reviewed his case and sent him home.

Siegfried is highly opinionated about many issues, not least on the topic of keeping dogs or any animals as pets. This mystifies James as Siegfried is forever surrounded by a pack of dogs, and not for any practical purpose other than he likes having them around.

People often wondered why Siegfried kept five dogs. Not only kept them but took them everywhere with him. Driving on his rounds it was difficult to see him at all among the shaggy heads and waving tails; and anybody approaching the car would recoil in terror from the savage barking and the bared fangs and glaring eyes framed in the windows.

'I cannot for the life of me understand,' Siegfried would declare, thumping his fist on his knee, 'why people keep dogs as pets. A dog should have a useful function. Let it be used for farm work, for shooting, for guiding; but why anybody should keep the things just hanging around the place beats me.'

It was a pronouncement he was continually making, often through a screen of flapping ears and lolling tongues as he sat in his car. His listener would look wonderingly from the huge greyhound to the tiny terrier, from the spaniel to the whippet to the Scottie; but nobody ever asked Siegfried why he kept his own dogs.

Siegfried's lack of self-awareness when it comes to his own sometimes outrageous behaviour continues unabated throughout the James Herriot stories, and living and working with such a larger-than-life character can be trying for the younger partner. Despite this, James enjoys the company of Siegfried and his younger brother Tristan and becomes accustomed to the noise, the madcap schemes and the great laughs they share when swapping stories about the day's rounds. In *Let Sleeping Vets Lie*, James looks back on the first two or three years of life at the practice and feels fortunate to be living with the two brothers, whom he considers friends, recognizing also that he had a lot to learn from Siegfried: 'As a city-bred youth trying to tell expert stock farmers how to treat their animals I had needed all his skill and guidance behind me.'

Donald Sinclair similarly had little awareness of how funny or unusual his behaviour could be, and never considered himself an eccentric in any way. But, like, Siegfried he was a fine vet and regularly offered sage advice to Alf, both in the care of their animal patients and in their dealings with clients. He also readily admitted to having made mistakes in his work, but was revered among the farming community and was particularly skilled when it came to horses. In fact he was very much a horseman, comfortable in the equine world and with horse owners in the region – those with racehorses or thoroughbreds trusted Donald with their prized steeds.

In *Vet in a Spin*, James looks back on his relationship with Siegfried, who remains a close friend and work colleague decades later. Although Siegfried has always been infuriating and something of a tyrant at times, his enthusiasm is infectious, he has immense charm and is always fizzing with ideas. Critically, though, he has a good heart and is a stalwart of the community and it is those traits which redeem him.

Even now, as we still jog along happily after thirty-five years, I wonder about it. I know I liked him instinctively when I first saw him in the garden at Skeldale House on that very first afternoon, but I feel there is another reason why we get on together.

Maybe it is because we are opposites. Siegfried's restless energy impels him constantly to try to alter things while I abhor change of any kind. A lot of people would call him brilliant, while not even my best friends would apply that description to me. His mind relentlessly churns out ideas of all grades – excellent, doubtful and very strange indeed. I, on the other hand, rarely have an idea of any sort. He likes hunting, shooting and fishing; I prefer football, cricket and tennis. I could go on and on – we are even opposite physical types – and yet, as I say, we get along.

This of course doesn't mean that we have never had our differences. Over the years there have been minor clashes on various points . . .

There was another time Siegfried had to take me to task. An old-age pensioner was leading a small mongrel dog along the passage on the end of a piece of string. I patted the consulting-room table.

'Put him up here, will you?' I said.

The old man bent over slowly, groaning and puffing.

'Wait a minute.' I tapped his shoulder. 'Let me do it.' I hoisted the little animal onto the smooth surface.

'Thank ye, sir.' The man straightened up and rubbed his back and leg. 'I 'ave arthritis bad and I'm not much good at liftin'. My name's Bailey and I live at t'council houses.'

'Right, Mr Bailey, what's the trouble?'

'It's this cough. He's allus at it. And 'e kind of retches at t'end of it.'

'I see. How old is he?'

'He were ten last month.'

'Yes . . .' I took the temperature and carefully auscultated the chest. As I moved the stethoscope over the ribs Siegfried came in and began to rummage in the cupboard.

'It's a chronic bronchitis, Mr Bailey,' I said. 'Many older dogs suffer from it just like old folks.'

He laughed. 'Aye, ah'm a bit wheezy myself sometimes.'

'That's right, but you're not so bad, really, are you?'

'Naw, naw.'

'Well neither is your little dog. I'm going to give him an injection and a course of tablets and it will help him quite a bit. I'm afraid he'll never quite get rid of this cough, but bring him in again if it gets very bad.'

He nodded vigorously. 'Very good, sir. Thank ye kindly, sir.'

As Siegfried banged about in the cupboard I gave the injection and counted out twenty of the new M&B 693 tablets.

The old man gazed at them with interest then put them in his pocket. 'Now what do ah owe ye, Mr Herriot?'

I looked at the ragged tie knotted carefully over the frayed shirt collar, at the threadbare antiquity of the jacket. His trouser knees had been darned but on one side I caught a pink glimpse of the flesh through the material.

'No, that's all right, Mr Bailey. Just see how he goes on.'

'Eh?'

'There's no charge.'

'But . . .'

'Now don't worry about it — it's nothing, really. Just see he gets his tablets regularly.'

'I will, sir, and it's very kind of you. I never expected . . .'

'I know you didn't, Mr Bailey. Goodbye for now and bring him back if he's not a lot better in a few days.'

The sound of the old man's footsteps had hardly died away when Siegfried emerged from the cupboard. He brandished a pair of horse-tooth forceps in my face. 'God, I've been ages hunting these down. I'm sure you deliberately hide things from me, James.'

I smiled but made no reply and as I was replacing my syringe on the trolley my colleague spoke again.

'James, I don't like to mention this, but aren't you rather rash, doing work for nothing?'

I looked at him in surprise. 'He was an old-age pensioner. Pretty hard up I should think.'

'Maybe so, but really, you know, you just cannot give your services free.'

'Oh but surely occasionally, Siegfried — in a case like this . . .'

'No, James, not even occasionally. It's just not practical.'

'But I've seen you do it — time and time again!'

'Me?' His eyes widened in astonishment. 'Never! I'm too aware of the harsh realities of life for that. Everything has become so frightfully expensive. For instance, weren't those M&B 693 tablets you were dishing out? Heaven help us, do you know those things are threepence each? It's no good — you must never work without charging.'

'But dammit, you're always doing it!' I burst out. 'Only last week there was that . . .'

Siegfried held up a restraining hand. 'Please, James, please. You imagine things, that's your trouble.'

I must have given him one of my most exasperated stares because he reached out and patted my shoulder.

'Believe me, my boy, I do understand. You acted from the highest possible motives and I have often been tempted to do the same. But you must be firm. These are hard times and one must be hard to survive. So remember in future — no more Robin Hood stuff, we can't afford it.'

I nodded and went on my way somewhat bemusedly, but I

soon forgot the incident and would have thought no more about it had I not seen Mr Bailey about a week later.

His dog was once more on the consulting-room table and Siegfried was giving it an injection. I didn't want to interfere so I went back along the passage to the front office and sat down to write in the day book. It was a summer afternoon, the window was open and through a parting in the curtain I could see the front steps.

As I wrote I heard Siegfried and the old man passing on their way to the front door. They stopped on the steps. The little dog, still on the end of its string, looked much as it did before.

'All right, Mr Bailey,' my colleague said. 'I can only tell you the same as Mr Herriot. I'm afraid he's got that cough for life, but when it gets bad you must come and see us.'

'Very good, sir,' the old man put his hand in his pocket. 'And what is the charge, please?'

'The charge, oh yes . . . the charge . . .' Siegfried cleared his throat a few times but seemed unable to articulate. He kept looking from the mongrel dog to the old man's tattered clothing and back again. Then he glanced furtively into the house and spoke in a hoarse whisper. 'It's nothing, Mr Bailey.'

'But Mr Farnon, I can't let ye . . .'

'Shh! Shh!' Siegfried waved a hand agitatedly in the old man's face. 'Not a word now! I don't want to hear any more about it.'

Having silenced Mr Bailey he produced a large bag.

'There's about a hundred M&B tablets in here,' he said, throwing an anxious glance over his shoulder. 'He's going to keep needing them, so I've given you a good supply.'

I could see my colleague had spotted the hole in the trouser knee because he gazed down at it for a long time before putting his hand in his jacket pocket.

'Hang on a minute.' He extracted a handful of assorted

chattels. A few coins fell and rolled down the steps as he prodded in his palm among scissors, thermometers, pieces of string, bottle openers. Finally his search was rewarded and he pulled out a banknote.

'Here's a quid,' he whispered and again nervously shushed the man's attempts to speak.

Mr Bailey, realizing the futility of argument, pocketed the money.

'Well, thank ye, Mr Farnon. Ah'll take t'missus to Scarborough wi' that.'

'Good lad, good lad,' muttered Siegfried, still looking around him guiltily. 'Now off you go.'

The old man solemnly raised his cap and began to shuffle painfully down the street.

'Hey, hold on, there,' my colleague called after him. 'What's the matter? You're not going very well.'

'It's this dang arthritis. Ah go a long way in a long time.'

'And you've got to walk all the way to the council houses?' Siegfried rubbed his chin irresolutely. 'It's a fair step.' He took a last wary peep down the passage then beckoned with his hand.

'Look, my car's right here,' he whispered. 'Nip in and I'll run you home.'

As well as taking an instant liking to Siegfried, James quickly feels at home at Skeldale House and becomes fond of its many features and the people who live within its walls. Every morning he walks out of the back of the house, through the high-walled garden, covered with wisteria, to the garage. To this day the garden at 23 Kirkgate remains intact, although it is half the size it once was, and now features a fine bronze statue of Alf Wight wearing his well-used Wellington boots. The wisteria has survived but the fruit trees have gone and sadly the acacia tree that Alf leaned upon as he dozed in the garden blew down one windy night. In *If Only They Could Talk* James already delights in his morning routine that takes him through the garden with its views of the fells beyond.

Down the narrow passage with its familiar, exciting smell of ether and carbolic and out into the high-walled garden which led to the yard where the cars were kept.

It was the same every morning but, to me, there was always the feeling of surprise. When I stepped out into the sunshine and the scent of the flowers it was as though I was doing it for the first time. The clear air held a breath of the nearby moorland; after being buried in a city for five years it was difficult to take it all in.

I never hurried over this part. There could be an urgent case waiting but I still took my time. Along the narrow part between the ivy-covered wall and the long offshoot of the house where the wisteria climbed, pushing its tendrils and its withered blooms into the very rooms. Then past the rockery where the garden widened to the lawn, unkempt and lost-looking but lending coolness and softness to the weathered brick. Around its borders flowers blazed in untidy profusion, battling with a jungle of weeds.

And so to the rose garden, then an asparagus bed whose fleshy fingers had grown into tall fronds. Further on were strawberries and raspberries. Fruit trees were everywhere, their branches dangling low over the path. Peaches, pears, cherries and plums were trained against the south wall where they fought for a place with wild-growing rambler roses.

In the years that Alf lived at Skeldale House, he developed a love for gardening and planted vegetable beds full of lettuces, onions, beans and asparagus, with masses of rhubarb, tomatoes trailing up the walls and strawberries in the summer. Manure from the local farms ensured the soil was rich, and Alf turned it over with the assistance of Wardman, an odd-job man who had come through the First World War and whom Donald had employed to help out in the garden, the garage and with any animals in the yard.

In the books, Wardman appears as Boardman, who is often lurking around the yard, tending the boiler or chortling with Tristan, who spends hours smoking his Woodbines or swapping jokes with the veteran, just as Brian Sinclair often did during his vacations. James describes the yard, Boardman's cubby hole and his memories of Skeldale House in grander days when it belonged to a doctor.

It was square and cobbled and the grass grew in thick tufts between the stones. Buildings took up two sides; the two garages, once coach houses, a stable and saddle room, a loose box and a pigsty. Against the free wall a rusty iron pump hung over a stone water trough.

Above the stable was a hay loft and over one of the garages a dovecot. And there was old Boardman. He, too, seemed to have been left behind from grander days, hobbling round on his lame leg, doing nothing in particular.

He grunted good morning from his cubby hole where he kept a few tools and garden implements. Above his head his reminder of the war looked down: a row of coloured prints of Bruce Bairnsfather cartoons. He had stuck them up when he came home in 1918 and there they were still, dusty and curled at the edges but still speaking to him of Kaiser Bill and the shell holes and muddy trenches.

Boardman washed a car sometimes or did a little work in the garden, but he was content to earn a pound or two and get back to his yard. He spent a lot of time in the saddle room, just sitting. Sometimes he looked round the empty hooks where the harness used to hang and then he would make a rubbing movement with his fist against his palm.

He often talked to me of the great days. 'I can see t'owd doctor now, standing on top step waiting for his carriage to come round. Big, smart-looking feller he was. Allus wore a top hat and frock coat, and I can remember him when I was a lad, standing there, pulling on 'is gloves and giving his hat a tilt while he waited.'

Boardman's features seemed to soften and a light came into his eyes as though he were talking more to himself than to me. 'The old house was different then. A housekeeper and six servants there were and everything just so. And a full-time gardener. There weren't a blade of grass out of place in them days and the flowers all in rows and the trees pruned, tidy like.'

Alongside Boardman and Mrs Hall, Siegfried also decides the veterinary practice needs someone to take charge of the bills. His pint-pot system, a large beer glass stuffed with banknotes and cheques, is less than satisfactory, and putting Tristan in charge of finances was only ever going to result in chaos. We learn that the new secretary, Miss Harbottle, is in her fifties and recently retired from a firm in Bradshaw where she was known for her efficiency. A big woman, her round face framed by gold-rimmed spectacles, she is introduced to James and Tristan.

I shook hands and was astonished at the power of Miss Harbottle's grip. We looked into each other's eyes and had a friendly trial of strength for a few seconds, then she seemed happy to call it a draw and turned away. Tristan was entirely

91

unprepared and a look of alarm spread over his face as his hand was engulfed; he was released only when his knees started to buckle.

Miss Harbottle proceeds to tour the office while Siegfried hovers behind. She examines with horror the ledger and day books, which are covered in illegible scrawl. She pulls open a drawer in a desk, out of which fall old seed packets, a few peas and some French beans. Crammed in another drawer are soiled calving ropes which somebody has forgotten to wash, while empty pale ale bottles clink in another drawer. When she asks to see the cashbox, Siegfried shows her the pint pot on the mantelpiece, with some of its contents spilled onto the hearth below.

Miss Harbottle clearly has her work set out for her and Siegfried is keen for her to start. The relationship, however, soon turns sour as Miss Harbottle grows increasingly frustrated with Siegfried's chaotic way of doing things.

Siegfried looked down at the square figure behind the desk. 'Good morning, Miss Harbottle, can I do anything for you?' The grey eyes glinted behind the gold-rimmed spectacles. 'You can, indeed, Mr Farnon. You can explain why you have once more emptied my petty cash box.'

'Oh, I'm so sorry. I had to rush through to Brawton last night and I found myself a bit short. There was really nowhere else to turn to.'

'But Mr Farnon, in the two months I have been here, we must have been over this a dozen times. What is the good of my trying to keep an accurate record of the money in the practice if you keep stealing it and spending it?'

'Well, I suppose I got into the habit in the old pint-pot days. It wasn't a bad system, really.'

'It wasn't a system at all. It was anarchy. You cannot run a business that way. But I've told you this so many times and each time you have promised to alter your ways. I feel almost at my wits' end.'

Miss Harbottle was based very loosely on Harold Wilson, a retired railway clerk whom Donald and Alf employed in 1949 to help with the practice paperwork and to balance the books. He, like Miss Harbottle, had a difficult relationship with Donald who found the presence of Harold increasingly irritating. Harold, however, valiantly persevered, bringing some order to the haphazard organization of the practice, and stayed on as a valued employee for ten years.

After a few months, the battle between Siegfried and Miss Harbottle intensifies as each combatant attempts to assert their authority in a variety of crafty ways, with Siegfried more often than not on the losing side.

Watching him go, I thought wonderingly of how things had built up since the secretary's arrival. It was naked war now and it gave life an added interest to observe the tactics of the two sides.

At the beginning it seemed that Siegfried must run out an easy winner. He was the employer; he held the reins and it appeared that Miss Harbottle would be helpless in the face of his obstructive strategy. But Miss Harbottle was a fighter and a resourceful one and it was impossible not to admire the way she made use of the weapons at her command.

In fact, over the past week the tide had been running in her favour. She had been playing Siegfried like an expert fisherman with a salmon; bringing him repeatedly back to her desk to answer footling questions. Her throat clearing had developed into an angry bark which could penetrate the full extent of the house. And she had a new weapon; she had taken to writing Siegfried's clerical idiocies on slips of paper; misspellings, errors in addition, wrong entries — they were all faithfully copied down.

Miss Harbottle used these slips as ammunition. She never brought one out when things were slack and her employer was hanging about the surgery. She saved them until he was under pressure, then she would push a slip under his nose and say 'How about this?'

She always kept an expressionless face at these times and it was impossible to say how much pleasure it gave her to see him cower back like a whipped animal. But the end was unvarying mumbled explanations and apologies from Siegfried and Miss Harbottle, radiating self-righteousness, correcting the entry.

As Siegfried went into the room I watched through the partly open door. I knew my morning round was waiting but I was impelled by morbid curiosity. Miss Harbottle, looking brisk and businesslike, was tapping an entry in the book with her pen while Siegfried shuffled his feet and muttered replies. He made several vain attempts to escape and, as the time passed, I could see he was nearing breaking point. His teeth were clenched and his eyes had started to bulge.

In the immediate post-war years Siegfried goes on to get married and lives with his wife a few miles outside Darrowby while James, Helen and their son Jim are still living in the practice headquarters. In reality, Donald had married in June 1943 while Alf was in the RAF and he and his new bride Audrey Adamson initially lived at 23 Kirkgate. (Donald had been briefly married before while he was a student at the Edinburgh Veterinary College but he lost his young wife to tuberculosis in the early 1930s.) Donald and Audrey would remain married for over fifty years and it was said that her calm temperament acted as the perfect foil to Donald's more impulsive nature.

When the James Herriot books were published many assumed that Alf had exaggerated the unruly tendencies of Donald to create the character of Siegfried. Donald himself was unhappy with his portrayal, declaring quite memorably after reading the first book: 'Alfred, this book is a test of our friendship!' In fact, many of those who knew Donald felt that Alf had underplayed his eccentricities – his behaviour was extraordinary and erratic in a myriad of ways, as reflected in the books. But he was at heart an immensely likeable and funny man, and, while he could be challenging, 'his many good qualities', as Alf's son Jim put it, 'far outweighed his less appealing ones'. Keen not to upset Donald, Alf deliberately played down his personality quirks in the remaining six books, although he still remains a key character right through to *Every Living Thing*.

By the time of *Every Living Thing*, set in the early 1950s, James, Helen and their two children decide to move out of Skeldale House into a more modern property, as they did in reality in 1953. Much as they love the place, it's a big house to look after and its high ceilings and draughty corridors make it impossible to heat.

We loved the old place but it had vast disadvantages for a young couple of moderate means. It was charming, graceful and undoubtedly a happy house in its atmosphere, but it was far too big and a veritable ice box in cold weather.

I looked up over the ivy-covered frontage at the big bedroom windows, then further to the next storey where there was a suite of rooms where, in the early days, we had had our bed-sitter. There was another storey if you counted the tiny rooms under the tiles; here there was a big bell mounted on the end of a spring which used to summon a little housemaid down to the ground floor in the early days of the century.

The old doctor who lived in Skeldale House before we took over had had six servants including a full-time housekeeper, but Helen looked after the whole place with the aid of a series of transient maids, most of whom soon grew tired of the hard work and the impossible inconvenience of the house.

On the day of the move, James finds that Skeldale House echoes with the life it once contained – the antics of three young bachelor vets, the squabbles between Siegfried and Tristan, the ever-present pack of dogs yelping at the door, children running down the corridors – a house that was noisy, chaotic but always happy. The lives of Siegfried and James are moving on, they are married men now and their domestic lives are no longer intertangled as they once were.

Leaving Skeldale had been a far greater wrench than I had ever imagined. After the van had taken the last of our things away I roamed through the empty rooms which had echoed to my children's laughter. The big sitting room where I had read the bedtime stories and where, before all that, Siegfried, Tristan and I had sprawled in bachelor contentment, seemed to reproach me with its ageless charm and grace. The handsome fireplace with its glass cupboard above, and the old pewter tankard which used to hold our cash still resting there, the French window opening onto the long, high-walled garden with its lawns, fruit trees, asparagus and strawberry beds — these things were part of a great surging ocean of memories.

Upstairs, I stood in the large alcoved room where Helen and I had slept and to where we had brought our children as babies to sleep in the cot which once stood in that corner. I clumped over the bare boards to the dressing room which Jimmy and Rosie had shared, almost hearing their giggles and teasings which were the beginning of each new day.

I climbed another flight to the little rooms under the eaves where Helen and I had started our married life, where a bench against the wall and a gas ring once served as our only cooking arrangements; then I walked to the window and looked over the tumbled roofs of the little town to the green fells and swallowed a huge lump in my throat. Dear old Skeldale. I was so glad it was going to be kept on as the practice house and I would walk through its doors every day, but my family was leaving and I wondered if we could ever be as happy again as we had been here.

∾

While both Alf and Donald continued to work at the Thirsk practice, Donald moved out with his wife Audrey in 1945. As Audrey came from a wealthy shipbuilding family, they were able to move into an elegant country estate, Southwoods Hall, in Thirlby near Thirsk, where Donald could indulge in the gentlemanly pursuits of hunting, shooting and fishing. Donald continued to work at 23 Kirkgate, although reduced his weekly hours, while Alf worked full-time with the help of assistants and eventually his son Jim.

Donald Sinclair was an extraordinary character, in life and on the page as Siegfried Farnon. Siegfried was always an essential part of the practice and of the world that existed inside Skeldale House. His presence in the James Herriot books adds vigour and humour to many of the stories, much of which reflect just how funny Donald was, often unconsciously so. Such is the case in *Every Living Thing* when Siegfried, who is still much admired by local farmers, treats Mr Hawley's calf.

The farmer, white hair straggling from under a tattered cap, watched anxiously as Siegfried bent over the prostrate calf in a pen in the corner of the cow house.

'What do ye make of it, Mr Farnon?' he asked. 'I've never seen owt like it.'

The appeal in his eyes was mingled with a deep faith. Siegfried was his hero, a wonder worker, the man who had brought off miracle cures for years, even before I had come to Darrowby. William Hawley was one of a breed of simple, unsophisticated farmers who still survived in the fifties but who have long since melted away under the glare of science and education.

Siegfried spoke gravely. 'Very strange indeed. No scour, no pneumonia, yet the little thing's flat out like this.'

Carefully and methodically he went over the little body with his stethoscope, auscultating heart, lungs and abdomen. He took the temperature, opened the mouth and peered at the tongue and throat, examined the eyes and ran his hand over the roan hairs of the coat. Then slowly he straightened up. His face was expressionless as he looked down at the motionless form.

Suddenly he turned to the old man. 'William,' he said, 'would you be so kind as to fetch me a piece of string.'

'Eh?'

'A piece of string, please.'

'String?'

'Yes, about this length.' Siegfried spread his arms wide. 'And quickly, please.'

'Right, right . . . I'll get ye some. Now where can I lay me hands on a bit that length?' Flustered, he turned to me. 'Can ye come and give me a hand, Mr Herriot?'

'Certainly.' I followed him as he hurried from the cow house and outside he clutched at my arm. It was clear he had only asked me to come with him to enlighten him.

'What does 'e want a piece of string for?' he asked in bewilderment.

I shrugged. 'I really have no idea, Mr Hawley.'

He nodded gleefully as though that was only what he expected. An ordinary vet couldn't possibly know what was in the mind of Mr Farnon, a man of legendary skill who was known to employ many strange things in the practice of his art — puffs of purple smoke to cure lame horses, making holes in jugular veins and drawing off buckets of blood to cure laminitis. Old William had heard all the stories and he was in no doubt that if anybody could restore his animal to health by means of a piece of string, it would be Mr Farnon.

But the maddening thing was that as we trotted round the buildings he couldn't find such a thing.

'Dang it,' he said. 'There's allus a coil of binder twine hangin' there, but it isn't there now! And I'm allus trippin' over bits o' string all over t'place, but not today. What'll he think of a farmer wi' no string?'

In a growing panic he rushed around and he was almost in tears when he saw a piece lying across a heap of sacks.

'How about this, Mr Herriot? Is it t'right length?'

'Just about right, I'd say.'

He grabbed it and ran as fast as his elderly limbs would carry him back to Siegfried.

'Here y'are, Mr Farnon,' he panted. 'Ah'm not too late, am I? He's still alive?'

'Oh yes, yes.' Siegfried took the string and held it dangling for a moment as he measured the length with his eye. Then, as we watched, wide-eyed, he quickly tied it round his waist. 'Thank you so much, William,' he murmured, 'that's much better. I couldn't work with that damned coat flapping open as I bent over. I lost a couple of buttons yesterday. Cow got her horn underneath them and tore them off — it's always happening to me.'

'But . . . but . . . the string . . .' The old man's face was a picture of woe. 'Ye can't do anything for my calf, then?'

'Of course I can. Whatever makes you think I can't?'

'Well . . . do ye know what ails him?'

'Yes, I do. He's got CCN.'

'What's that?'

'Cerebrocortical necrosis. It's a brain disease.'

'It's a terrible big name. And his brain? It'll be a hopeless case?'

'Not a bit. I'm going to inject vitamin B into his vein. It usually works like a charm. Just hold his head for a moment. You see how it's bent over his back? That's called opisthotonos — typical of this condition.'

Siegfried quickly carried out the injection and got to his feet. 'One of us will be passing your door tomorrow, so we'll look in. I'd like to bet he'll be a lot better.'

It was I who called next day and indeed the calf was up and eating. William Hawley was pleased.

'Must have been wonderful stuff Mr Farnon gave 'im,' he said.

To him it was another miracle, but in his manner I sensed something of the deflation I had seen the day before when Siegfried tied up his coat. His favourite vet had done the trick again, but I knew that in his heart there was still the wistful regret that he hadn't done it with that piece of string.

Chapter 4

TRISTAN FARNON
and OTHER ASSISTANTS

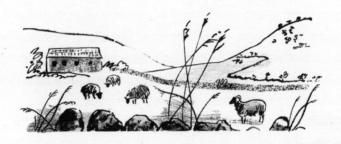

I huddled deeper in the blankets as the strident brreeng-brreeng, brreeng-brreeng of the telephone echoed through the old house.

It was three weeks since Tristan's arrival and life at Skeldale House had settled into a fairly regular pattern. Every day began much the same with the phone ringing between seven and eight o'clock after the farmers had had the first look at their stock. There was only one phone in the house. It rested on a ledge in the tiled passage downstairs. Siegfried had impressed on me that I shouldn't get out of bed for these early calls. He had delegated the job to Tristan; the responsibility would be good for him. Siegfried had been emphatic about it.

I listened to the ringing. It went on and on — it seemed to get louder. There was neither sound nor movement from Tristan's room and I waited for the next move in the daily drama. It came, as always, with a door crashing back on its hinges, then Siegfried rushed out onto the landing and bounded down the stairs three at a time.

A long silence followed and I could picture him shivering in the draughty passage, his bare feet freezing on the tiles as he listened to the farmer's leisurely account of the animal's symptoms. Then the ting of the phone in its rest and the mad pounding of feet on the stairs as Siegfried made a dash for his brother's room. Next a wrenching sound as the door was flung open, then a yell of rage. I detected a note of triumph; it meant Tristan had been caught in bed – a definite victory for Siegfried and he didn't have many victories. Usually, Tristan exploited his quick-dressing technique and confronted his brother fully dressed. It gave him a psychological advantage to be knotting his tie when Siegfried was still in pyjamas.

But this morning Tristan had overplayed his hand; trying to snatch the extra few seconds, he was caught between the sheets. I listened to the shouts. 'Why didn't you answer the bloody phone like I told you? Don't tell me you're deaf as well as idle! Come on, out of it, out, out!'

But I knew Tristan would make a quick comeback. When he was caught in bed he usually scored a few points by being halfway through his breakfast before his brother came in.

Later, I watched Siegfried's face as he entered the dining room and saw Tristan munching his toast happily, his *Daily Mirror* balanced against the coffee pot. It was as if he had felt a sudden twinge of toothache.

Life is never dull at Skeldale House, especially when Siegfried's younger brother Tristan is around. Conflict is the norm between the two brothers as Siegfried attempts to instil in Tristan a sense of responsibility by doling out a variety of jobs around the house. Tristan, however, shirks from any kind of hard labour, preferring to prop up the bar at the Drovers' Arms or to catnap in his favourite armchair, preferably without Siegfried knowing about it. It's not that Tristan's mind isn't sharp – he'll often finish the *Telegraph* crossword while others are still wrestling with the first clue – it's just that his main goal in life is to enjoy himself and he'll go to great lengths to ensure he does.

In the early books, Tristan, who is five years younger than Siegfried, is studying veterinary medicine in Edinburgh and returns to Skeldale during his holidays but often stays long after he should have resumed his studies. Easily distracted, he is constantly failing his exams – much to the annoyance of Siegfried, who is footing his tuition bills. Like Tristan, Brian Sinclair, on whom Tristan is based, took a good few years to pass his exams, graduating in 1943 from the Royal Veterinary College in Edinburgh, ten years after beginning his training.

James frequently finds himself caught in the crossfire between the brothers, which invariably ends up with a furious Siegfried banishing Tristan from the house and practice. James is at first alarmed by this although he soon learns that the sacking is a regular occurrence and par for the course when the Farnon brothers live under the same roof.

Siegfried finally located the book he was looking for, took it down from the shelf and began to leaf through it unhurriedly. Then, without looking up, he said quietly: 'Well, how did the exams go?'

Tristan swallowed carefully and took a deep breath. 'Did all right in parasitology,' he replied in a flat monotone.

Siegfried didn't appear to have heard. He had found something interesting in his book and settled back to read. He took his time over it, then put the book on the shelf. He began again the business of going along the titles; still with his back to his brother, he spoke again in the same soft voice.

'How about pathology?'

Tristan was on the edge of his chair now, as if ready to make a run for it. His eyes darted from his brother to the bookshelves and back again. 'Didn't get it,' he said tonelessly.

There was no reaction from Siegfried. He kept up his patient search for his book, occasionally pulling a volume out, glancing at it and replacing it carefully. Then he gave up the hunt, lay back in the chair with his arms dangling almost to the floor and looked at Tristan. 'So you failed pathology,' he said conversationally.

I was surprised to hear myself babbling with an edge of hysteria in my voice. 'Well now, that's pretty good, you know. It puts him in the final year and he'll be able to sit path at Christmas. He won't lose any time that way and, after all, it's a tough subject.'

Siegfried turned a cold eye on me. 'So you think it's pretty good, do you?' There was a pause and a long silence which was broken by a totally unexpected bellow as he rounded on his brother. 'Well, I don't! I think it is bloody awful! It's a damned disgrace, that's what it is. What the hell have you been doing all this term, anyway? Boozing, I should think, chasing women, spending my money, anything but working. And now you've got the bloody nerve to walk in here and tell me you've failed pathology. You're lazy, that's your trouble, isn't it? You're bloody bone idle!'

He was almost unrecognizable. His face was darkly flushed and his eyes glared. He yelled wildly again at his brother. 'But I've had enough this time. I'm sick of you. I'm not going to work my fingers to the bloody bone to keep you up there idling your time away. This is the end. You're sacked, do you hear me? Sacked once and for all. So get out of here — I don't want to see you around any more. Go on, get out!'

Aghast at having to witness the fracas between the brothers, James is relieved when Siegfried sends him on a call. It's nearly dark when he returns and, on driving into the practice yard, he spots a figure in the gloom. It turns out to be Tristan.

'Sorry about the way things turned out,' I said awkwardly.

The tip of the cigarette glowed brightly as Tristan took a long pull. 'No, no, that's all right. Could have been a lot worse, you know.'

'Worse? Well, it's bad enough, isn't it? What are you going to do?'

'Do? What do you mean?'

'Well, you've been kicked out, haven't you? Where are you going to sleep tonight?'

'I can see you don't understand,' Tristan said. He took his cigarette from his mouth and I saw the gleam of very white teeth as he smiled. 'You needn't worry, I'm sleeping here and I'll be down to breakfast in the morning.'

'But how about your brother?'

'Siegfried? Oh, he'll have forgotten all about it by then.'

'Are you sure?'

'Dead sure. He's always sacking me and he always forgets. Anyway, things turned out very well. The only tricky bit back there was getting him to swallow that bit about the parasitology.'

I stared at the shadowy form by my side. Again, there was a rustling as the rooks stirred in the tall trees then settled into silence.

'The parasitology?'

'Yes. If you think back, all I said was that I had done all right. I wasn't any more specific than that.'

'Then you mean . . .?'

Tristan laughed softly and thumped my shoulder.

'That's right, I didn't get parasitology. I failed in both. But don't worry, I'll pass them at Christmas.'

Once Siegfried has simmered down from their various arguments, he'll continue to provide Tristan with more chores around the house – ranging from washing cars to mixing up medicines in the practice dispensary – all in a bid to keep his younger brother busy. Tristan, however, usually has other ideas and is nothing if not imaginative in avoiding his assignments.

He interpreted his role rather differently from his brother and, while resident in Darrowby, he devoted a considerable amount of his acute intelligence to the cause of doing as little as possible. Tristan did, in fact, spend much of his time sleeping in a chair. When he was left behind to dispense when we went out on our rounds he followed an unvarying procedure. He half filled a sixteen-ounce bottle with water, added a few drachms of chlorodyne and a little ipecacuanha, pushed the cork in and took it through to the sitting room to stand by his favourite chair. It was a wonderful chair for his purpose: old-fashioned and high-backed with wings to support the head.

He would get out his *Daily Mirror*, light a Woodbine and settle down till sleep overcame him. If Siegfried rushed in on him he grabbed the bottle and started to shake it madly, inspecting the contents at intervals. Then he went through to the dispensary, filled up the bottle and labelled it.

It was a sound, workable system but it had one big snag. He never knew whether it was Siegfried or not when the door opened and often I walked in and found him half lying in his chair, staring up with startled, sleep-blurred eyes while he agitated his bottle.

Most evenings found him sitting on a high stool at the bar counter of the Drovers' Arms, conversing effortlessly with the barmaid. At other times he would be out with one of the young nurses from the local hospital, which he seemed to regard as an agency to provide him with female company. All in all, he managed to lead a fairly full life.

When Mrs Hall the housekeeper is away for a week, Siegfried decides that Tristan must help with the cooking and housework. It soon becomes apparent that his culinary repertoire consists of just one meal – sausages and mash – which, much to the annoyance of Siegfried, he serves up every day. Tristan is also something of a liability in the kitchen, particularly when he uses cotton wool soaked in ether to light the fire. James and Siegfried are horrified to hear a sudden 'whuff' noise rushing down the corridors, rattling the windows of the house. On dashing to the kitchen, they discover Tristan flat on his back on the floor amid pots and pans. Siegfried rages that ether is 'bloody well explosive! It's a wonder you didn't blow the whole place up!'

Tristan proceeds to clear up with a mop and bucket but, as soon as Siegfried heads out for the morning rounds, he stops and heads to his favourite armchair in the sitting room. Having had enough of the hot stove, Tristan explains to James that he has decided to roast the potatoes in the sitting room fire, ready for lunchtime. Siegfried returns, sits at the dining table, and is presented with an 'amorphous dark grey mass liberally speckled with black foreign bodies of varying size':

'What in the name of God,' he enquired with ominous quiet, 'is this?'

His brother swallowed. 'Sausage and mash,' he said lightly.

Siegfried gave him a cold look. 'I am referring to this.' He poked warily at the dark mound.

'Well, er, it's the potatoes.' Tristan cleared his throat. 'Got a little burned, I'm afraid.'

My boss made no comment. With dangerous calm he spooned some of the material onto his plate, raised a forkful and began to chew slowly. Once or twice he winced as a particularly tough fragment of carbon cracked between his molars, then he closed his eyes and swallowed.

For a moment he was still, then he grasped his midriff with both hands, groaned and jumped to his feet.

'No, that's enough!' he cried. 'I don't mind investigating poisonings on the farms but I object to being poisoned myself in my own home!' He strode away from the table and paused at the door. 'I'm going over to the Drovers' for lunch.'

Tristan clearly has little interest in cooking or housework, preferring instead to cook up schemes to amuse himself. On picking up the phone at Skeldale House, he will sometimes answer using a ludicrous foreign accent – 'Allo, plis, oo is dis?' – farmers later mentioning to James that 'some foreign feller' had answered the phone when they called. When Siegfried comes up with the idea of putting magazines in the practice waiting room, Tristan smuggles in a German naturist magazine, complete with full-frontal nudity, just so he can catch out a worthy local citizen having a quick peek. The prank predictably backfires on him when Mr Mount, the father of a girl whom Tristan has been seeing, is caught red-handed and subsequently forbids Tristan from seeing his daughter Deborah any more.

Brian Sinclair was similarly an energetic prankster and would often answer the phone with a silly accent or call in from a public phone box pretending to be a local farmer in need of an urgent visit. Not content with playing pranks on Alf and their clients, Brian also took his mischief further afield. He once dressed in white sheets and after nightfall took himself off to Pannal Bank near Harrogate where he pretended to be the 'Pannal ghost'. Flitting across the bank in a ghostly manner, he would take great pleasure in seeing motorists making hasty U-turns and revving away. Such antics were recreated in *Let Sleeping Vets Lie* when James is scared half to death by the sudden appearance of a phantom monk dressed in a brown habit, which turns out to be Tristan up to his usual tricks. He subsequently learns that Tristan is behind the much-talked-of 'Raynes ghost' – a mysterious cowled figure often seen heading into the woods near Raynes Abbey.

Alf was often the victim of Brian's pranks, as James is in *If Only They Could Talk* when Tristan phones and imitates the gruff Yorkshire accent of Mr Sims.

Saturday night, 10.30 p.m. and I was writing up my visits when the phone rang. I swore, crossed my fingers and lifted the receiver.

'Hello, Herriot speaking.'

'Oh, it's you, is it?' growled a dour voice in broadest Yorkshire. 'Well, ah want Mr Farnon.'

'I'm sorry, Mr Farnon is out. Can I help you?'

'Well, I 'ope so, but I'd far raither 'ave your boss. This is Sims of Beal Close.'

(Oh no, please, no, not Beal Close on a Saturday night. Miles up in the hills at the end of a rough lane with about eight gates.)

'Yes, Mr Sims, and what is the trouble?'

'Ah'll tell you, there is some trouble an' all. I 'ave a grand big show 'oss here. All of seventeen hands. He's cut 'isself badly

on the hind leg, just above the hock. I want him stitched immediately.'

(Glory be! Above the hock! What a charming place to have
to stitch a horse. Unless he's very quiet, this is going to be a
real picnic.)

'How big is the wound, Mr Sims?'

'Big? It's a gurt big thing about a foot long and bleedin' like
'ell. And this 'oss is as wick as an eel. Could kick a fly's eye
out. Ah can't get near 'im nohow. Goes straight up wall when
he sees anybody. By gaw, I tell you I had 'im to t'blacksmith
t'other day and feller was dead scared of 'im. Twiltin' gurt 'oss
'e is.'

(Damn you, Mr Sims, damn Beal Close and damn your twiltin'
gurt 'oss.)

'Well, I'll be along straight away. Try to have some men
handy just in case we have to throw him.'

'Throw 'im? Throw 'im? You'd never throw this 'oss. He'd
kill yer first. Anyways, I 'ave no men here so you'll 'ave to
manage on your own. Ah know Mr Farnon wouldn't want a
lot of men to help 'im.'

(Oh lovely, lovely. This is going to be one for the diary.)

'Very well, I'm leaving now, Mr Sims.'

'Oh, ah nearly forgot. My road got washed away in the floods
yesterday. You'll 'ave to walk the last mile and a half. So get a
move on and don't keep me waiting all night.'

(This is just a bit much.)

'Look here, Mr Sims, I don't like your tone. I said I would
leave now and I will get there just as soon as I can.'

'You don't like ma tone, eh? Well, ah don't like useless young
apprentices practising on my good stock, so ah don't want no
cheek from you. You know nowt about t'damn job, any road.'

(That finally does it.)

'Now just listen to me, Sims. If it wasn't for the sake of the horse I'd refuse to come out at all. Who do you think you are, anyway? If you ever try to speak to me like that again . . .'

'Now, now, Jim, get a grip on yourself. Take it easy, old boy. You'll burst a blood vessel if you go on like this.'

'Who the devil . . .?'

'Ah, ah, Jim, calm yourself now. That temper of yours, you know. You'll really have to watch it.'

'Tristan! Where the hell are you speaking from?'

'The kiosk outside the Drovers'. Five pints inside me and feeling a bit puckish. Thought I'd give you a ring.'

'By God, I'll murder you one of these days if you don't stop this game. It's putting years on me. Now and again isn't so bad, but this is the third time this week.'

'Ah, but this was by far the best, Jim. It was really wonderful. When you started drawing yourself up to your full height – it nearly killed me. Oh God, I wish you could have heard yourself.' He trailed off into helpless laughter.

And then my feeble attempts at retaliation; creeping, trembling, into some lonely phone box.

'Is that young Mr Farnon?' in a guttural croak. 'Well, this is Tilson of High Wood. Ah want you to come out here immediately. I 'ave a terrible case of . . .'

'Excuse me for interrupting, Jim, but is there something the matter with your tonsils? Oh, good. Well, go on with what you were saying, old lad. Sounds very interesting.'

Tristan delights in escorting young ladies to local dances and is a dedicated beer drinker and pub dweller. The bon viveur will also happily tag along to any social get-together, as Siegfried rages in *Vet in a Spin* when Tristan has clearly been carousing until the early hours: 'If there's a good booze-up going on anywhere, you'll find it.'

Brian and Alf similarly spent many convivial evenings together at nearby pubs or escorting young women to local dances or the cinema. Like Tristan, Brian had a repertoire of party tricks which he would perform with gusto, especially after a little lubrication. On the night that Tristan and James take nurses Brenda and Connie to a dance in the village of Poulton – as featured in Chapter 2 – they first head to a local pub. After downing a few pints, Tristan treats them to his legendary 'mad conductor' and is so absorbed in his outlandish performance that he almost knocks himself out.

Tristan raised his arms and gazed imperiously over his imaginary orchestra, taking in the packed rows of strings, the woodwind, brass and tympani in one sweeping glance. Then with a violent downswing he led them into the overture. Rossini, this time, I thought, or maybe Wagner as I watched him throwing his head about, bringing in the violins with a waving clenched fist or exhorting the trumpets with a glare and a trembling, outstretched hand.

It was somewhere near the middle of the piece that the rot always set in and I watched enthralled as the face began to twitch and the lips to snarl. The arm waving became more and more convulsive, then the whole body jerked with uncontrollable spasms. It was clear that the end was near – Tristan's eyes were rolling, his hair hung over his face and he had lost control of the music which crashed and billowed about him. Suddenly he grew rigid, his arms fell to his sides and he crashed to the floor.

I was joining in the applause and laughter when I noticed that Tristan was very still. I bent over him and found that he had struck his head against the heavy oak leg of the settle and was almost unconscious. The nurses went quickly into action. Brenda expertly propped up his head while Connie ran for a basin of hot water and a cloth. When he opened his eyes they were bathing a tender lump above his ear. Mr Peacock hovered anxiously in the background. 'Ista all right? Can ah do anything?'

Tristan sat up and sipped weakly at his beer. He was very pale. 'I'll be all right in a minute and there is something you can do. You can bring us one for the road and then we must be getting on to this dance.'

Brian's 'mad conductor' performance was just as legendary in real life, as was his manic laughter which, like a baddie in a pantomime, he boomed out with theatrical glee. After attending the publication party of *Let Sleeping Vets Lie* in London, Alf's son Jim remembers the streets echoing with Brian's deranged laughter as they walked back to their hotel in the early hours. He and Alf were entirely used to his tomfoolery, whereas anyone who didn't know him must have thought it very strange behaviour!

In the books, James develops a close friendship with Tristan, despite his sometimes strange behaviour, agreeing that he is something of a 'rum lad' (a typical Yorkshire term for someone who is a bit peculiar or mischievous) but who is 'very sound. His humour and zest for life had lightened my days.' Tristan continues to work as an assistant at the Darrowby practice and by the time of *Let Sleeping Vets Lie* he is in his final year. He is quick to learn, seemingly able to absorb information without any effort on his part, so that eventually by the time of *Vet in Harness*, Tristan graduates as a veterinary surgeon.

James is glad of Tristan's help at the practice. The local farmers had always liked Tristan when he did the occasional visit as a student and the young vet soon proves himself adept at the job. Positive comments start to come in thick and fast, many of which emphasize Tristan's commitment to his work: 'He meks some queer noises but he does try. I think he'd kill 'isself afore he'd give up.' As James discovers, it's clear that Tristan has developed a unique way of dealing with their clients, often putting on a kind of theatrical performance that elicits admiration from even the most hard-bitten types. On one call-out James joins Tristan as he calves a cow belonging to Mr Dowson, a hard and apparently emotionless character. He arrives just as Tristan is inserting his arm into a large red cow, while the farmer is holding the tail.

He braced himself and reached as far forward as he could, and just then the cow's flanks bulged as she strained hard against him. This is never very nice; the powerful contractions of the uterus squeeze the arm relentlessly between calf and pelvis and you have to grit your teeth till it passes off.

Tristan, however, went a little further.

'Ooh! Aah! Ouch!' he cried. Then as the animal still kept up the pressure he went into a gasping groan. When she finally relaxed he stood there quite motionless for a few seconds, his head hanging down as though the experience had drained him of all his strength.

The farmer drew on his pipe and regarded him impassively. Throughout the years I had known Mr Dowson I had never seen any particular emotion portrayed in those hard eyes and craggy features. In fact it had always seemed to me that I could have dropped down dead in front of him and he wouldn't even blink.

My colleague continued his struggle and the cow, entering into the spirit of the game, fought back with a will. Some animals will stand quietly and submit to all kinds of internal interference but this was a strainer; every movement of the arm within her was answered by a violent expulsive effort. I had been through it a hundred times and I could almost feel the grinding pressure on the wrist, the helpless numbing of the fingers.

Tristan showed what he thought about it all by a series of heart-rending sounds. His repertoire was truly astounding and he ranged from long harrowing moans through shrill squeals to an almost tearful whimpering.

At first Mr Dowson appeared oblivious to the whole business, puffing smoke, glancing occasionally through the byre door, scratching at the bristle on his chin. But as the minutes passed his eyes were dragged more and more to the suffering creature before him until his whole attention was riveted on the young man.

And in truth he was worth watching because Tristan added to his vocal performance an extraordinary display of facial contortions. He sucked in his cheeks, rolled his eyes, twisted his lips, did everything in fact but wiggle his ears. And there was no doubt he was getting through to Mr Dowson. As the noises and grimaces became more extravagant the farmer showed signs of growing uneasiness; he darted anxious glances at my colleague and occasionally his pipe trembled violently. Like me, he clearly thought some dreadful climax was at hand.

As if trying to bring matters to a head, the cow started to build up to a supreme effort. She straddled her legs wide, grunted deeply and went into a prolonged heave. As her back arched Tristan opened his mouth wide in a soundless protest then little panting cries began to escape him. This, I thought, was his most effective ploy yet; a long-drawn 'Aah . . . aah . . .

aah . . .' creeping gradually up the scale and building increasing tension in his audience. My toes were curling with apprehension when, with superb timing, he released a sudden piercing scream.

That was when Mr Dowson cracked. His pipe had almost wobbled from his mouth but now he stuffed it into his pocket and rushed to Tristan's side.

'Ista all right, young man?' he enquired hoarsely.

My colleague, his face a mask of anguish, did not reply.

The farmer tried again. 'Will ah get you a cup o' tea?'

For a moment Tristan made no response, then, eyes closed, he nodded dumbly.

Mr Dowson scampered eagerly from the byre and within minutes returned with a steaming mug. After that I had to shake my head to dispel the feeling of unreality. It couldn't be true, this vision of the hard-bitten farmer feeding the tea to the young man in sips, cradling the lolling head in a horny hand. Tristan was still inside the cow, still apparently semiconscious with pain but submitting helplessly to the farmer's ministrations.

With a sudden lunge he produced one of the calf's legs and as he flopped against the cow's rump he was rewarded with another long gulp of tea. After the first leg the rest wasn't so bad and the second leg and the calf itself soon followed.

As the little creature landed wriggling on the floor Tristan collapsed on his knees beside it and extended a trembling hand towards a pile of hay, prepared to give the new arrival a rub down.

Mr Dowson would have none of it.

'George!' he bellowed to one of his men in the yard. 'Get in 'ere and wisp this calf!' Then solicitously to Tristan, 'You maun come into t'house, lad, and have a drop o' brandy. You're about all in.'

The dream continued in the farm kitchen and I watched

disbelievingly as my colleague fought his way back to health and strength with the aid of several stiff measures of Martell Three Star. I had never had treatment like this and a wave of envy swept over me as I wondered whether it was worth adopting Tristan's system.

But I still have never found the courage to try it.

Once Tristan has graduated, however, he doesn't stay long at the Darrowby practice because, like many others during the war, he is army bound and leaves soon after James joins the RAF. James volunteered earlier than Tristan, when there was no need for vets in the military but, by the time Tristan signs up they are crying out for medics to doctor horses, mules and other animals in the Far East. It's no surprise, James muses, that Tristan landed on his feet: 'The timing suggested that the gods were looking after him as usual. In fact I think the gods love people like Tristan who sway effortlessly before the winds of fate and spring back with a smile, looking on life always with blithe optimism.' Tristan ends the war as Captain Farnon of the Royal Army Veterinary Corps. He has also married and goes on to join the Ministry of Agriculture as an Infertility Investigations Officer. 'He left a sad gap in our lives, but fortunately we still saw him and his wife regularly,' writes James, and the two young men remain good friends, despite spending less time in other's company.

Their paths, however, cross in *The Lord God Made Them All* after James calls in the services of a sterility advisory officer. As featured in Chapter 7, James attempts to use for the first time an artificial vagina (AV) to retrieve a semen sample from a bull but instead ends up using the AV to fight off the incensed animal. The next day, on returning to the yard, James sees a familiar figure ahead, blowing out clouds of cigarette smoke

– it turns out be Tristan who is the sterility officer come to his aid. James explains to him the whole sorry incident with the bull and Tristan cannot quite believe how much danger James had put himself in. As James continues to tell Tristan what happened, Tristan begins to laugh so much 'tears coursed down his cheeks and feeble little moans issued from his mouth'. Tristan clearly is still as animated as ever, although he appears a little more businesslike when they return to see the bull together. Tristan confidently attends to the bull, but things start to go wrong when, unbeknown to him, the farmer has filled the AV with boiling water, causing the animal to emit a deafening bellow when Tristan plunges its penis into the contraption.

Tristan, slightly pop-eyed, managed to jam the AV over the penis as it hurtled past him but as he did so the velocity of the charge caused the animal to lose his footing so that the bull slid on his back clean underneath the cow. The AV was jerked from Tristan's grasp and soared high into the air. Mr Hartley followed it, open-mouthed, as it described a graceful parabola before landing on a pile of straw at the other end of the yard. As the bull scrambled to his feet Tristan strolled unhurriedly towards the straw. The glass tube was still attached to the cylinder and my friend held it up at eye level.

'Ah yes,' he murmured. 'A nice 3 cc sample.'

The farmer came puffing up. 'You've got what you wanted, 'ave you?'

'Yes indeed,' Tristan replied airily. 'Exactly what I wanted.'

The farmer shook his head wonderingly. 'By 'ell, it's a complicated sort o' business, isn't it?'

'Ah well.' Tristan shrugged his shoulders. 'It can be just a little at times, it can be. Anyway, I'll get my microscope from the car and examine the sample.'

It didn't take long and soon afterwards we were all having a cup of tea in the kitchen. My colleague put down his cup and reached for a scone. 'That's a fine fertile bull you have there, Mr Hartley.'

'Eee, that's champion.' The farmer rubbed his hands. 'I paid a fair bit o' brass for 'im and it's grand to know he's up to scratch.' He looked across at the young man with undisguised admiration. 'You've done a grand job and I'm right grateful to you.' As I sipped my tea the thought occurred to me that despite the passage of years things hadn't changed. Just as that glass tube had landed on a soft bed of straw, Tristan always landed on his feet.

Brian Sinclair similarly worked for the Royal Army Veterinary Corps in India and then, like Tristan, worked for the Ministry of Agriculture in Inverness, Scotland, until 1949 after which he returned to Leeds, Yorkshire. By then he had a wife, Sheila, having realized during the war that she was the girl for him when at a pub in Kilburn, she laughed so hard at one of his jokes that dandelion and burdock came spurting out of her nose. Sheila and Brian went on to have three daughters and remained good friends with Joan and Alf in later years. Brian was always very happy to be featured in the Herriot books and even consulted with Alf on the first book, providing some useful additions to the storylines as well as suggestions for some of the colourful dialogue Siegfried would mete out to him when he was particularly enraged.

Tristan was not the only student to work at Skeldale House; a variety of other young men – still all men in those days – helped out during their vacations, the profession attracting a broad range of characters. They vary in capability but James generally finds working with them a rewarding process, as he describes in *Let Sleeping Vets Lie*.

I always liked having a student with us. These young men had to see at least six months' practice on their way through college and most of their vacations were spent going round with a vet.

We, of course, had our own resident student in Tristan but he was in a different category; he didn't have to be taught anything – he seemed to know things, to absorb knowledge without apparent effort or indeed without showing interest. If you took Tristan to a case he usually spent his time on the farm sitting in the car reading his *Daily Mirror* and smoking Woodbines.

There were all types among the others – some from the country, some from the towns, some dull-witted, some bright – but as I say, I liked having them.

For one thing, these visiting students were good company in the car. A big part of a country vet's life consists of solitary driving and it was a relief to be able to talk to somebody. It was wonderful, too, to have a gate-opener. Some of the outlying farms were approached through long, gated roads – one which always struck terror into me had eight gates – and it is hard to convey the feeling of sheer luxury when somebody else leaped out and opened them.

And there was another little pleasure; asking the students questions. My own days of studying and examinations were still fresh in my memory and on top of that I had all the vast experience of nearly three years of practice. It gave me a feeling of power to drop casual little queries about the cases we saw and watch the lads squirm as I had so recently squirmed myself. I suppose that even in those early days I was forming a pattern for later life; unknown to myself I was falling into the way of asking a series of my own pet questions as all examiners are liable to do and many years later I overheard one youngster asking another, 'Has he grilled you on the causes of fits in calves yet? Don't worry, he will.' That made me feel suddenly old but there was compensation on another occasion when a newly qualified ex-student rushed up to me and offered to buy me all the beer I could drink. 'You know what the examiner asked me in the final oral? The causes of fits in calves! By God I paralysed him — he had to beg me to stop talking.'

And students were useful in other ways. They ran and got things out of the car boot, they pulled a rope at calvings, they were skilled assistants at operations, they were a repository for my worries and doubts; it isn't too much to say that during their brief visits they revolutionized my life.

In the same chapter, James eagerly awaits his next protégé, a student recommended by the Ministry of Agriculture as a first-class student, who is arriving by train at Darrowby station. On meeting, however, it's soon clear this young man is very different to anyone they've had before at the practice.

'My name is Carmody.'

'Ah yes, good. How are you?' We shook hands and I took in the fine check suit and tweedy hat, the shining brogues and pigskin case. This was a very superior student, in fact a highly impressive young man. About a couple of years younger than myself but with a mature air in the set of his broad shoulders and the assurance on his strong, high-coloured face.

Unlike other students, Richard Carmody is not particularly impressed when James shows him round the surgery, although he shows a glimmer of approval when taking in the garden and the fell views beyond. The next morning, James takes Carmody to visit a lame calf, the young student now dressed in a smart hacking jacket and flannels. After the call, Carmody coolly tells James he thinks his diagnosis is wrong. Taken aback, James makes a mental note to keep Carmody well away from Siegfried, who would unhesitatingly hurl him out of the car at such an affront. Then, following a visit to a cow with slow fever (acetonaemia), James casually questions Carmody on the causes of the condition. Carmody confidently rattles off all the latest scientific theories, leaving James a little dumbfounded.

I slumped lower in my seat and decided not to ask Carmody any more questions and as the stone walls flipped past the windows I began to face up to the gradually filtering perception that this was a superior being next to me. It was depressing to ponder on the fact that not only was he big, good-looking, completely sure of himself but brilliant as well. Also, I thought bitterly, he had every appearance of being rich.

Carmody remains remarkably assured throughout the morning until the two men head to their last call before lunch where, having just opened the farm gate, the young vet's composure is put to the test.

Apparently from nowhere an evil-looking little black cur dog glided silently out, sank its teeth with dedicated venom into Carmody's left buttock and slunk away.

Not even the most monolithic dignity can survive being bitten deeply and without warning in the backside. Carmody screamed, leaped in the air clutching his rear, then swarmed to the top of the gate with the agility of a monkey.

By the afternoon, Carmody has recovered some of his poise and asks James, with a touch of arrogance, whether he can perform some injections. James then tasks him with a variety of difficult and dirty jobs: chasing a litter of pigs around a pen so they splatter filth all over him; treating an unwilling old carthorse with Istin drenching liquid, most of which ends up on his expensive clothes; and finally taking some blood samples from a large white sow. James takes pleasure in seeing all of this, surprised to detect a vein of sadism in his make-up.

> Extracting a few ccs of blood from the ear vein of a struggling pig is a job which makes most vets shudder and it was clearly a dirty trick to ask a student to do it, but the memory of his coldly confident request at the beginning of the afternoon seemed to have stilled my conscience.

The two young vets then visit a bullock that has a tumour on its jaw, which, when a halter rope is placed over his head, bolts 'like a black thunderbolt' across a field, with Carmody hanging on for dear life.

> He took a last few soaring, swooping steps then he was down on his face. But he didn't let go. The bullock, going better than ever, had turned towards us now, dragging the inert form apparently without effort, and I winced as I saw it was headed straight for a long row of cowpats.
>
> It was when Carmody was skidding face down through the third heap of muck that I suddenly began to like him. And when he finally did have to release his hold and lay for a moment motionless on the grass I hurried over to help him up. He thanked me briefly then looked calmly across the field at a sight

which is familiar to every veterinary surgeon — his patient thundering out of sight across the far horizon.

The student was almost unrecognizable. His clothes and face were plastered with filth except where the saffron streaks of the Istin showed up like war paint, he smelt abominably, he had been bitten in the backside, nothing had really gone right for him all day yet he was curiously undefeated. I smiled to myself. It was no good judging this bloke by ordinary standards; I could recognize the seeds of greatness when I saw them.

Carmody stays with the Darrowby practice for two weeks, after which, not unsurprisingly, he qualifies with top marks before gaining a PhD and further degrees and qualifications. The character of Carmody was in fact based on the assistant Oliver Murphy who worked at 23 Kirkgate in 1956 for four months. Like Carmody, he was serious, with a great academic mind, but Alf found him pleasant to work with and local farmers admired his dogged perseverance under trying circumstances. He returned one day caked in mud having chased wild bullocks around a yard, even hanging upside down from a beam in a rodeo-style attempt to catch one.

Another two assistants would feature in the books, although in reality over thirty assistants worked at the Thirsk practice, all of them providing a rich array of stories for the James Herriot books. Alf gave his students a lot of support and they in turn learned a huge amount and provided invaluable help during busy periods, particularly during tuberculin testing.

The assistant John Crooks features in the last two books. Having worked with the practice during university vacations, he is almost part of the family when he joins them as an assistant. He soon proves himself a capable veterinary surgeon and stays with the practice for three years – a period on which James looks back fondly.

> As John settled into the practice, I found a miraculous easing of my life. It was rather wonderful to have an assistant, especially a good one like him. I had always liked him, but when I got a call to a calving heifer at three o'clock in the morning and was able to pass it on to him and turn over and go back to sleep, I could feel the liking deepening into a warm affection.

John eventually marries a local teacher, Heather, and the two live at the Darrowby practice before setting up a practice in Beverley. 'Before he departed,' writes James, 'he paid us the charming compliment of "filling" a bottle with the air from Skeldale House to be released in his new surgery with the object of transferring some of our atmosphere.' The real John Crooks – the only assistant in the Herriot books to retain his real name – did exactly this when he left the practice. He too was a self-assured and immensely likeable man, and he and his wife, Heather (her real name also), remained good friends with Alf and his family. After setting up a practice in Beverley, Yorkshire, he rose to become president of the British Veterinary Association in 1983, but he never forgot the support and invaluable advice he received from Alf and Donald, and looked back on his days in Thirsk as some of the happiest of his life.

A few days after John leaves, the new assistant Calum Buchanan arrives. Tall and sporting a walrus moustache, he walks down the platform of Darrowby station with a giant lurcher by his side. Also draped over his shoulder is a large hairy animal, which James is surprised to discover is his pet badger Marilyn.

At Skeldale House, Siegfried looks aghast as the young graduate wolfs down an entire fruit cake; Siegfried pushes James into an empty office: 'What the hell have we got here, James? An assistant with a blasted badger round his neck! And a dog as big as a donkey!'

While clearly an unusual fellow, Calum has glowing references from his university and soon shows how capable he is as a veterinary surgeon, performing a caesarean on a heifer on his very first call-out and then meticulously cleaning his instruments afterwards. Before long, people are requesting the services of 'the vet wi' t'badger'.

'Can I speak to the vet wi' t'badger?'

As I handed the phone to our new assistant, it struck me that this request was becoming common and it did me good to hear it. It meant that Calum was being accepted by the farmers. I didn't mind at all if some of them wanted him instead of me. What I dreaded hearing was 'Don't send that young bugger!' which I had heard about from some of my neighbouring vets when they employed new assistants.

We had been so lucky with John Crooks who had been an outstanding asset to our practice and it seemed to be asking too much of fate for a second top-class man to come along. All the new graduates were better educated than I had been but there were other reasons why a few didn't make the grade. Some of them just couldn't face the long rough and tumble of general practice with its antisocial hours, others lacked the ability to get on with the clients, and one or two were academically bright but unpractical.

Calum, to my vast relief, seemed to be slotting into the job effortlessly but, just as John and Tristan had been different from each other, so was he from them. Very different. His ever-present badger fascinated people, his tall, walrus-moustached appearance, eager friendliness and unusual outlook on life made him interesting to both farm and small animal clients but, most important of all, he knew his stuff. He was a fine vet.

Calum is also a keen ornithologist and naturalist, and even convinces James to join him on a trip to look for deer, the two rising before dawn and riding two shire horses into the woods as if in some kind of Narnia fantasy. As Siegfried predicts, however, Calum continually adds to his menagerie of pets, soon bringing into the house two Dobermann dogs, Maggie and Anna, alongside a variety of other wild creatures.

It was around the time when Calum's third badger arrived that an uncanny sense of the inevitable began to settle on me.

The new badger was called Bill and Calum didn't say much about his unheralded advent. He did mention it in an off-hand way to me, but prudently failed to take Siegfried into his confidence. I think he realized that there wasn't much point in upsetting my partner further — it seemed only reasonable to assume that Siegfried was getting a little punch-drunk with the assorted creatures milling around and wouldn't even notice.

I was discussing the day's work with my colleagues in the doorway of the dispensary when Siegfried ducked down. 'What the hell was that?' he exclaimed as a large feathery body whizzed past, just missing our heads.

'Oh, it's Calum's owl,' I said.

Siegfried stared at me. 'That owl? I thought it was supposed to be ill.' He turned to our assistant. 'Calum, what's that owl doing here? You brought it in days ago and it looks fit enough now, so take it back where it came from. I like birds, as you know, but not rocketing round in our surgery like bloody eagles — could frighten the life out of the clients.'

The young man nodded. 'Yes . . . yes . . . she's almost recovered. I expect to take her back to the wood very soon.' He pocketed his list of visits and left.

I didn't say anything, but it seemed certain to me that once Calum had got his hands on an owl of his very own he wasn't going to part with it in a hurry. I foresaw some uncomfortable incidents.

'And listen to those fox cubs!' Siegfried went on. 'What a racket they're making!' The yapping, snarling and barking echoed along the passage from the back of the house. There was no doubt they were noisy little things. 'What does Calum want them in here for?'

'I'm not sure . . . He did say something, but I can't quite recall . . .'

'Well,' Siegfried grunted, 'I just hope he'll remove them as soon as the problem is over.'

Later that day, Siegfried and I were setting a dog's fractured radius when Calum walked into the operating room. Marilyn, as usual, was on his shoulder, but today she had company; seated comfortably in the crook of the young man's arms was a little monkey.

Siegfried looked up from his work. He stopped winding the plaster of Paris bandage and his mouth fell open. 'Oh, my God, no! This is too much! Not a bloody monkey now! It's like living in a bloody zoo.'

'Yes,' replied Calum with a pleased smile. 'His name is Mortimer.'

'Never mind his name!' Siegfried growled. 'What the hell is he doing here?'

'Oh, don't worry, this isn't a pet — in a way, he's a patient.'

Siegfried's eyes narrowed. 'What do you mean — in what way? Is he ill?'

'Well, not exactly . . . Diana Thurston has asked me to look after him while she's away on holiday.'

'And you said yes, of course! No hesitation! That's just what we need here — bloody monkeys roaming the place on top of everything else!'

Calum looked at him gravely. 'Well, you know, I was in a difficult position. Colonel Thurston is a very nice man and one of our biggest clients — large farm, hunting horses and umpteen dogs. I couldn't very well refuse.'

My partner recommenced his winding. The plaster was setting and I could see he wanted time to think. 'Well, I see your point,' he said after a few moments. 'It wouldn't have looked so good.' He glanced up at Calum. 'But it's definitely just while Diana's on holiday?'

'Oh, absolutely, I promise you.' The young man nodded vigorously. 'She's devoted to the little chap and she'll pick him up as soon as she returns.'

'Oh, well, I suppose it'll be all right.' Siegfried shot a hunted look at the monkey which, open-mouthed, teeth bared and chattering, was apparently laughing at him.

We lifted the sleeping dog from the table and carried him to one of the recovery kennels. My partner seemed indisposed to speak and I didn't break the silence. I had no desire to discuss Calum's latest acquisition because I happened to know that Diana Thurston wasn't just going to Scarborough for a fortnight — she was off to Australia for six months.

I was called out that evening and went to the surgery for extra drugs. As I walked along the passage I could hear a babel of animal sounds from the end of the house and, on opening the door to the back room, I found Calum among his friends.

The three badgers were nosing around the food bowls, the owl flapped lazily onto a high shelf. Storm, vast and amiable, waved his tail in welcome, while the Dobermanns regarded me contemplatively. Mortimer the monkey, clearly already under Calum's spell, leaped from a table into the young man's arms and grinned at me. In a corner, the fox cubs kept up their strange yapping and growling and I noticed two cages containing a couple of rabbits and a hare – apparently new arrivals.

Looking round the room I realized that Siegfried had been right from the very beginning. The menagerie was now firmly installed. And as I opened the door to leave I wondered just how big it was going to grow.

Calum was modelled on Brian Nettleton, an assistant who joined the Thirsk practice in 1957. He proved to be one of the most capable veterinary surgeons to work there and was immensely popular with the clients. His large stature matched his personality, and he too carried around a badger which always accompanied him when he frequented the local pubs. He had a great affinity with animals of all types and, as featured in *Every Living Thing*, he would cook up large vats of hideous-smelling tripe for his badgers while owls swooped up and down the corridor and foxes ran around the garden. A lover of nature, he was less bound by routine and frequently disappeared off into the wilds. It was Alf's son Jim who joined him on the early-morning trips, and Brian always knew exactly where they could see animals in their own habitat. He was also very musical and played the piano accordion; he once bought Alf's daughter a squeeze box in a jumble sale, teaching her slightly risqué songs thereafter. The 'vet wi' t'badger' – adored by Alf's family, the local farmers and the regulars in the Drovers' Arms – was as unforgettable in life as he was on the page.

Chapter 5

ROMANCE *and* FAMILY LIFE

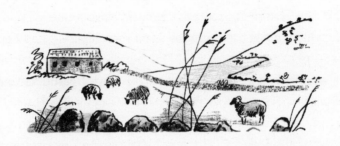

A voice answered 'Come in,' and I opened the door into a huge, stone-flagged kitchen with hams and sides of bacon hanging from hooks in the ceiling. A dark girl in a check blouse and green linen slacks was kneading dough in a bowl. She looked up and smiled.

'Sorry I couldn't let you in. I've got my hands full.' She held up her arms, floury-white to the elbow.

'That's all right. My name is Herriot. I've come to see a calf. It's lame, I understand.'

'Yes, we think he's broken his leg. Probably got his foot in a hole when he was running about. If you don't mind waiting a minute, I'll come with you. My father and the men are in the fields. I'm Helen Alderson, by the way.'

She washed and dried her arms and pulled on a pair of short Wellingtons. 'Take over this bread, will you, Meg,' she said to an old woman who came through from an inner room. 'I have to show Mr Herriot the calf.'

Outside, she turned to me and laughed. 'We've got a bit of

a walk, I'm afraid. He's in one of the top buildings. Look, you can just see it up there.' She pointed to a squat, stone barn, high on the fell-side. I knew all about these top buildings; they were scattered all over the high country and I got a lot of healthy exercise going round them. They were used for storing hay and other things and as shelters for the animals on the hill pastures.

I looked at the girl for a few seconds. 'Oh, that's all right, I don't mind. I don't mind in the least.'

James has driven to the Alderson farm of Heston Grange to see to a calf. There, he is met by the farmer's daughter, Helen Alderson, who immediately catches his attention, and he is more than happy to spend a few more minutes in her company as they walk up a hill. In a barn, he finds a trembling calf, which, he confirms, has a fractured radius and ulna. He applies a wet bandage to its leg, waits for it to dry and the calf immediately trots away and happily reunites with his mother. Pleased with his success, the two leave the barn and take in the view below.

We sat down on the warm grass of the hillside, a soft breeze pulled at the heads of the moorland flowers, somewhere a curlew cried. Darrowby and Skeldale House and veterinary practice seemed a thousand miles away.

'You're lucky to live here,' I said. 'But I don't think you need me to tell you that.'

'No, I love this country. There's nowhere else quite like it.' She paused and looked slowly around her. 'I'm glad it appeals to you too — a lot of people find it too bare and wild. It almost seems to frighten them.'

I laughed. 'Yes, I know, but as far as I'm concerned I can't help feeling sorry for all the thousands of vets who don't work in the Yorkshire Dales.'

I began to talk about my work, then almost without knowing, I was going back over my student days, telling her of the good times, the friends I had made and our hopes and aspirations.

I surprised myself with my flow of talk — I wasn't much of a chatterbox usually — and I felt I must be boring my companion. But she sat quietly looking over the valley, her arms around her green-clad legs, nodding at times as though she understood. And she laughed in all the right places.

I wondered too, at the silly feeling that I would like to forget all about the rest of the day's duty and stay up here on this sunny hillside. It came to me that it had been a long time since I had sat down and talked to a girl of my own age. I had almost forgotten what it was like.

I didn't hurry back down the path and through the scented pine wood but it seemed no time at all before we were walking across the wooden bridge and over the field to the farm.

I turned with my hand on the car door. 'Well, I'll see you in a month.' It sounded like an awful long time.

The girl smiled. 'Thank you for what you've done.' As I started the engine she waved and went into the house.

'Helen Alderson?' Siegfried said later over lunch. 'Of course I know her. Lovely girl.'

Tristan, across the table, made no comment, but he laid down his knife and fork, raised his eyes reverently to the ceiling and gave a long, low whistle. Then he started to eat again.

Siegfried went on. 'Oh yes, I know her very well. And I admire her. Her mother died a few years ago and she runs the whole place. Cooks and looks after her father and a younger brother and sister.' He spooned some mashed potatoes onto his plate. 'Any men friends? Oh, half the young bloods in the district are chasing her but she doesn't seem to be going steady with any of them. Choosy sort, I think.'

James's first encounter with Helen has gone well – they can talk easily to each other; she is clearly a very capable young woman and they both count themselves lucky to live and work in the Dales. Back at Skeldale House, James scans the day book regularly, in the hope he can visit the farm again, but is sorry to see the Aldersons seem to have 'lamentably healthy stock'. Instead, he makes do with joining the Darrowby Music Society, having seen Helen going into its meetings. There, with heart thudding, he summons up the courage to ask her out. She agrees and a date is set for Saturday evening.

James is desperate to impress Helen when they meet and he plans to take her to a dinner dance at the grand Reniston Hotel in Brawton. Dressed in a tight-fitting and hopelessly outdated dinner jacket and suit, James turns up at the Alderson farm to pick Helen up. He is shown to the kitchen by Helen's grinning younger brother, who clearly finds the situation funny, as does Helen's little sister, who has a fixed smirk on her face as she sits at the table doing her homework. Mr Alderson beckons James to sit with him by the fire as he reads the *Farmer and Stockbreeder*.

After about a year I heard footsteps on the stairs, then Helen came into the room. She was wearing a blue dress – the kind, without shoulder straps, that seems to stay up by magic. Her dark hair shone under the single pressure lamp which lit the kitchen, shadowing the soft curves of her neck and shoulders. Over one white arm she held a camel-hair coat.

I felt stunned. She was like a rare jewel in the rough setting of stone flags and whitewashed walls. She gave me her quiet, friendly smile and walked towards me. 'Hello, I hope I haven't kept you waiting too long.'

I muttered something in reply and helped her on with her coat. She went over and kissed her father, who didn't look up but waved his hand vaguely. There was another outburst of giggling from the table. We went out.

In the car I felt unusually tense and for the first mile or two had to depend on some inane remarks about the weather to keep a conversation going. I was beginning to relax when I drove over a little hump-backed bridge into a dip in the road. Then the car suddenly stopped. The engine coughed gently and then we were sitting silent and motionless in the darkness. And there was something else; my feet and ankles were freezing cold. 'My God!' I shouted. 'We've run into a bit of flooded road. The water's right into the car.' I looked round at Helen. 'I'm terribly sorry about this – your feet must be soaked.'

But Helen was laughing. She had her feet tucked up on the seat, her knees under her chin. 'Yes, I am a bit wet, but it's no good sitting about like this. Hadn't we better start pushing?'

Wading out into the black icy waters was a nightmare but there was no escape. Mercifully it was a little car and between us we managed to push it beyond the flooded patch. Then by torchlight I dried the plugs and got the engine going again.

Helen shivered as we squelched back into the car. 'I'm afraid I'll have to go back and change my shoes and stockings. And so will you. There's another road back through Fensley. You take the first turn on the left.'

Back at the farm, Mr Alderson was still reading the *Farmer and Stockbreeder* and kept his finger on the list of pig prices while he gave me a baleful glance over his spectacles. When he learned that I had come to borrow a pair of his shoes and socks he threw the paper down in exasperation and rose, groaning, from his chair. He shuffled out of the room and I could hear him muttering to himself as he mounted the stairs.

Helen followed him and I was left alone with the two young children. They studied my sodden trousers with undisguised delight. I had wrung most of the surplus water out of them but the final result was remarkable. Mrs Hall's knife-edge crease reached to just below the knee, but then there was chaos. The trousers flared out at that point in a crumpled, shapeless mass and as I stood by the fire to dry them a gentle steam rose about me. The children stared at me, wide-eyed and happy. This was a big night for them.

Mr Alderson reappeared at length and dropped some shoes and rough socks at my feet. I pulled on the socks quickly but shrank back when I saw the shoes. They were a pair of dancing slippers from the early days of the century and their cracked patent leather was topped by wide, black silk bows.

I opened my mouth to protest but Mr Alderson had dug himself deep into his chair and had found his place again among the pig prices. I had the feeling that if I asked for another pair of shoes Mr Alderson would attack me with the poker. I put the slippers on.

We had to take a roundabout road to avoid the floods but I kept my foot down and within half an hour we had left the steep sides of the Dale behind us and were heading out on to the rolling plain. I began to feel better. We were making good time and the little car, shuddering and creaking, was going well. I was just thinking that we wouldn't be all that late when the steering wheel began to drag to one side.

I had a puncture most days and recognized the symptoms immediately. I had become an expert at changing wheels and with a word of apology to Helen was out of the car like a flash. With my rapid manipulation of the rusty jack and brace the

136

wheel was off within three minutes. The surface of the crumpled tyre was quite smooth except for the lighter, frayed parts where the canvas showed through. Working like a demon, I screwed on the spare, cringing inwardly as I saw that this tyre was in exactly the same condition as the other. I steadfastly refused to think of what I would do if its frail fibres should give up the struggle.

By day, the Reniston dominated Brawton like a vast medieval fortress, bright flags fluttering arrogantly from its four turrets, but tonight it was like a dark cliff with a glowing cavern at street level where the Bentleys discharged their expensive cargoes. I didn't take my vehicle to the front entrance but tucked it away quietly at the back of the car park. A magnificent commissionaire opened the door for us and we trod noiselessly over the rich carpeting of the entrance hall.

We parted there to get rid of our coats, and in the men's cloakroom I scrubbed frantically at my oily hands. It didn't do much good; changing that wheel had given my fingernails a border of deep black which defied ordinary soap and water. And Helen was waiting for me.

I looked up in the mirror at the white-jacketed attendant hovering behind me with a towel. The man, clearly fascinated by my ensemble, was staring down at the wide-bowed pierrot shoes and the rumpled trouser bottoms. As he handed over the towel he smiled broadly as if in gratitude for this little bit of extra colour in his life.

I met Helen in the reception hall and we went over to the desk. 'What time does the dinner dance start?' I asked.

The girl at the desk looked surprised. 'I'm sorry, sir, there's no dance tonight. We only have them once a fortnight.'

I turned to Helen in dismay but she smiled encouragingly. 'It doesn't matter,' she said. 'I don't really care what we do.'

'We can have dinner, anyway,' I said. I tried to speak cheerfully but a little black cloud seemed to be forming just above my head. Was anything going to go right tonight?

The evening limps on and there's confusion when a waiter asks if they are staying, and James doesn't realize he means overnight at the hotel. When they are finally led to their table, James is convinced the whole evening has been a disaster, is thoroughly miserable and is as hot as hell in his ghastly suit.

Everything was in French and in my numbed state the words were largely meaningless, but somehow I ordered the meal and, as we ate, I tried desperately to keep a conversation going. But long deserts of silence began to stretch between us; it seemed that only Helen and I were quiet among all the surrounding laughter and chatter.

Worst of all was the little voice which kept telling me that Helen had never really wanted to come out with me anyway. She had done it out of politeness and was getting through a boring evening as best she could.

The journey home was a fitting climax. We stared straight ahead as the headlights picked out the winding road back into the Dales. We made stumbling remarks, then the strained silence took over again. By the time we drew up outside the farm my head had begun to ache.

We shook hands and Helen thanked me for a lovely evening. There was a tremor in her voice and in the moonlight her face was anxious and withdrawn. I said goodnight, got into the car and drove away.

Alf Wight's first date with the real Helen Alderson – Joan Danbury – was similarly disastrous. They weren't on their own, though. A cattle dealer friend of Alf and Brian Sinclair, Malcolm Johnson, knew a few ladies in Thirsk, including Joan. He asked her one day whether she and any friends would like to come along to a dance at a nearby village of Sandhutton. She had never met Alf or Brian but Malcolm assured her they were good fun and Joan agreed that she and two friends would join them. They drove in one of the practice cars, a battered little Ford with holes in the footwell, which promptly ground to a halt in a flooded road, forcing them all to return to 23 Kirkgate once they'd got the car started again. They eventually got to the dance, then returned to the practice house where they chatted further and Brian entertained them all with his usual funny stories and tomfoolery.

Like Helen, Joan, who had dark hair and deep blue eyes, had many admirers but she wasn't a farmer's daughter. She was a secretary at a corn merchant's in Thirsk and her father a government official then working in York. She had grown up in Thirsk, her family moving to the town from the Cotswolds in Gloucestershire when she was eight years old. She had had a few boyfriends before meeting Alf but she instantly took a liking to the young vet and when he asked to see her again, she agreed. While Alf had a solid profession, well revered amongst the rural community, he certainly wasn't as wealthy as some of the richer farmers Joan had dated but she was attracted to Alf, enjoyed his company and they shared a similar sense of humour. Alf had had the odd girlfriend at school and veterinary college, and he and Brian had taken a few young women out to dances locally, but none would captivate him as much as Joan.

In *It Shouldn't Happen to a Vet* Helen, thankfully, has not been put off by their disastrous first date, although a subsequent cinema trip also proves less than romantic. James is accosted by a farmer, they are ogled at by the local blacksmith's daughter and the cinema shows an ancient Western instead of the film they came to see. Helen, however, is able to see the funny side of the situation – an important trait when spending time with James. When Gobber Newhouse, sozzled after a session in the pub, plonks himself near them and proceeds to clonk James round the back of the head accidentally, Helen breaks into laughter.

> I had never seen a girl laugh like this. It was as though it was something she had wanted to do for a long time. She abandoned herself utterly to it, lying back with her head on the back of the seat, legs stretched out in front of her, arms dangling by her side. She took her time and waited until she had got it all out of her system before she turned to me.
>
> She put her hand on my arm. 'Look,' she said faintly. 'Next time, why don't we just go for a walk?'

While the date hadn't gone exactly to plan, James is at least relieved there will be a next time and they continue to spend more time together. They walk for miles in the hills, Helen occasionally comes on evening calls with James or they go to dances in the village institutes locally. As James puts it: 'There wasn't anything spectacular to do in Darrowby, but there was a complete lack of strain, a feeling of being self-sufficient in a warm existence of our own that made everything meaningful and worthwhile.'

James is clearly besotted and, on the insistence of Siegfried to throw aside his usual cautious ways, he proposes to Helen, who agrees and an early date for a wedding is set. Alf and Joan's wedding, held on a cold winter's morning on 5 November 1941, at St Mary Magdalene church in Thirsk was a similarly small affair. The bride and groom had little money to lavish on a bigger wedding and many couples chose to have more modest nuptials during the wartime years. In addition, neither set of parents attended: Joan's father Horace was ill and there were some difficulties with Alf's parents, who were concerned that Alf was marrying too early, before he was financially secure. Alf's mother Hannah, who ran a successful wedding dress business, had also hoped for a grander wedding and perhaps a daughter-in-law from a better background. Alf, nonetheless, stood firm in his determination to marry Joan and his father was eventually won over by her, but his mother's continuing disapproval would cause Alf uneasiness in later years. Alf had always felt a great deal of affection and respect for his mother – she was very much the driving force in the family, with great ambitions for her son – but their relationship was a complex one.

Five people attended the wedding, including Donald Sinclair who was the best man, exclaiming 'amen' at regular intervals, just as Siegfried does in *It Shouldn't Happen to a Vet*. They were married by Canon Young, whom Alf remembers shivering with the cold, glad when it was all over and they could head outside into the frosty sunshine.

I can't remember much about the wedding. It was a 'quiet do' and my main recollection is of desiring to get it all over with as soon as possible. I have only one vivid memory; of Siegfried, just behind me in the church, booming 'Amen' at regular intervals throughout the ceremony – the only time I have ever heard a best man do this.

It was an incredible relief when Helen and I were ready to drive away and when we were passing Skeldale House Helen grasped my hand.

'Look!' she cried excitedly. 'Look over there!'

Underneath Siegfried's brass plate, which always hung slightly askew on the iron railings, was a brand-new one. It was of the modern Bakelite type with a black background and bold white letters which read 'J. Herriot, MRCVS, Veterinary Surgeon', and it was screwed very straight and level on the metal.

The newlyweds drive out of Darrowby, James swelling with pride not only to have Helen, his wife, by his side but knowing also that the brass plate means he is now a bona fide partner at the practice alongside Siegfried. After driving and walking in the hills for a few hours, both of them in a bit of a daze, they head to the Wheatsheaf inn where they spend the first night of their honeymoon, after being fed a delicious meal of soup, stew and gooseberry pie and cream. The wedding has come at a busy time for the practice and James has agreed that he and Helen will spend a working honeymoon undertaking tuberculin testing. Helen causes surprise when she wears slacks (trousers) on the morning after their wedding, just as Joan often did, which was still very much a novelty in rural Yorkshire in the late 1930s.

I particularly enjoyed, too, our very first morning when I took Helen to do the test at Allen's. As I got out of the car I could see Mrs Allen peeping round the curtains in the kitchen window. She was soon out in the yard and her eyes popped when I brought my bride over to her. Helen was one of the pioneers of slacks in the Dales and she was wearing a bright purple pair this morning which would in modern parlance knock your eye out. The farmer's wife was partly shocked, partly fascinated but she soon found that Helen was of the same stock as herself and within seconds the two women were chattering busily. I judged from Mrs Allen's vigorous head-nodding and her ever-widening smile that Helen was putting her out of her pain by explaining all the circumstances. It took a long time and finally Mr Allen had to break into the conversation.

'If we're goin' we'll have to go,' he said gruffly and we set off to start the second day of the test.

We began on a sunny hillside where a group of young animals had been penned. Jack and Robbie plunged in among the beasts while Mr Allen took off his cap and courteously dusted the top of the wall.

'Your missus can sit 'ere,' he said.

I paused as I was about to start measuring. My missus! It was the first time anybody had said that to me. I looked over at Helen as she sat cross-legged on the rough stones, her notebook on her knee, pencil at the ready, and as she pushed back the shining dark hair from her forehead she caught my eye and smiled; and as I smiled back at her I became aware suddenly of the vast, swelling glory of the Dales around us, and of the Dales scent of clover and warm grass, more intoxicating than any wine. And it seemed that my first two years at Darrowby had been leading up to this moment; that the first big step of my life was being completed right here with Helen smiling at me and the memory, fresh in my mind, of my new plate hanging in front of Skeldale House.

I might have stood there indefinitely, in a sort of trance, but Mr Allen cleared his throat in a marked manner and I turned back to the job in hand.

'Right,' I said, placing my calipers against the beast's neck. 'Number thirty-eight, seven millimetres and circumscribed.' I called out to Helen, 'Number thirty-eight, seven, C.'

'Thirty-eight, seven, C,' my wife repeated as she bent over her book and started to write.

Alf and Joan Wight also spent the first two days of their honeymoon tuberculin testing, partly to keep up with the busy workload at the practice but also because they had little spare money to spend on a holiday. They nonetheless had a wonderful time, staying at the old Wheatsheaf inn at Caperby, where, Alf remembers, they ate like royalty, the owner Mrs Kilburn and her niece Gladys producing an array of Yorkshire fare, from home-cured ham and Wensleydale cheese to roast beef and Yorkshire puddings.

By the time of *Let Sleeping Vets Lie*, James has settled into life as a married man, relishing in particular the utter bliss of returning to a warm bed after a bitterly cold farm visit in the middle of the night.

As I crawled into bed and put my arm around Helen it occurred to me, not for the first time, that there are few pleasures in this world to compare with snuggling up to a nice woman when you are half frozen.

There weren't any electric blankets in the thirties. Which was a pity because nobody needed the things more than country vets. It is surprising how deeply bone-marrow cold a man can get when he is dragged from his bed in the small hours and made to strip off in farm buildings when his metabolism is at a low ebb. Often the worst part was coming back to bed; I often lay exhausted for over an hour, longing for sleep but kept awake until my icy limbs and feet had thawed out.

But since my marriage such things were but a dark memory. Helen stirred in her sleep — she had got used to her husband leaving her in the night and returning like a blast from the North Pole — and instinctively moved nearer to me. With a sigh of thankfulness I felt the blissful warmth envelop me and almost immediately the events of the last two hours began to recede into unreality.

Alf and Joan spent the early years of married life living on the top two floors of 23 Kirkgate, the basic kitchen on the very top floor, where water had to be carried in jugs from the ground floor, and on the floor below was their bed-sitting room. Despite the primitive conditions, Joan enjoyed looking after the house and became an excellent cook – causing Alf for the first time in his life to put on extra weight, despite the physicality of the job. By July 1942 the happy news came that they were expecting their first child although just a few months later, in November that year, Alf was called up for training in the RAF.

Throughout his time away, Alf and Joan exchanged letters on a daily basis. Clearly anxious about his wife's condition, Alf even experienced bizarre stomach pains as the birth approached, which impelled him to travel to Thirsk to see Joan, without getting authorization to do so.

James is similarly vexed at being separated from Helen and in *Vets Might Fly*, on his third absence without leave, arrives just after Helen has given birth to their son Jimmy.

I took my first look at my son. Little Jimmy was brick red in colour and his face had a bloated, dissipated look. As I hung over him he twisted his tiny fists under his chin and appeared to be undergoing some mighty internal struggle. His face swelled and darkened as he contorted his features, then from deep among the puffy flesh his eyes fixed me with a baleful glare and he stuck his tongue out of the corner of his mouth.

'My God!' I exclaimed.

The nurse looked at me, startled. 'What's the matter?'

'Well, he's a funny-looking little thing, isn't he?'

'What!' She stared at me furiously. 'Mr Herriot, how can you say such a thing? He's a beautiful baby!'

I peered into the cot again. Jimmy greeted me with a lopsided leer, turned purple and blew a few bubbles.

'Are you sure he's all right?' I said.

There was a tired giggle from the bed but Nurse Brown was not amused.

'All right! What exactly do you mean?' She drew herself up stiffly.

I shuffled my feet. 'Well, er — is there anything wrong with him?'

I thought she was going to strike me. 'Anything . . . how dare you! Whatever are you talking about? I've never heard such nonsense!' She turned appealingly towards the bed, but Helen, a weary smile on her face, had closed her eyes.

I drew the enraged little woman to one side. 'Look, Nurse, have you by chance got any others on the premises?'

'Any other what?' she asked icily.

'Babies — new babies. I want to compare Jimmy with another one.'

Her eyes widened. 'Compare him! Mr Herriot, I'm not going to listen to you any longer — I've lost patience with you!'

'I'm asking you, Nurse,' I repeated. 'Have you any more around?'

There was a long pause as she looked at me as though I was something new and incredible. 'Well — there's Mrs Dewburn in the next room. Little Sidney was born about the same time as Jimmy.'

'Can I have a look at him?' I gazed at her appealingly.

She hesitated, then a pitying smile crept over her face. 'Oh you . . . you . . . just a minute, then.'

She went into the other room and I heard a mumble of voices. She reappeared and beckoned to me.

Mrs Dewburn was the butcher's wife and I knew her well. The face on the pillow was hot and tired like Helen's.

'Eee, Mr Herriot, I didn't expect to see you. I thought you were in the army.'

'RAF, actually, Mrs Dewburn. I'm on – er – leave at the moment.'

I looked in the cot. Sidney was dark red and bloated, too, and he, also, seemed to be wrestling with himself. The inner battle showed in a series of grotesque facial contortions culminating in a toothless snarl.

I stepped back involuntarily. 'What a beautiful child,' I said.

'Yes, isn't he lovely,' said his mother fondly.

'He is indeed, gorgeous.' I took another disbelieving glance into the cot. 'Well, thank you, very much, Mrs Dewburn. It was kind of you to let me see him.'

'Not at all, Mr Herriot, it's nice of you to take an interest.' Outside the door I took a long breath and wiped my brow. The relief was tremendous. Sidney was even funnier than Jimmy.

When I returned to Helen's room Nurse Brown was sitting on the bed and the two women were clearly laughing at me. And of course, looking back, I must have appeared silly. Sidney Dewburn and my son are now two big, strong, remarkably good-looking young men, so my fears were groundless.

The little nurse looked at me quizzically. I think she had forgiven me.

'I suppose you think all your calves and foals are beautiful right from the moment they are born?'

'Well yes,' I replied. 'I have to admit it – I think they are.'

In reality, Alf was similarly shocked to see his son for the first time when he visited Joan at the Sunnyside Nursing Home in Thirsk. It was Nurse Bell, not Nurse Brown, who had to show him another little baby, just to calm his fears about the appearance of little Jimmy, only then to waft the new father out of his wife's room. Joan and Jimmy stayed at Sunnyside for fourteen days – which was the norm in those days for women who had given birth. Confined to bed, Joan always maintained this made for the best holiday of her life!

In *The Lord God Made Them All* Jimmy is now four and regularly joins his father on his rounds. James clearly loves spending time with his young son, and Jimmy is an enthusiastic helper, showing early on his interest in pursuing his father's profession.

'Hello! Hello!' I bellowed.

'Hello! Hello!' little Jimmy piped just behind me.

I turned and looked at my son. He was four years old now and had been coming on my rounds with me for over a year. It was clear that he considered himself a veteran of the farmyards, an old hand versed in all aspects of agricultural lore.

This shouting was a common habit of mine. When a vet arrived on a farm it was often surprisingly difficult to find the farmer. He might be a dot on a tractor half a mile across the fields, on rare occasions he might be in the house, but I always hoped to find him among the buildings and relied on a few brisk shouts to locate him.

Certain farms in our practice were for no apparent reason distinctive in that you could never find anybody around. The house door would be locked and we would scour the barns, cow houses and fold yards while our cries echoed back at us from the unheeding walls. Siegfried and I used to call them the 'no-finding' places and they were responsible for a lot of wasted time.

Jimmy had caught on to the problem quite early and there

was no doubt he enjoyed the opportunity to exercise his lungs a bit. I watched him now as he strutted importantly over the cobbles, giving tongue every few seconds. He was also making an unnecessary amount of noise by clattering on the rough stones with his new boots.

Those boots were his pride, the final recognition of his status as veterinary assistant. When I first began to take him round with me his first reaction was the simple joy of a child at being able to see animals of all kinds, particularly the young ones – the lambs, foals, piglets, calves – and the thrill of discovery when he came upon a huddle of kittens in the straw or found a bitch with pups in a loose box.

Before long, however, he began to enlarge his horizons. He wanted to get into the action. The contents of my car boot were soon as familiar to him as his toy box at home, and he delighted in handing out the tins of stomach powder, the electuaries and red blisters, the white lotion and the still revered long cartons of Universal Cattle Medicine. Finally he began to forestall me by rushing back to the car for calcium and flutter valve as soon as he saw a recumbent cow. He had become a diagnostician as well.

I think the thing he enjoyed most was accompanying me on an evening call, if Helen would allow him to postpone his bedtime. He was in heaven driving into the country in the darkness, training my torch on a cow's teat while I stitched it.

The farmers were kind, as they always are with young people. Even the most uncommunicative would grunt, 'Ah see you've got t'apprentice with ye,' as we got out of the car.

During the long drives to farms, little Jimmy also takes the opportunity to assail his father with a constant barrage of questions, along the lines of 'What is the fastest train – the

Blue Peter or the *Flying Scotsman*?' which James does his best to answer. In reality, Jim Wight also joined his father Alf on farm visits from an early age and proved equally curious and also coveted the thick hobnailed boots that farmers wore. By opening gates and carrying equipment, Jim was a useful helper and the time he spent with his father driving around on rounds from the age of two until he started secondary school undoubtedly resulted in him also becoming a veterinary surgeon. Alf was pleased he showed an early interest in veterinary practice – it was after all a way of life that fascinated him – and he was always encouraging and patient with his son. However, he never pressured Jim into following his career and in fact always warned him that he'd never be a wealthy man as a rural vet and advised him only to pursue the profession if he was really sure it was what he wanted.

Jimmy could be a little mischievous at times and such is the case one afternoon in *The Lord God Made Them All* when James is in the consulting room looking at Mr Garrett's sheepdog. Jim Wight well remembers this incident, which occurred when he was around six or seven. Jim was never a very naughty child but he did get into the occasional scrape, often when ranging around with his gang of friends, scrumping for apples or swimming in rivers. But in this story, he is on his own – just as his father is preparing to inject an anaesthetic, he glimpses his son up to no good in the garden.

It was when I was filling the syringe that a knee came into view at the corner of the window. I felt a pang of annoyance. Jimmy surely couldn't be climbing up the wisteria. It was dangerous and I had expressly forbidden it. The branches of the beautiful creeper curled all over the back of the house and though they were as thick as a man's leg near ground level they became quite slender as they made their way up past the bathroom window to the tiles of the roof.

James, nonetheless, must focus on what he is doing – finding and removing a thorn or some kind of foreign body from the pad of the sheepdog's foot, with the use of a scalpel. At first he thinks he's probably mistaken about Jimmy but then realizes the little blighter is on the wisteria but there's nothing he can do other than give him a quick glare.

I was drawing the scalpel across at right angles to my first cut when from the corner of my eye I spotted two feet dangling just below the top of the window. I tried to concentrate on my job but the feet swung and kicked repeatedly, obviously for my benefit. At last they disappeared, which could only mean that their owner was ascending to the dangerous regions. I dug down a little deeper and swabbed with cotton wool.

Ah yes, I could see something now, but it was very deep, probably the tip of a thorn which had broken off well below the surface. I felt the thrill of the hunter as I reached for forceps and just then the head showed itself again, upside down this time.

My God, he was hanging by his feet from the branches and the face was positively leering. In deference to my client I had been trying to ignore the by-play from outside but this was too much. I leaped at the glass and shook my fist violently. My fury must have startled the performer because the face vanished instantly and I could hear faint sounds of feet scrambling upwards.

That was not much comfort either. Those top branches might not support a boy's weight. I forced myself back to my task.

'Sorry, Mr Garrett,' I said. 'Will you hold the leg up again, please.'

He replied with a thin smile and I pushed my forceps into the depths. They grated on something hard. I gripped, pulled gently, and, oh lovely, lovely, out came the pointed, glistening head of a thorn. I had done it.

It was one of the tiny triumphs which lighten vets' lives and I was beaming at my client and patting his dog's head when I heard the crack from above. It was followed by a long howl of terror then a small form hurtled past the window and thudded with horrid force into the garden.

I threw down the forceps and shot out of the room, along the passage and through the side door into the garden. Jimmy was already sitting up among the wallflowers and I was too relieved to be angry.

'Have you hurt yourself?' I gasped, and he shook his head.

I lifted him to his feet and he seemed to be able to stand all right. I felt him over carefully. There appeared to be no damage.

I led him back into the house. 'Go along and see Mummy,' I said, and returned to the consulting room.

I must have been deathly pale when I entered because Mr Garrett looked startled. 'Is he all right?' he asked.

'Yes, yes, I think so. But I do apologize for rushing out like that. It was really too bad of me to . . .'

Mr Garrett laid his hand on my shoulder. 'Say no more, Mr Herriot, I have children of my own.' And then he spoke the words which have become engraven on my heart. 'You need nerves of steel to be a parent.'

On 9 May 1947, Alf and Joan's second child, Rosie, was born, much to their delight. The afternoon before, Alf and Joan had been at the cinema in Harrogate where Joan began to experience the early pains of labour. They headed back to Thirsk and by 6 a.m. the following morning, Joan announced Rosie was definitely on her way. 'Shaking with panic', as Alf put it, he whisked her into the Sunnyside Nursing Home and after a few more hours of 'floor pacing and repeated attempts to read the newspaper upside down' Dr Addison phoned to announce, 'A sister for Jimmy!' In *The Lord God Made Them All*, James muses on the blessing of a new life while walking his dog Sam.

> After I had seen my patient, I took a walk on the high tops along a favourite path of beaten earth on the hill's edge with Sam trotting at my heels. I looked away over the rolling patchwork of the plain sleeping in the sun's haze and at the young bracken on the hillside springing straight and green from last year's dead brown stalks. Everywhere new life was calling out its exultant message, and it was so apt with my new little daughter lying down there in Darrowby.
>
> We had decided to call her Rosemary. It is such a pretty name and I still love it, but it didn't last long. It became Rosie at a very early stage and, though I did make one or two ineffectual stands, it has remained so to this day. She is now Doctor Rosie in our community.

Rosie, like Jimmy before, also delighted in accompanying her father on farm visits and became extremely adept in helping out Alf was similarly happy to take little Rosie on his rounds, experiencing for the second time, as James writes, 'the intense pleasure of showing them the farm animals and seeing their growing wonder at the things of the countryside; the childish chatter which never palled, the fun and the laughter which lightened my days'. Rosie and Jimmy both learn that there can be dangers involved in veterinary work; Jim becomes wary of sows, whereas Rosie is lucky she escapes unharmed when a large cow comes careering towards her.

I leaned from the pen. 'Rosie, will you bring me my scissors, the cotton wool and that bottle of peroxide.'

The farmer watched wonderingly as the tiny figure trotted to the car and came back with the three things. 'By gaw, t'little lass knows 'er way around.'

'Oh yes,' I said, smiling. 'I'm not saying she knows where everything is in the car, but she's an expert on the things I use regularly.'

Rosie handed me my requirements and I reached over the door. Then she retreated to her place at the end of the passage.

I began my work on the abscess. Since the tissue was necrotic the cow couldn't feel anything as I snipped and swabbed, but that didn't stop the hind leg from pistoning out every few seconds. Some animals cannot tolerate any kind of interference and this was one of them.

I finished at last with a nice wide clean area onto which I trickled the hydrogen peroxide. I had a lot of faith in this old remedy as a penetrative antiseptic when there was a lot of pus about, and I watched contentedly as it bubbled on the skin surface. The cow, however, did not seem to enjoy the sensation because she made a sudden leap into the air, tore the rope from the farmer's hands, brushed me to one side and made for the door.

The door was closed but it was a flimsy thing and she went straight through it with a splintering crash. As the hairy black monster shot into the passage I desperately willed her to turn left but to my horror she went right and after a wild scraping of her feet on the cobbles began to thunder down towards the dead end where my little daughter was standing.

It was one of the worst moments of my life. As I dashed towards the broken door I heard a small voice say 'Mama'. There was no scream of terror, just that one quiet word. When I left the pen Rosie was standing with her back against the end wall of the passage and the cow was stationary, looking at her from a distance of two feet.

The animal turned when she heard my footsteps then whipped round in a tight circle and galloped past me into the yard.

I was shaking when I lifted Rosie into my arms. She could easily have been killed and a jumble of thoughts whirled in my brain. Why had she said 'Mama'? I had never heard her use the word before – she always called Helen 'Mummy' or 'Mum'. Why had she been apparently unafraid? I didn't know the answers. All I felt was an overwhelming thankfulness. To this day I feel the same whenever I see that passage.

The incident with Rosie was a real one but, at the age of three, she was too small to remember it but well remembers her father telling it to her and the family in later years. When driving around with her father, Rosie loved also to sing in the back of the car and if Jim was there, he would whistle, harmonizing with his sister's tunes. And just as Jimmy liked to quiz his father with a myriad of random questions, Rosie liked to have her father quiz her on her interest in wildflowers and the natural world, no doubt inspired by the hedgerows and wild beauty of North Yorkshire that they sped past.

Rosie solemnly opened the three gates on the way back, then she looked up at me expectantly. I knew what it was – she wanted to play one of her games. She loved being quizzed just as Jimmy had loved to quiz me.

I took my cue and began. 'Give me the names of six blue flowers.'

She coloured quickly in satisfaction because of course she knew. 'Field scabious, harebell, forget-me-not, bluebell, speedwell, meadow cranesbill.'

'Clever girl,' I said. 'Now let's see — how about the names of six birds?'

Again the blush and the quick reply. 'Magpie, curlew, thrush, plover, yellowhammer, rook.'

'Very good indeed. Now name me six red flowers.' And so it went on, day after day, with infinite variations. I only half realized at the time how lucky I was. I had a demanding, round-the-clock job and yet I had the company of my children at the same time. So many men work so hard to keep the home going that they lose touch with the families who are at the heart of it, but it never happened to me.

Both Jimmy and Rosie, until they went to school, spent most of their time with me round the farms. With Rosie, as her school-days approached, her attitude, always solicitous, became distinctly maternal. She really couldn't see how I was going to get by without her and by the time she was five she was definitely worried.

'Daddy,' she would say seriously. 'How are you going to manage when I'm at school? All those gates to open and having to get everything out of the boot by yourself. It's going to be awful for you.'

I used to try to reassure her, patting her head as she looked up at me in the car. 'I know, Rosie, I know. I'm going to miss you, but I'll get along somehow.'

Her response was always the same. A relieved smile and then the comforting words. 'But never mind, Daddy, I'll be with you every Saturday and Sunday. You'll be all right then.'

Having seen Alf at work and the pleasure he took from veter-inary practice it's no surprise that both children wanted to be veterinary surgeons when they grew up. Alf had no qualms about Jim following in his footsteps but he had concerns about Rosie doing the same, as he writes in *Every Living Thing*:

Our practice was ninety per cent large animal work and although I loved the work I was always being kicked, knocked about and splashed with various kinds of filth. With all its charms and rewards it was a dirty and often dangerous job. On several occasions, I was called to help out in neighbouring practices where the vet had sustained a broken limb, and I had myself been lame for weeks when a huge carthorse whacked my thigh with his iron-shod hoof.

As a result Alf talked Rosie out of veterinary practice but during the writing of *Every Living Thing* (published in 1992) he wonders whether he did the right thing, considering the high percentage of women who now do the job. He acknowledges that much has changed in the profession, not least that small animals have now taken up more than half of vets' work and there's far less wrestling with large farm animals. Alf instead persuaded Rosie to become a doctor of humans, a career in which she flourished, studying medicine at the University of Cambridge before working as a partner in a successful GP practice in Thirsk.

In *The Lord God Made Them All*, James and six-year-old Rosie are visiting a farm, where they chat to Grandma Clarke, a local woman in her late eighties who had lived a long life of toil but from whom goodness seems to flow.

'How old are ye now, Rosie?' she asked as she presented the chocolate.

'Thank you, I'm six,' my daughter replied.

Grandma looked down at the smiling face, at the sturdy tanned legs in their blue shorts and sandals. 'Well, you're a grand little lass.' For a moment she rested her work-roughened hand against the little girl's cheek, then she returned to her chair. They didn't make much of a fuss, those old Yorkshire folk, but to me the gesture was like a benediction.

The old lady picked up her knitting again. 'And how's that lad o' yours. How's Jimmy?'

'Oh, he's fine, thank you. Ten years old now. He's out with some of his pals this morning.'

'Ten, eh? Ten and six . . . ten and six . . .' For a few seconds her thoughts seemed far away as she plied her needles, then she looked at me again. 'Maybe ye don't know it, Mr Herriot, but this is the best time of your life.'

'Do you think so?'

'Aye, there's no doubt about it. When your children are young and growin' up around ye — that's when it's best. It's the same for everybody, only a lot o' folk don't know it and a lot find out when it's too late. It doesn't last long, you know.'

'I believe I've always realized that, Mrs Clarke, without thinking about it very much.'

'Reckon you have, young man.' She gave me a sideways smile. 'You allus seem to have one or t'other of your bairns with you on your calls.'

As I drove away from the farm the old lady's words stayed in my mind. They are still in my mind, all these years later, when Helen and I are soon to celebrate our Ruby Wedding of forty years of marriage. Life has been good to us and is still good to us. We are lucky — we have had so many good times — but I think we both agree that Grandma Clarke was right about the very best time of all.

Chapter 6

PEOPLE *of the* DALES

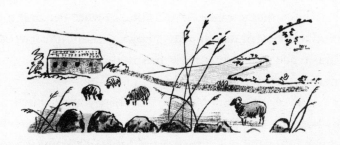

'Hello, 'ello, 'ello! Who's this we've got then? New chap eh?
Now we're going to learn summat!' He still had his hands inside
his braces and was grinning wider than ever.

'My name is Herriot,' I said.

'Is it now?' Phin cocked his head and surveyed me, then he
turned to three young men standing by. 'Hasn't he a nice smile,
lads? He's a real Happy Harry!'

He turned and began to lead the way across the yard. 'Come
on, then, and we'll see what you're made of. I 'ope you know
a bit about calves because I've got some here that are right
dowly.'

Phin Calvert, owner of a fine dairy herd in the Dales, extends
a typical greeting to the young James Herriot. It's clear that
James must prove himself to the hard-working farmers around
Darrowby, especially as Siegfried before him has already earned
their respect. While Phin Calvert is suspicious of James and
pokes a little fun at him, other farmers – the gruff, silent types

159

– are less talkative on first meeting and will only thaw a little when they know they can trust the young vet with their animals.

Early on in *If Only They Could Talk*, James sums up how daunting it is to turn up to a case and to witness the disappointment on a farmer's face when he realizes James, and not the much-revered Siegfried, will be attending to their animals. Despite this, James soon becomes familiar with the many qualities and quirks of the Dales people, many of whom are unfailingly generous with their hospitality, even to James the 'furriner'.

But I had to admit they were fair. I got no effusive welcomes and when I started to tell them what I thought about the case they listened with open scepticism, but I found that if I got my jacket off and really worked at the job they began to thaw a little. And they were hospitable. Even though they were disappointed at having me they asked me into their homes. 'Come in and have a bit o' dinner,' was a phrase I heard nearly every day. Sometimes I was glad to accept and I ate some memorable meals with them.

Often, too, they would slip half a dozen eggs or a pound of butter into the car as I was leaving. This hospitality was traditional in the Dales and I knew they would probably do the same for any visitor, but it showed the core of friendliness which lay under the often unsmiling surface of these people and it helped.

I was beginning to learn about the farmers and what I found I liked. They had a toughness and a philosophical attitude which was new to me. Misfortunes which would make the city dweller want to bang his head against a wall were shrugged off with 'Aye, well, these things happen.'

Alfred Wight was similarly under the microscope when he first joined the Thirsk practice working alongside Donald Sinclair. The arrival of a new vet does not go unnoticed in rural practice and Alf certainly felt he was being watched and assessed by local farmers. Not only were many of them inscrutable in their manner – making it difficult for the young vet to understand what they were thinking – but they also spoke in a broad Yorkshire dialect using words that would have been entirely alien to the Glaswegian vet. Understanding what a farmer meant by a cow being a bit 'dowly' was just the start of the process.

Gradually, however, Alf got to grips with this new world and language and soon became accepted and well liked in the community. Just as the locals were interested in him, Alf was similarly fascinated by the array of people he met – and would write about them with great affection in his books. Alf also delighted in their humour and peculiar way with words, as Dales farmer Dick Rudd illustrates in *It Shouldn't Happen to a Vet*.

Dick believed in veterinary advice for everything so I was a frequent visitor at Birch Tree Farm. After every visit there was an unvarying ritual; I was asked into the house for a cup of tea and the whole family downed tools and sat down to watch me drink it. On weekdays the eldest girl was out at work and the boys were at school but on Sundays the ceremony reached its full splendour with myself sipping the tea and all nine Rudds sitting around in what I can only call an admiring circle. My every remark was greeted with nods and smiles all round. There is no doubt it was good for my ego to have an entire family literally hanging on my words, but at the same time it made me feel curiously humble.

I suppose it was because of Dick's character. Not that he was unique in any way – there were thousands of small farmers just like him – but he seemed to embody the best qualities of the Dalesman: the indestructibility, the tough philosophy, the unthinking generosity and hospitality. And there were the things that were Dick's own: the integrity which could be read always in his steady eyes and the humour which was never very far away. Dick was no wit but he was always trying to say ordinary things in a funny way. If I asked him to get hold of a cow's nose for me he would say solemnly 'Ah'll endeavour to do so,' or I remember when I was trying to lift a square of plywood which was penning a calf in a corner he said, 'Just a minute till ah raise portcullis.' When he broke into a smile a kind of radiance flooded his pinched features.

The resilience of the Dales people was not just confined to the men: Mrs Dalby in *Let Sleeping Vets Lie* showed just how tough a widow could be under the most difficult of circumstances. Having recently lost her husband Billy Dalby to cancer, she is left with three young sons and a farm to run, which neighbouring farmers assume will fail without a man to run it. However, they underestimate Mrs Dalby's strength of character which is soon tested when she almost loses her entire herd of cattle to husk (also known as lungworm or parasitic bronchitis, a disease caused by the presence of parasites in the lungs. Vaccines now protect animals from the disease). In the face of near disaster, Mrs Dalby battles on and twenty years later, as James muses in the same book, she and the family are thriving, even buying a neighbouring farm and land. Throughout it all, she never complains of the struggle and grinding toil and is unfailingly hospitable to James.

The general opinion was that Mrs Dalby should sell up and get out. You needed a man to run this place and anyway Prospect

House was a bad farm. Neighbouring farmers would stick out their lower lips and shake their heads when they looked at the boggy pastures on the low side of the house with the tufts of spiky grass sticking from the sour soil or at the rocky outcrops and scattered stones on the hillside fields. No, it was a poor place and a woman would never make a go of it.

Everybody thought the same thing except Mrs Dalby herself. There wasn't much of her, in fact she must have been one of the smallest women I have ever seen — around five feet high — but there was a core of steel in her. She had her own mind and her own way of doing things.

I remember when Billy was still alive I had been injecting some sheep up there and Mrs Dalby called me into the house.

'You'll have a cup of tea, Mr Herriot?' She said it in a gracious way, not casually, her head slightly on one side and a dignified little smile on her face.

And when I went into the kitchen I knew what I would find; the inevitable tray. It was always a tray with Mrs Dalby. The hospitable Dales people were continually asking me in for some kind of refreshment — a 'bit o' dinner' perhaps, but if it wasn't midday there was usually a mug of tea and a scone or a hunk of thick-crusted apple pie — but Mrs Dalby invariably set out a special tray. And there it was today with a clean cloth and the best china cup and saucer and side plates with sliced buttered scones and iced cakes and malt bread and biscuits. It was on its own table away from the big kitchen table.

'Do sit down, Mr Herriot,' she said in her precise manner. 'I hope that tea isn't too strong for you.'

Her speech was what the farmers would call 'very proper' but it went with her personality which to me embodied a determination to do everything as correctly as possible.

'Looks perfect to me, Mrs Dalby.' I sat down feeling

somewhat exposed in the middle of the kitchen with Billy smiling comfortably from an old armchair by the fire and his wife standing by my side.

She never sat down with us but stood there, very erect, hands clasped in front of her, head inclined, ceremoniously attending to my every wish. 'Let me fill your cup, Mr Herriot,' or 'Won't you try some of this custard tart?'

More often than not, farmers and the local people of the Dales are welcoming to James and Siegfried, knowing that they depend on the two vets for the welfare of their animals. Small farmers Mr and Mrs Horner express their gratitude, like Mrs Dalby and many like her, in the form of food. After a difficult but successful calving, Mr Horner ushers James into the kitchen where he is presented with a treat much prized by the locals, fatty bacon, along with a pungent pickle known as piccalilli. James, however, has a pathological loathing of fat and combined with a powerfully strong piccalilli, the meal becomes something of a trial for him.

'Will you sit down along o' my husband and have a bit o' breakfast?' she asked.

There is nothing like an early calving to whet the appetite and I nodded readily. 'That's very kind of you, I'd love to.'

It is always a good feeling after a successful delivery and I sighed contentedly as I sank into a chair and watched the old lady set out bread, butter and jam in front of me. I sipped my tea and as I exchanged a word with the farmer I didn't see what she was doing next. Then my toes curled into a tight ball as I found two huge slices of pure white fat lying on my plate.

Shrinking back in my seat I saw Mrs Horner sawing at a

great hunk of cold boiled bacon. But it wasn't ordinary bacon, it was one hundred per cent fat without a strip of lean anywhere. Even in my shocked state I could see it was a work of art; cooked to a turn, beautifully encrusted with golden crumbs and resting on a spotless serving dish . . . but fat.

She dropped two similar slices on her husband's plate and looked at me expectantly.

My position was desperate. I could not possibly offend this sweet old person but on the other hand I knew beyond all doubt that there was no way I could eat what lay in front of me. Maybe I could have managed a tiny piece if it had been hot and fried crisp, but cold, boiled and clammy . . . never. And there was an enormous quantity; two slices about six inches by four and at least half an inch thick with the golden border of crumbs down one side. The thing was impossible.

Mrs Horner sat down opposite me. She was wearing a flowered mob cap over her white hair and for a moment she reached out, bent her head to one side and turned the dish with the slab of bacon a little to the left to show it off better. Then she turned to me and smiled. It was a kind, proud smile.

There have been times in my life when, confronted by black and hopeless circumstances, I have discovered in myself undreamed-of resources of courage and resolution. I took a deep breath, seized knife and fork and made a bold incision in one of the slices, but as I began to transport the greasy white segment to my mouth I began to shudder and my hand stayed frozen in space. It was at that moment I spotted the jar of piccalilli.

Feverishly I scooped a mound of it onto my plate. It seemed to contain just about everything; onions, apples, cucumber and other assorted vegetables jostling each other in a powerful mustard-vinegar sauce. It was the work of a moment to smother

165

my loaded fork with the mass, then I popped it into my mouth, gave a couple of quick chews and swallowed. It was a start and I hadn't tasted a thing except the piccalilli.

'Nice bit of bacon,' Mr Horner murmured.

'Delicious!' I replied, munching desperately at the second forkful. 'Absolutely delicious!'

'And you like ma piccalilli too!' The old lady beamed at me. 'Ah can tell by the way you're slappin' it on!' She gave a peal of delighted laughter.

'Yes indeed.' I looked at her with streaming eyes. 'Some of the best I've ever tasted.'

Looking back, I realize it was one of the bravest things I have ever done. I stuck to my task unwaveringly, dipping again and again into the jar, keeping my mind a blank, refusing grimly to think of the horrible thing that was happening to me. There was only one bad moment, when the piccalilli, which packed a tremendous punch and was never meant to be consumed in large mouthfuls, completely took my breath away and I went into a long coughing spasm. But at last I came to the end. A final heroic crunch and swallow, a long gulp at my tea and the plate was empty. The thing was accomplished.

And there was no doubt it had been worth it. I had been a tremendous success with the old folks. Mr Horner slapped my shoulder.

'By gaw, it's good to see a young feller enjoyin' his food! When I were a lad I used to put it away sharpish, like that, but ah can't do it now.' Chuckling to himself, he continued with his breakfast.

His wife showed me the door. 'Aye, it was a real compliment to me.' She looked at the table and giggled. 'You've nearly finished the jar!'

'Yes, I'm sorry, Mrs Horner,' I said, smiling through my tears and trying to ignore the churning in my stomach. 'But I just couldn't resist it.'

Contrary to my expectations I didn't drop down dead soon afterwards but for a week I was oppressed by a feeling of nausea which I am prepared to believe was purely psychosomatic.

At any rate, since that little episode I have never knowingly eaten fat again. My hatred was transformed into something like an obsession from then on.

And I haven't been all that crazy about piccalilli either.

While generosity abounds in the Dales, so too does thriftiness. Farmers are often careful with their money and those unable or reluctant to part with their cash resent having to pay vet bills, only calling a veterinary surgeon in as a very last resort when all other home-spun remedies have failed. The odd farmer also delights in crafty schemes to save or make themselves a bit of money – as is the case with Mr Cranford and others like him who blatantly bend the rules when it comes to insurance claims.

Cranford was a hard man, a man who had cast his life in a mould of iron austerity. A sharp bargainer, a win-at-all-cost character and, in a region where thrift was general, he was noted for meanness. He farmed some of the best land in the lower Dale, his shorthorns won prizes regularly at the shows but he was nobody's friend. Mr Bateson, his neighbour to the north, summed it up: 'That feller 'ud skin a flea for its hide.' Mr Dickon, his neighbour to the south, put it differently: 'If he gets haud on a pound note, by gaw it's a prisoner.'

This morning's meeting had had its origin the previous day. A phone call mid-afternoon from Mr Cranford. 'I've had a cow struck by lightning. She's laid dead in the field.'

I was surprised. 'Lightning? Are you sure? We haven't had a storm today.'

'Maybe you haven't, but we have 'ere.'

'Mmm, all right, I'll come and have a look at her.'

Driving to the farm, I couldn't work up much enthusiasm for the impending interview. This lightning business could be a bit of a headache. All farmers were insured against lightning stroke — it was usually part of their fire policy — and after a severe thunderstorm it was common enough for the vets' phones to start ringing with requests to examine dead beasts.

The insurance companies were reasonable about it. If they received a certificate from the vet that he believed lightning to be the cause of death they would usually pay up without fuss.

In cases of doubt they would ask for a post-mortem or a second opinion from another practitioner. The difficulty was that there are no diagnostic post-mortem features to go on; occasionally a bruising of the tissues under the skin, but very little else. The happiest situation was when the beast was found with the tell-tale scorch marks running from an ear down the leg to earth into the ground. Often the animal would be found under a tree which itself had obviously been blasted and torn by lightning. Diagnosis was easy then.

Ninety-nine per cent of the farmers were looking only for a square deal and if their vet found some other clear cause of death they would accept his verdict philosophically. But the odd one could be very difficult.

I had heard Siegfried tell of one old chap who had called him out to verify a lightning death. The long scorch marks on the carcass were absolutely classic and Siegfried, viewing them, had been almost lyrical. 'Beautiful, Charlie, beautiful, I've never seen more typical marks. But there's just one thing.' He put an arm round the old man's shoulder. 'What a great pity you let the candle grease fall on the skin.'

The old man looked closer and thumped a fist into his palm. 'Dang it, you're right, maister! Ah've mucked t'job up. And ah took pains ower it an' all — been on for dang near an hour.' He walked away muttering. He showed no embarrassment, only disgust at his own technological shortcomings.

While Mr Cranford grows increasingly frustrated with James when he refuses to collude with the farmer's bogus insurance claims, there is the odd family who positively despise James, Siegfried and any vet. Principal of these are the Sidlows, who are unwavering in their contempt of vets. In their view, veterinary surgeons are parasites of the agricultural community who know nothing about animals and are out to rob farmers of their hard-earned money. This viewpoint is only confirmed when in *Every Living Thing* James has the audacity to turn up in a new-looking car.

'You call yourself a vet, but you're nowt but a robber!'

Mrs Sidlow, her fierce little dark eyes crackling with fury, spat out the words and as I looked at her, taking in the lank, black hair framing the haggard face with its pointed chin, I thought, not for the first time, how very much she resembled a witch. It was easy to imagine her throwing a leg over a broomstick and zooming off for a quick flip across the moon.

'All t'country's talkin' about you and your big bills,' she continued. 'I don't know how you get away with it, it's daylight robbery — robbin' the poor farmers and then you come out here bold as brass in your flash car.'

That was what had started it. Since my old vehicle was dropping to bits I had splashed out on a second-hand Austin

10. It had done twenty thousand miles but had been well main-tained and looked like new with its black bodywork shining in the sun and the very sight of it had sparked off Mrs Sidlow.

The purchase of a new car was invariably greeted with a bit of leg-pulling by most of the farmers. 'Job must be payin' well,' they would say with a grin. But it was all friendly, with never a hint of the venom which seemed to be part of the Sidlow menage.

The Sidlows hated vets. Not just me, but all of them and that was quite a few because they had tried every practice for miles around and had found them all wanting. The trouble was that Mr Sidlow himself was quite simply the only man in the district who knew anything about doctoring sick animals – his wife and all his grown-up family knew this as an article of faith and whenever illness struck any of his cattle, it was natural that father took over. It was only when he had exhausted his supply of secret remedies that the vet was called in. I personally had seen only dying animals on that farm and had been unable to bring them back to life, so the Sidlows were invariably confirmed in their opinion of me along with the rest of my profession.

Today I had been viewing with the old feeling of hopelessness an emaciated little beast huddled in a dark corner of the fold yard taking its last few breaths after a week of pneumonia while the family stood around breathing hostility, shooting the usual side glances at me from their glowering faces. I had been trailing wearily back to my car on the way out when Mrs Sidlow had spotted me from the kitchen window and catapulted into the yard.

'Aye, it's awright for you,' she went on. 'We 'ave to work hard to make a livin' on this spot and then such as you come and take our money away from us without doin' anythin' for it. Ah know what it is, your idea is to get rich quick!'

Only my long training that the customer is always right stopped me from barking back. Instead I forced a smile.

'Mrs Sidlow,' I said, 'I assure you that I'm anything but rich. In fact, if you could see my bank balance, you would see what I mean.'

'You're tellin' me you haven't much money?'

'That's right.'

She waved towards the Austin and gave me another searing glare. 'So this fancy car's just a lot o' show on nowt!'

I had no answer. She had me both ways — either I was a fat cat or a stuck-up poseur.

As I drove away up the rising road I looked back at the farm with its substantial house and wide sprawl of buildings. There were five hundred lush acres down there, lying in the low country at the foot of the Dale. The Sidlows were big, prosperous farmers with none of the worries of the hill men who struggled to exist on the bleak smallholdings higher up, and it was difficult to understand why my imagined affluence should be such an affront to them.

Another distinctly unfriendly client is the local scrap merchant and second-hand car dealer Walt Barnett. A hard-edged character, he keeps some livestock and horses, but calls James in to take a look at his ailing cat, Fred. James is surprised to discover there's a sentimental side to the cheerless Walt Barnett, proving that even he has a heart and that animals can sometimes bring out the best in people.

When Walt Barnett asked me to see his cat I was surprised. He had employed other veterinary surgeons ever since Siegfried had mortally offended him by charging him ten pounds for castrating a horse, and that had been a long time ago. I was

171

surprised, too, that a man like him should concern himself with the ailments of a cat.

A lot of people said Walt Barnett was the richest man in Darrowby – rolling in brass which he made from his many and diverse enterprises. He was mainly a scrap merchant, but he had a haulage business, too, and he was a dealer in second-hand cars, furniture – anything, in fact, that came his way. I knew he kept some livestock and horses around his big house outside the town, but there was money in these things and money was the ruling passion of his life. There was no profit in cat-keeping.

Another thing which puzzled me as I drove to his office was that owning a pet indicated some warmth of character, a vein of sentiment, however small. It just didn't fit in with his nature.

I picked my way through the litter of the scrapyard to the wooden shed in the corner from which the empire was run. Walt Barnett was sitting behind a cheap desk and he was exactly as I remembered him, the massive body stretching the seams of his shiny navy-blue suit, the cigarette dangling from his lips, even the brown trilby hat perched on the back of his head. Unchanged, too, was the beefy red face with its arrogant expression and hostile eyes.

'Over there,' he said, glowering at me and poking a finger at a black and white cat sitting among the papers on the desk.

It was a typical greeting. I hadn't expected him to say 'Good morning' or anything like that, and he never smiled. I reached across the desk and tickled the animal's cheek, and was rewarded with a rich purring and an arching of the back against my hand. He was a big tom, long-haired and attractively marked with a white breast and white paws, and though I have always had a predilection for tabbies I took an immediate liking to this cat. He exuded friendliness. 'Nice cat,' I said. 'What's the trouble?'

James eventually discovers that somebody had cruelly put an elastic band first around the cat's legs and then his neck. As James explains, the police are aware that this cruelty occurs but they rarely catch the culprits in the act. A year later Fred falls ill, not by poisoning as Walt Barnett first suspects, but from an outbreak of the highly contagious virus, cat distemper. Fred sadly dies from the condition, much to the distress of his owner.

Fred was still and as I approached I saw with a dull feeling of inevitability that he was not breathing. I put my stethoscope over his heart for a few moments and then looked up.

'I'm afraid he's dead, Mr Barnett.'

The big man did not change expression. He reached slowly across and rubbed his forefinger against the dark fur in that familiar gesture. Then he put his elbows on the desk and covered his face with his hands.

I did not know what to say, but watched helplessly as his shoulders began to shake and tears welled between the thick fingers. He stayed like that for some time, then he spoke.

'He was my friend,' he said.

I still could find no words and the silence was heavy in the room until he suddenly pulled his hands from his face.

He glared at me defiantly. 'Aye, ah know what you're thinkin'. This is that big tough bugger, Walt Barnett, cryin' his eyes out over a cat. What a joke! I reckon you'll have a bloody good laugh later on.'

Evidently he was sure that what he considered a display of weakness would lower my opinion of him, and yet he was so wrong. I have liked him better ever since.

James and Siegfried come across many other local people who are just as sentimental about their animals, even if they're bred to feed their families or as farm livestock. With the size of farms on the increase, Siegfried in *It Shouldn't Happen to a Vet* reads out an article claiming that the larger the farm, the less affection there is for the animals. The two vets agree that, sadly, this is likely to be the case.

As I sat at breakfast I looked out at the autumn mist dissolving in the early sunshine. It was going to be another fine day but there was a chill in the old house this morning, a shiveriness as though a cold hand had reached out to remind us that summer had gone and the hard months lay just ahead.

'It says here,' Siegfried said, adjusting his copy of the *Darrowby and Houlton Times* with care against the coffee pot, 'that farmers have no feeling for their animals.' I buttered a piece of toast and looked across at him.

'Cruel, you mean?'

'Well, not exactly, but this chap maintains that to a farmer, livestock are purely commercial – there's no sentiment in his attitude towards them, no affection.'

'Well, it wouldn't do if they were all like poor Kit Bilton, would it? They'd all go mad.'

Kit was a lorry driver who, like so many of the working men of Darrowby, kept a pig at the bottom of his garden for family consumption. The snag was that when killing time came, Kit wept for three days. I happened to go into his house on one of these occasions and found his wife and daughter hard at it cutting up the meat for pies and brawn while Kit huddled miserably by the kitchen fire, his eyes swimming with tears. He was a huge man who could throw a twelve-stone sack of meal on to his wagon with a jerk of his arms, but he seized my hand in his and sobbed at me, 'I can't bear it, Mr Herriot. He was like a Christian was that pig, just like a Christian.'

'No, I agree.' Siegfried leaned over and sawed off a slice of Mrs Hall's home-baked bread. 'But Kit isn't a real farmer. This article is about people who own large numbers of animals. The question is, is it possible for such men to become emotionally involved? Can the dairy farmer milking maybe fifty cows become really fond of any of them or are they just milk-producing units?'

'It's an interesting point,' I said, 'and I think you've put your finger on it with the numbers. You know there are a lot of our farmers up in the high country who have only a few stock. They always have names for their cows — Daisy, Mabel, I even came across one called Kipperlugs the other day. I do think these small farmers have an affection for their animals but I don't see how the big men can possibly have.'

One small farmer who is undoubtedly sentimental about his animals is Mr Dakin. In *Vets Might Fly*, James is sent to stitch up the udder of Blossom the cow, who lives in a cobbled byre with six other cows, all of whom have names. Blossom is very old and her drooping udder needs repeated stitching. It's clear she's reached the end of her productive life and Mr Dakin reluctantly agrees to send her for slaughter. Dodson the drover is called in and James is there when he takes Blossom away. He and Mr Dakin then attend to one of the other cows which needs its afterbirth removing. When they have finished, James and Mr Dakin are suddenly alerted to another sound.

From somewhere on the hillside I could hear the clip-clop of a cow's feet. There were two ways to the farm and the sound came from a narrow track which joined the main road half a mile beyond the other entrance. As we listened a cow rounded a rocky outcrop and came towards us.

It was Blossom, moving at a brisk trot, great udder swinging, eyes fixed purposefully on the open door behind us.

'What the hangment . . .?' Mr Dakin burst out, but the old cow brushed past us and marched without hesitation into the stall which she had occupied for all those years. She sniffed enquiringly at the empty hay rack and looked round at her owner.

Mr Dakin stared back at her. The eyes in the weathered face were expressionless but the smoke rose from his pipe in a series of rapid puffs.

Mr Dodson the drover comes running after Blossom but Mr Dakin blocks his approach. He then fastens a chain around Blossom's neck and fills her rack with hay.

'What's to do, Mr Dakin?' the drover cried in bewilderment. 'They're waiting for me at t'mart!'

The farmer tapped out his pipe on the half door and began to fill it with black shag from a battered tin. 'Ah'm sorry to waste your time, Jack, but you'll have to go without 'er.'

'Without 'er . . .? But . . .?'

'Aye, ye'll think I'm daft, but that's how it is. T'awd lass has come 'ome and she's stoppin' 'ome.' He directed a look of flat finality at the drover.

Dodson nodded a couple of times then shuffled from the byre. Mr Dakin followed and called after him, 'Ah'll pay ye for your time, Jack. Put it down on ma bill.'

He returned, applied a match to his pipe and drew deeply.

'Mr Herriot,' he said as the smoke rose around his ears, 'do you ever feel when summat happens that it was meant to happen and that it was for t'best?'

'Yes, I do, Mr Dakin. I often feel that.'

'Aye well, that's how I felt when Blossom came down that hill.' He reached out and scratched the root of the cow's tail. 'She's allus been a favourite and by gaw I'm glad she's back.'

'But how about those teats? I'm willing to keep stitching them up, but . . .'

'Nay, lad, ah've had an idea. Just came to me when you were tekkin' away that cleansin' and I thowt I was ower late.'

'An idea?'

'Aye.' The old man nodded and tamped down the tobacco with his thumb. 'I can put two or three calves on to 'er instead of milkin' 'er. The old stable is empty — she can live in there where there's nobody to stand on 'er awd tits.'

I laughed. 'You're right, Mr Dakin. She'd be safe in the stable and she'd suckle three calves easily. She could pay her way.'

'Well, as ah said, it's matterless. After all them years she doesn't owe me a thing.' A gentle smile spread over the seamed face. 'Main thing is, she's come 'ome.'

The tale of Blossom was inspired by a couple of incidents related to Alf, including one concerning a cow belonging to local Pauline Parlour, which ended up back at her family farm, and another by the dairy farmer and friend of Alf, Arthur Dand. Arthur had an aged cow which he reluctantly agreed to send for slaughter. When the slaughterman began to take her away in his truck, the sight and sound of his cow, giving a sad bellow, was too much for Arthur and he raced after the truck, retrieved his cow and brought her back home. As he said to Jim: 'She may be no use to me any more, but she's going to spend the rest of her days right here!'

When an animal had reached the end of its life, it was either sent to a slaughterhouse or, if it was deemed unfit for human consumption, to a knacker's yard where the knackerman would slaughter and strip the carcass, selling the meat for pet food. Bones would also be sent to knife manufacturers for handles or rendered down to make fertilizer, hides sent to local tanneries, and oils might be used for soap or even by local football clubs to soften their boots or the cricket club to rub into their bats. In *If Only They Could Talk*, Jeff Mallock presides over the Darrowby knacker's yard. He lives there, amid the rotting carcasses and stinking filth, with his wife Mrs Mallock and their eight children, all of whom seem to be in the peak of health.

In Darrowby the name Mallock had a ring of doom. It was the graveyard of livestock, of farmers' ambitions, of veterinary surgeons' hopes. If ever an animal was very ill somebody was bound to say: 'I reckon she'll be off to Mallock's afore long,' or 'Jeff Mallock'll have 'er in t'finish.' And the premises fitted perfectly into the picture: a group of drab, red-brick buildings standing a few fields back from the road with a stumpy chimney from which rolled endlessly a dolorous black smoke.

It didn't pay to approach Mallock's too closely unless you had a strong stomach, so the place was avoided by the towns-people, but if you ventured up the lane and peeped through the sliding metal doors you could look in on a nightmare world. Dead animals lay everywhere. Most of them were dismembered and great chunks of meat hung on hooks, but here and there you could see a bloated sheep or a greenish, swollen pig which not even Jeff could bring himself to open.

Skulls and dry bones were piled to the roof in places and brown mounds of meat meal stood in the corners. The smell was bad at any time but when Jeff was boiling up the carcasses it was indescribable. The Mallock family bungalow stood in the middle of the buildings and strangers could be pardoned if they expected a collection of wizened gnomes to dwell there. But Jeff was a pink-faced, cherubic man in his forties, his wife plump, smiling and comely. Their family ranged from a positively beautiful girl of nineteen down to a robust five-year-old boy. There were eight young Mallocks and they had spent their lifetimes playing among tuberculous lungs and a vast spectrum of bacteria from salmonella to anthrax. They were the healthiest children in the district.

It was said in the pubs that Jeff was one of the richest men in town but the locals, as they supped their beer, had to admit that he earned his money. At any hour of the day or night he would rattle out into the country in his ramshackle lorry, winch on a carcass, bring it back to the yard and cut it up. A dog food dealer came twice a week from Brawton with a van and bought the fresh meat. The rest of the stuff Jeff shovelled into his boiler to make the meat meal which was in great demand for mixing in pig and poultry rations. The bones went for making fertilizer, the hides to the tanner and the nameless odds and ends were collected by a wild-eyed individual known only as the 'ket feller'. Sometimes, for a bit of variety, Jeff would make long slabs of strange-smelling soap which found a brisk sale for scrubbing shop floors. Yes, people said, there was no doubt Jeff did all right. But, by gaw, he earned it.

The story no doubt resonates with Alf's own visits to knackers' yards. He visited his first one as a student, while working at a practice in Dumfries, Scotland, and the experience remained imprinted in his mind. On entering, the putrefying stink of dead and decomposing animals immediately overwhelmed him, causing him to vomit up his breakfast on the floor. All the while a slaughterman looked upon him while sat on a carcass munching a sandwich and drinking tea out of a cup smeared with fat and blood stains.

While the Mallocks are a particularly hardy family, James also comes across another robust character in the form of Roddy Travers. James spots him walking along the moorland roads, pushing a pram containing his dog and his only belongings. Clearly living rough, he moves around the Yorkshire countryside and earns his keep by doing odd jobs on farms, helping out with ditching, hedging, looking after stock and drystone walling. Instead of hedges or fences, countless miles of drystone walls enclose the fields and border the roads throughout the fells of the Yorkshire Dales. They are built without mortar using an ancient and very skilled technique of fitting boulders and angular stones together, and in the wild weather of the moorland are in regular need of repair.

I suppose it isn't unusual to see a man pushing a pram in a town, but on a lonely moorland road the sight merits a second glance. Especially when the pram contains a large dog.

That was what I saw in the hills above Darrowby one morning and I slowed down as I drove past. I had noticed the strange combination before – on several occasions over the last few weeks – and it was clear that man and dog had recently moved into the district.

As the car drew abreast of him the man turned, smiled and raised his hand. It was a smile of rare sweetness in a very brown face. A forty-year-old face, I thought, above a brown neck which bore neither collar nor tie, and a faded striped shirt lying open over a bare chest despite the coldness of the day.

I couldn't help wondering who or what he was. The outfit of scuffed suede golf jacket, corduroy trousers and sturdy boots didn't give much clue. Some people might have put him down as an ordinary tramp, but there was a businesslike energetic look about him which didn't fit the term.

I wound the window down and the thin wind of a Yorkshire March bit at my cheeks.

'Nippy this morning,' I said.

The man seemed surprised. 'Aye,' he replied after a moment. 'Aye, reckon it is.'

I looked at the pram, ancient and rusty, and at the big animal sitting upright inside it. He was a lurcher, a cross-bred greyhound, and he gazed back at me with unruffled dignity.

'Nice dog,' I said.

'Aye, that's Jake.' The man smiled again, showing good regular teeth. 'He's a grand 'un.'

I waved and drove on. In the mirror I could see the compact figure stepping out briskly, head up, shoulders squared, and, rising like a statue from the middle of the pram, the huge brindled form of Jake.

I didn't have to wait long to meet the unlikely pair again. I was examining a carthorse's teeth in a farmyard when on the hillside beyond the stable I saw a figure kneeling by a drystone wall. And by his side, a pram and a big dog sitting patiently on the grass.

'Hey, just a minute.' I pointed at the hill. 'Who is that?'

The farmer laughed. 'That's Roddy Travers. D'you ken 'im?'

'No, no I don't. I had a word with him on the road the other day, that's all.'

'Aye, on the road.' He nodded knowingly. 'That's where you'd see Roddy, right enough.'

'But what is he? Where does he come from?'

'He comes from somewhere in Yorkshire, but ah don't rightly know where and ah don't think anybody else does. But I'll tell you this — he can turn 'is hand to anything.'

181

'Yes,' I said, watching the man expertly laying the flat slabs of stone as he repaired a gap in the wall. 'There's not many can do what he's doing now.'

'That's true. Wallin' is a skilled job and it's dying out, but Roddy's a dab hand at it. But he can do owt – hedgin', ditchin', lookin' after stock, it's all the same to him.'

I lifted the tooth rasp and began to rub a few sharp corners off the horse's molars. 'And how long will he stay here?'

'Oh, when he's finished that wall he'll be off. Ah could do with 'im stoppin' around for a bit but he never stays in one place for long.'

'But hasn't he got a home anywhere?'

'Nay, nay.' The farmer laughed again. 'Roddy's got nowt. All 'e has in the world is in that there pram.'

The character of Roddy Travers was based on a roving handyman known to everyone in the district, Freddy Manners. He did everything from gardening and sharpening knives to general farm work and was one of many such types who travelled around doing odd jobs for people. He also had a big greyhound dog called Joe, which Donald bought from him and was one of the pack dogs that greeted Alf when he first arrived at the practice in Thirsk.

The Dales are filled with a wide assortment of folk and not all of them are gruff, rugged types, as James discovers when he meets Roland Partridge. Despite being a son of a small farmer, he lives as an artist, having eschewed the gritty life of farming – and dispensing with the broad Yorkshire accent – for a more creative and modest existence in Darrowby.

You could hardly expect to find a more unlikely character in Darrowby than Roland Partridge. The thought came to me for the hundredth time as I saw him peering through the window which looked onto Trengate just a little way up the other side of the street from our surgery.

He was tapping the glass and beckoning to me and the eyes behind the thick spectacles were wide with concern. I waited and when he opened the door I stepped straight from the street into his living room because these were tiny dwellings with only a kitchen in the rear and a single small bedroom overlooking the street above. But when I went in I had the familiar feeling of surprise. Because most of the other occupants of the row were farm workers and their furnishings were orthodox; but this place was a studio.

An easel stood in the light from the window and the walls were covered from floor to ceiling with paintings. Unframed canvases were stacked everywhere and the few ornate chairs and the table with its load of painted china and other bric-à-brac added to the artistic atmosphere.

The simple explanation was, of course, that Mr Partridge was in fact an artist. But the unlikely aspect came into it when you learned that this middle-aged velvet-jacketed aesthete was the son of a small farmer, a man whose forebears had been steeped in the soil for generations.

'I happened to see you passing there, Mr Herriot,' he said. 'Are you terribly busy?'

'Not too busy, Mr Partridge. Can I help you?'

He nodded gravely. 'I wondered whether you could spare a moment to look at Percy. I'd be most grateful.'

'Of course,' I replied. 'Where is he?'

He was ushering me towards the kitchen when there was a bang on the outer door and Bert Hardisty the postman burst in. Bert was a rough-hewn character and he dumped a parcel unceremoniously on the table.

'There y'are, Rolie!' he shouted and turned to go.

Mr Partridge gazed with unruffled dignity at the retreating back. 'Thank you very much indeed, Bertram, good day to you.'

Here was another thing. The postman and the artist were both Darrowby born and bred, had the same social background, had gone to the same school, yet their voices were quite different. Roland Partridge, in fact, spoke with the precise, well-modulated syllables of a barrister at law.

We went into the kitchen. This was where he cooked for himself in his bachelor state. When his father died many years ago he had sold the farm immediately. Apparently his whole nature was appalled by the earthy farming scene and he could not get out quickly enough. At any rate he had got sufficient money from the sale to indulge his interests and he had taken up painting and lived ever since in this humble cottage, resolutely doing his own thing. This had all happened long before I came to Darrowby and the dangling lank hair was silver now. I always had the feeling that he was happy in his way because I couldn't imagine that small, rather exquisite figure plodding around a muddy farmyard.

Mr Partridge's dog Percy has a large tumour on one of his testicles, which grows so large that he is subjected to ridicule by some of the locals, until Mr Partridge eventually allows James to remove it. A while later, he brings Percy into the surgery again and James is disappointed to see the tumour has spread. He decides to try a new hormonal treatment, Stilboestrol, which seems to stop the tumour growing, although either the drug or the dog's tumour gives Percy the attributes of a bitch on heat and half the dogs in the neighbourhood start to hang around Mr Partridge's house. Thankfully, the growth disappears and never returns, as is also the case with the local dogs, and over the years James is happy to see Mr Partridge and Percy pass his window in good health, their dignity very much restored.

Unlike Mr Partridge, some clients can be far less articulate when they come into the practice and it can be a struggle to understand what the problem is. Some locals turn up at Skeldale House on the way back from the pub and are too sozzled to make any sense. Others are incredibly vague about their animal's ailments or agonize over whether they want a vet to visit, their anxiety centred upon the impending bill. And if an animal has a problem with anything vaguely sexual or a natural function, then some clients are too embarrassed to give any real detail, especially if it's a man and a woman is in the vicinity. Mr Pinkerton, who comes into the practice with his dog, has that very problem.

Mr Pinkerton, a smallholder, was sitting in the office next to Miss Harbottle's desk. By his side sat his farm collie.

'Well, what can I do for you, Mr Pinkerton?' I asked as I closed the door behind me.

The farmer hesitated. 'It's me dog — 'e isn't right.'

'What do you mean? Is he ill?' I bent down and stroked the shaggy head and as the dog leaped up in delight his tail began to beat a booming tom-tom rhythm against the side of the desk.

'Nay, nay, he's right enough in 'imself.' The man was clearly ill at ease.

'Well, what's the trouble? He looks the picture of health to me.'

'Aye, but ah'm a bit worried. Ye see it's 'is . . .' He glanced furtively towards Miss Harbottle. 'It's 'is pencil.'

'What d'you say?'

A faint flush mounted in Mr Pinkerton's thin cheeks. Again he shot a terrified glance at Miss Harbottle. 'It's 'is . . . pencil. There's summat matter with 'is pencil.' He indicated by the merest twitch of his forefinger somewhere in the direction of the animal's belly.

I looked. 'I'm sorry, but I can't see anything unusual.'

'Ah, but there is.' The farmer's face twisted in an agony of embarrassment and he pushed his face close to mine. 'There's summat there,' he said in a hoarse whisper. 'Summat comin' from 'is . . .'is pencil.'

I got down on my knees and had a closer look, and suddenly all became clear.

'Is that what you mean?' I pointed to a tiny blob of semen on the end of the prepuce.

He nodded dumbly, his face a study of woe.

I laughed. 'Well you can stop worrying. That's nothing abnormal. You might call it an overflow. He's just a young dog, isn't he?'

'Aye, nobbut eighteen months.'

'Well, that's it. He's just too full of the joys. Plenty of good food and maybe not a lot of work to do, eh?'

'Aye, he gets good grub. Nowt but the best. And you're right — I 'aven't much work for him.'

'Well, there you are.' I held out a hand. 'Just cut down his diet and see he gets more exercise and this thing will sort itself out.'

Most of James's clients consider him a capable vet, but there are a few farmers who, despite his best efforts, have a low opinion of him, principally because every time he visits them, something always seems to go wrong. Alf himself experienced what seem to be jinxed places, which he called 'bogey farms', where animals promptly died or inexplicable events happened. Such is the case in *Every Living Thing* when a series of minor accidents afflicts James whenever he visits the Hardwicks.

My clients' opinion of me varied widely, and although there were the odd one or two who thought I was brilliant, a large majority looked on me as a steady, reliable vet, while a few regarded me as of strictly limited ability. But I really think that only one family nourished the private conviction that I was not quite right in the head.

They were the Hardwicks, and it was a pity because they were some of my favourite people.

After a quick visit to the Hardwicks' farm to check on some calves he'd treated, James returns to his car and discovers that his dog, Dinah, has pushed down the doorknobs, accidentally locking the car from the inside. Apologizing, James has to ask one of the Hardwick brothers to drive him to Darrowby so he can retrieve the spare key. Subsequent trips involve him inadvertently picking up Mrs Hardwick's reading glasses and then turning up at the farm when he is meant to be at another one down the road. When he is next called to the Hardwicks', to examine a cow that can't get up, his embarrassment is now acute.

'She's got a dislocated hip, Seb,' I said. 'There's nothing broken, but the head of the femur is right out of its socket.'

'Are ye sure?' The farmer looked at me doubtfully.

'Absolutely positive. Here, feel this prominence. In fact, you can just about see it sticking up there.'

Seb didn't bother to take his hands out of his pockets. 'Well, ah don't know. I thought she'd maybe just strained 'erself. Maybe you could give me summat to rub on 'er — that might put her right.'

'No, I assure you. There's no doubt in my mind.'

'Awright, then, what do we do?'

'Well, we'll have to try to pull the joint back into place. It's not easy, but since it has only just happened I'd say there was a good chance of success.'

The farmer sniffed. 'Very well, then. On ye go.'

'I'm sorry,' I said, smiling, 'but it's quite a big job and I can't do it by myself. In fact, you and I can't do it. We'll need some help.'

'Help? I haven't got no 'elp. Josh is right over on the far field.'

'Well, I'm really sorry about that, but you'll have to get him back. And I hate to say it, but we'll also need one of your neighbours to lend a hand. And he'd better be a big strong chap, too.'

'Bloody 'ell!' Seb stared at me. 'What's all this for?'

'I know it seems a big fuss to you, but although she's only a young beast, she's big and strong and in order to get the joint back in place we have to overcome the muscular resistance. It needs a right good pull, I can tell you. I've done a lot of these jobs and I know.'

He nodded. 'Ah well, I'll go and see if Charlie Lawson can come over. You'll wait 'ere, then?'

'No, I'll have to go back to the surgery for the chloroform muzzle.'

'Chloroform! What the 'ell next?'

'I told you about the muscular resistance. We need to put her to sleep to overcome that.'

188

'Now, look 'ere, Mr Herriot.' The farmer lifted a portentous forefinger. 'Are ye sure we have to go through all this carry-on? Don't ye think we could just rub summat on? A bit of embrocation, maybe?'

'I'm sorry, Seb, it's all necessary.'

He turned and strode out of the cow house, muttering, while I hurried across to my car.

On the journey to Darrowby and back, two thoughts were uppermost in my mind. This was one of the tricky jobs in veterinary practice but, when successful, it was spectacular. A hopelessly lame animal would rise and walk away, good as new. And I did feel I badly needed something to resuscitate my reputation on this farm.

When I returned with the muzzle, Josh and Charlie Lawson were waiting in the yard with Seb. 'Now, Mr Herriot,' 'Now then, Mr Herriot,' but they looked at me sceptically, and I could tell that the other brother had been voicing his doubts.

'It's good of you gentlemen to rally round,' I said cheerfully. 'I hope you're all feeling strong. It's a tough job, this.' Charlie Lawson grinned and rubbed his hands. 'Aye, we'll do our best.'

'OK, now.' I looked down at the heifer. 'We'd better move her nearer the door. You'll get a stronger pull that way. Then we'll get the chloroform muzzle on and rope the leg. You'll haul away while I put pressure on the joint. But first let's roll her over.'

As the farmers pushed against the animal's side, I tried to tuck the lame leg underneath her. As she rolled over there was a loud click, and after a rapid look around her she rose to her feet and walked out through the door.

The four of us watched her as she ambled across the yard and through a gate into the field. She was perfectly sound. Not the slightest trace of lameness.

'Well, I've never seen that happen before,' I gasped. 'The rolling movement and the pressure on the joint must have clicked it back. Would you believe it!'

The three farmers gave me a level stare. It was clear that they didn't believe it.

Retreating to my car, I heard Seb confiding to the other two. 'Might as well have rubbed summat on it.' And as I drove away past the heifer grazing contentedly on the green hillside, Siegfried's words at the beginning of our partnership came back to me. 'Our profession offers unparalleled opportunities for making a chump of yourself.'

How true that was. How true it would always be. But why, why, *why* did it have to happen this time at the Hardwicks'?

Chapter 7

CATTLE

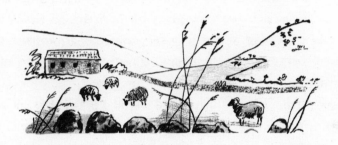

They didn't say anything about this in the books, I thought, as the snow blew in through the gaping doorway and settled on my naked back.

I lay face down on the cobbled floor in a pool of nameless muck, my arm deep inside the straining cow, my feet scrabbling for a toehold between the stones. I was stripped to the waist and the snow mingled with the dirt and the dried blood on my body. I could see nothing outside the circle of flickering light thrown by the smoky oil lamp which the farmer held over me.

No, there wasn't a word in the books about searching for your ropes and instruments in the shadows; about trying to keep clean in a half-bucket of tepid water; about the cobbles digging into your chest. Nor about the slow numbing of the arms, the creeping paralysis of the muscles as the fingers tried to work against the cow's powerful expulsive efforts.

There was no mention anywhere of the gradual exhaustion, the feeling of futility and the little far-off voice of panic.

If Only They Could Talk begins with a gruelling calving, James having crawled out of his bed at 2 a.m. before heading across a snowy moorland, only to spend the next few hours with his arm inside a straining cow. This was the reality of veterinary practice in rural Yorkshire where cattle-farming predominated, and the likes of James Herriot were frequently called out to attend to calvings and the host of complications that can ensue when a cow gives birth. Stripped to the waist in a cold cow byre, veterinary surgeons had to work hard to find feet, bring heads round and do all they could to deliver a healthy calf.

James and Siegfried are called in all year round to attend to cattle, and a veterinary practice in rural Yorkshire relies upon its regular income – one of the reasons why Alf Wight had a great affection for the bovine race in general. Some cattle were raised for beef but vets saw more of the dairy cows which needed to calve at least once a year so they could continue to produce milk.

Prior to arriving in Yorkshire, Alf had had some practical experience of working with cows, having spent his university vacations in Dumfries in the south-west of Scotland. There, he looked after Galloway cattle and on one occasion was given the opportunity to remove the afterbirth from a cow chained up in a rickety old henhouse. When he gently tugged at the hanging mass, the cow bellowed, broke through its chain, smashed through the window, taking one side of the henhouse with her, with the remainder collapsing on top of the men standing there. They all survived intact although the incident at least prepared Alf for the physical rigours of bovine care in later years.

Returning to *If Only They Could Talk* and James, still with his arm in the cow, must summon every ounce of strength he has to deliver the calf, while the dour farmers look on, more concerned about the welfare of their prized cow than that of the young veterinary surgeon.

My mind went back to that picture in the obstetrics book. A cow standing in the middle of a gleaming floor while a sleek veterinary surgeon in a spotless parturition overall inserted his arm to a polite distance. He was relaxed and smiling, the farmer and his helpers were smiling, even the cow was smiling. There was no dirt or blood or sweat anywhere.

That man in the picture had just finished an excellent lunch and had moved next door to do a bit of calving just for the sheer pleasure of it, as a kind of dessert. He hadn't crawled shivering from his bed at two o'clock in the morning and bumped over twelve miles of frozen snow, staring sleepily ahead till the lonely farm showed in the headlights. He hadn't climbed half a mile of white fell-side to the doorless barn where his patient lay.

I tried to wriggle my way an extra inch inside the cow. The calf's head was back and I was painfully pushing a thin, looped rope towards its lower jaw with my fingertips. All the time my arm was being squeezed between the calf and the bony pelvis. With every straining effort from the cow the pressure became almost unbearable, then she would relax and I would push the rope another inch. I wondered how long I would be able to keep this up. If I didn't snare that jaw soon I would never get the calf away. I groaned, set my teeth and reached forward again.

Another little flurry of snow blew in and I could almost hear the flakes sizzling on my sweating back. There was sweat on my forehead too, and it trickled into my eyes as I pushed.

There is always a time at a bad calving when you begin to wonder if you will ever win the battle. I had reached this stage.

Little speeches began to flit through my brain. 'Perhaps it would be better to slaughter this cow. Her pelvis is so small and narrow that I can't see a calf coming through,' or 'She's a good fat animal and really of the beef type, so don't you think it would pay you better to get the butcher?' or perhaps 'This is a very bad presentation. In a roomy cow it would be simple enough to bring the head round but in this case it is just about impossible.'

Of course, I could have delivered the calf by embryotomy — by passing a wire over the neck and sawing off the head. So many of these occasions ended with the floor strewn with heads, legs, heaps of intestines. There were thick textbooks devoted to the countless ways you could cut up a calf.

But none of it was any good here, because this calf was alive. At my furthest stretch I had got my finger as far as the commissure of the mouth and had been startled by a twitch of the little creature's tongue. It was unexpected because calves in this position are usually dead, asphyxiated by the acute flexion of the neck and the pressure of the dam's powerful contractions. But this one had a spark of life in it and if it came out it would have to be in one piece.

I went over to my bucket of water, cold now and bloody, and silently soaped my arms. Then I lay down again, feeling the cobbles harder than ever against my chest. I worked my toes between the stones, shook the sweat from my eyes and for the hundredth time thrust an arm that felt like spaghetti into the cow; alongside the little dry legs of the calf, like sandpaper tearing against my flesh, then to the bend in the neck and so to the ear and then, agonizingly, along the side of the face towards the lower jaw which had become my major goal in life.

It was incredible that I had been doing this for nearly two hours; fighting as my strength ebbed to push a little noose round that jaw. I had tried everything else — repelling a leg, gentle traction with a blunt hook in the eye socket, but I was back to the noose.

James must struggle on with the calving in the presence of the farmer Mr Dinsdale, 'a long, sad, silent man of few words' along with his equally silent son, both of them watch the vet's efforts with deepening gloom. Worst of all, however, is the presence of 'Uncle', Mr Dinsdale's brother, a farmer who keeps up a non-stop stream of comments, while eulogizing about his wonderful vet Mr Broomfield. As Uncle blethers on about Mr Broomfield's Herculean strength, James, now exhausted, considers tipping the bucket of water over Uncle's head, then running down the hill and driving away 'from Yorkshire, from Uncle, from the Dinsdales, from this cow'.

Instead, I clenched my teeth, braced my legs and pushed with everything I had; and with a sensation of disbelief I felt my noose slide over the sharp little incisor teeth and into the calf's mouth. Gingerly, muttering a prayer, I pulled on the thin rope with my left hand and felt the slipknot tighten. I had hold of that lower jaw.

At last I could start doing something. 'Now hold this rope, Mr Dinsdale, and just keep a gentle tension on it. I'm going to repel the calf and if you pull steadily at the same time, the head ought to come round.'

'What if the rope comes off?' asked Uncle hopefully.

I didn't answer. I put my hand in against the calf's shoulder and began to push against the cow's contractions. I felt the small body moving away from me. 'Now a steady pull, Mr Dinsdale, without jerking.' And to myself, 'Oh God, don't let it slip off.'

The head was coming round. I could feel the neck straightening against my arm, then the ear touched my elbow. I let go the shoulder and grabbed the little muzzle. Keeping the teeth away from the vaginal wall with my hand, I guided the head till it was resting where it should be, on the fore limbs.

Quickly I extended the noose till it reached behind the ears. 'Now pull on the head as she strains.'

'Nay, you should pull on the legs now,' cried Uncle.

'Pull on the bloody head rope, I tell you!' I bellowed at the top of my voice and felt immediately better as Uncle retired, offended, to his bale.

With traction the head was brought out and the rest of the body followed easily. The little animal lay motionless on the cobbles, eyes glassy and unseeing, tongue blue and grossly swollen.

'It'll be dead. Bound to be,' grunted Uncle, returning to the attack.

I cleared the mucus from the mouth, blew hard down the throat and began artificial respiration. After a few pressures on the ribs, the calf gave a gasp and the eyelids flickered. Then it started to inhale and one leg jerked.

Uncle begrudgingly accepts that the calf is alive – 'I'd have thowt it'd sure to be dead after you'd messed about all that time.' James positions the calf by its mother who licks it methodically and within a minute it is trying to sit up. James grins at what always feels like a miracle of life, although he is exhausted, with every muscle aching and his mouth parched from thirst.

A long, sad figure hovered near. 'How about a drink?' asked Mr Dinsdale.

I could feel my grimy face cracking into an incredulous smile. A vision of hot tea well laced with whisky swam before me. 'That's very kind of you, Mr Dinsdale, I'd love a drink. It's been a hard two hours.'

'Nay,' said Mr Dinsdale looking at me steadily, 'I meant for the cow.'

Calving a cow often made for a dramatic event, especially in the pre-war days when caesareans were not generally an option for veterinary surgeons. In essence, the calf needed to come out the way nature intended, and if there were complications, the fate of the calf and its mother – not to mention the reputation of the vet – could hang in the balance. James is more than aware of this when in *It Shouldn't Happen to a Vet* he attends to the calving of the Aldersons' pet Jersey cow Candy. Not only does James want to make a good impression on Mr Alderson, as these were early days and he was his prospective father-in-law, but James also knows just how special a cow this is to the family.

She was the house cow, a pretty little Jersey and Mr Alderson's particular pet. She was the sole member of her breed in the herd but whereas the milk from the shorthorns went into the churns to be collected by the big dairy, Candy's rich yellow offering found its way onto the family porridge every morning or appeared heaped up on trifles and fruit pies or was made into butter, a golden creamy butter to make you dream.

James examines Candy, hoping the problem is something simple. It's not a good sign, however, when he hears Candy has been labouring for hours, with nothing to show for it. He feels inside but can only find an empty vagina and a small, ridged opening, beyond which he can feel the feet and head of a calf.

My spirits plummeted. Torsion of the uterus. There was going to be no easy victory for me here.

I sat back on my heels and turned to the farmer. 'She's got a twisted calf bed. There's a live calf in there all right, but there's no way out for it — I can barely get my hand through.'

'Aye, I thought it was something peculiar.' Mr Alderson rubbed his chin and looked at me doubtfully. 'What can we do about it, then?'

'We'll have to try to correct the twist by rolling the cow over while I keep hold of the calf. It's a good job there's plenty of us here.'

'And that'll put everything right, will it?'

I swallowed. I didn't like these jobs. Sometimes rolling worked and sometimes it didn't and in those days we hadn't quite got round to performing caesareans on cows. If I was unsuccessful I had the prospect of telling Mr Alderson to send Candy to the butcher. I banished the thought quickly.

With two men holding the front and hind legs and Mr Alderson holding Candy's head, James pushes his hand inside, grab's the calf's foot and they roll the cow onto her side. After James's arm is almost crushed, they roll her back on the other side, James lying face down and holding grimly on. Nothing happens and they try once more and then, finally, everything magically unravels. Candy gives a determined push and out pops the calf, wet and wriggling. As Alf writes, 'After every delivery there is a feeling of relief but in this case it was overwhelming.' With Candy the cow saved, James decides this is a good moment to approach Mr Alderson about his intended proposal to his daughter.

Such life-or-death events – with all the emotions that go with them – are commonplace for veterinary surgeons, as it was for Alf in practice. Sometimes there was simply no viable way to extract a live calf and it was the job of the vet always to make firm and sometimes difficult decisions quickly. Jim remembers his father telling him about a time when his old college friend Eddie Straiton came to work at the Thirsk practice and they were called to a calving. They both came to the decision that attempting to extract a large calf out of the cow in question would likely kill the mother. They advised the farmer that the best option was to slaughter the cow so he at least would receive a good price for her carcass. Another man who had been observing the proceedings, however, suggested he ''ave a go'. He then inserted his arm into the cow's vagina and, using a knife, produced the decomposing calf bit by bit. Alf and Eddie, now utterly dejected, left feeling that they had failed, their reputation and careers in tatters. Their decision, however, would be vindicated when they later discovered the cow died almost instantly afterwards and that the farmer in question had wished he'd listened to the two young veterinary surgeons.

By the time of *The Lord God Made Them All*, set in the years just after the war, caesareans are beginning to be done on cows or at least taught to students in veterinary colleges. In fact, veterinary medicine and procedures had advanced considerably since Alf had been at college and he knew that some of the students who worked at the practice had a little more knowledge about the latest methods. The assistant Norman Beaumont who features in *The Lord God Made Them All* suggests they do a caesarean on a small cow named Bella who is unable to give birth to her large calf. James agrees this would be a good case for the new procedure but needs Norman to guide him through it.

We do these jobs under a local anaesthetic nowadays, and in most cases the cow lies quietly on her side or even stands during the operation. The animal can't feel anything, of course, but I have a few extra grey hairs round my ears which owe their presence to the occasional wild cow suddenly rearing up halfway through and taking off with me in desperate pursuit trying to keep her internal organs from flopping on the ground.

But that was all in the future. On this first occasion I had no such fears. I cut through skin, muscle layers and peritoneum and was confronted by a protruding pink and white mass of tissue.

I poked at it with my finger. There was something hard inside. Could it be the calf?

'What's that?' I hissed.

'Eh?' Norman, kneeling by my side, jumped convulsively. 'What do you mean?'

'That thing. Is it the rumen or the uterus? It's pretty low down, it could be the uterus.'

The student swallowed a couple of times. 'Yes . . . yes . . . that's the uterus all right.'

'Good.' I smiled in relief and made a bold incision. A great gout of impacted grass welled out, followed by a burst of gas and an outflow of dirty brown fluid.

'Oh Christ!' I gasped. 'It's the rumen. Look at all that bloody mess!' I groaned aloud as the filthy tide surged away down and out of sight into the abdominal cavity. 'What the hell are you playing at, Norman?'

I could feel the young man's body trembling against mine.

'Don't just sit there!' I shouted. 'Thread me one of those needles. Quick! Quick!'

Norman bounded to his feet, rushed over to the bale and returned with a trailing length of catgut extended in shaking

200

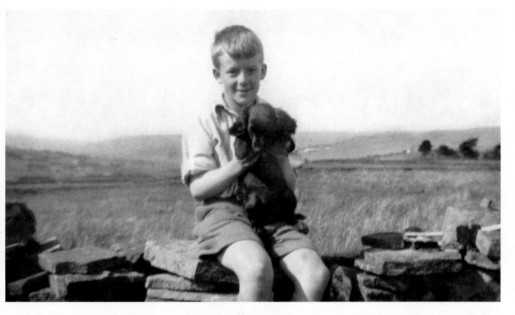

Dad, aged twelve, with his first dog Don the Irish setter.

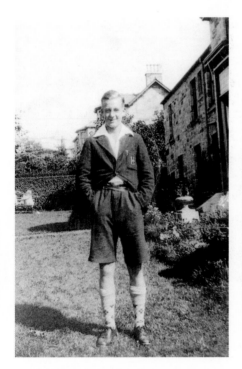

Sixteen years old, in the Hillhead
High school uniform.

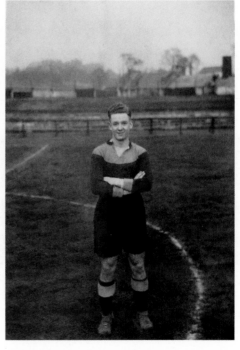

Playing for the veterinary college
football team.

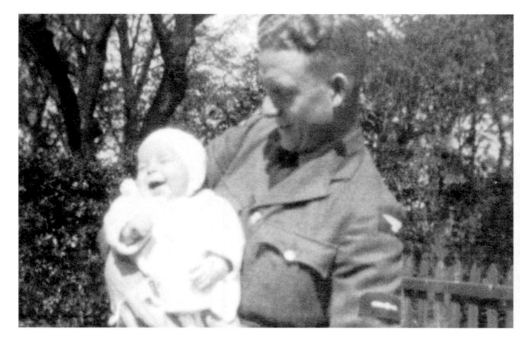

Dad in his RAF uniform with a very young Jim.

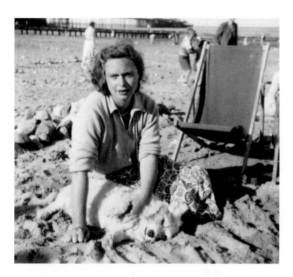

Mum, Joan, with our first dog Danny.

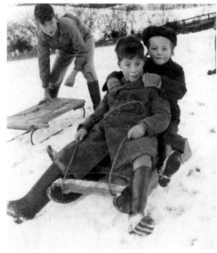

Us on a sledge at Hood Grange
on Sutton Bank.

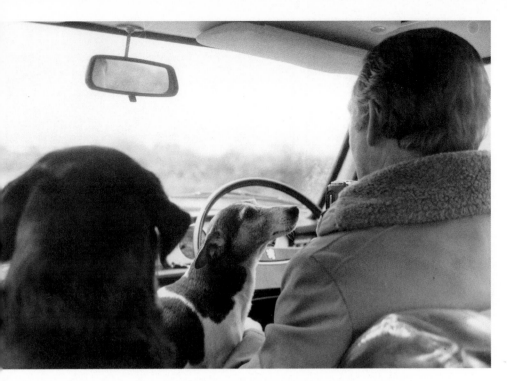

Dan the black Labrador and Hector the Jack Russell. Hector was his favourite dog. Both loved to ride in the front of the car.

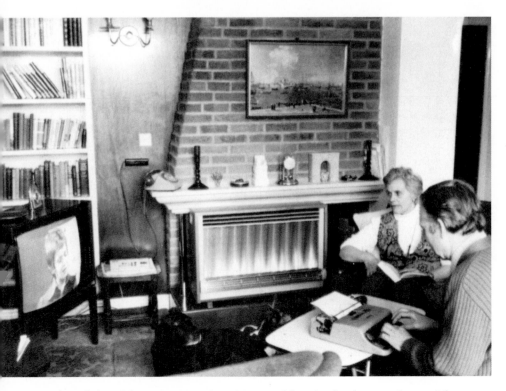

Dad with his Olivetti typewriter. He would write in the evenings with the telly on and Mum by his side.

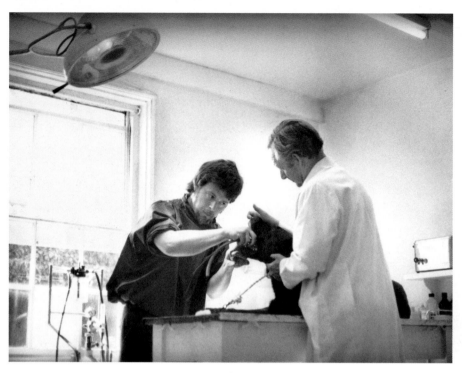

Jim helping Dad with a small dog at the Thirsk veterinary practice.

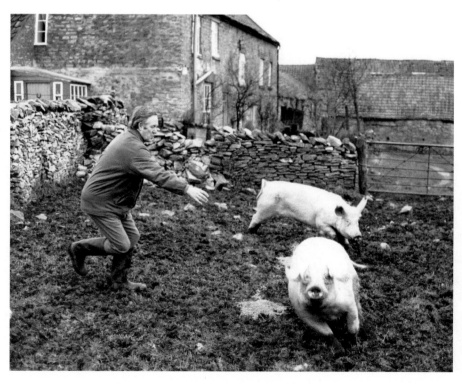

This wouldn't be the way he'd catch the pigs on the job but he was having some fun for the cameras here!

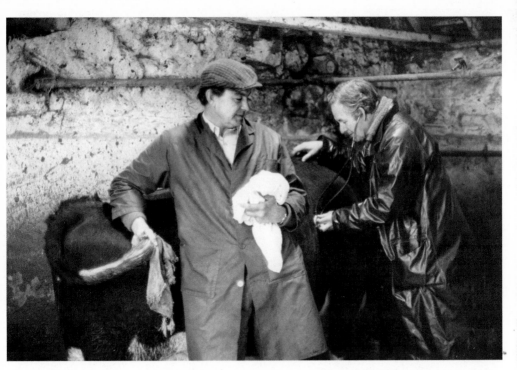

With Arthur Dand – one of Dad's favourite farmers and the person who thought up the title *If Only They Could Talk*.

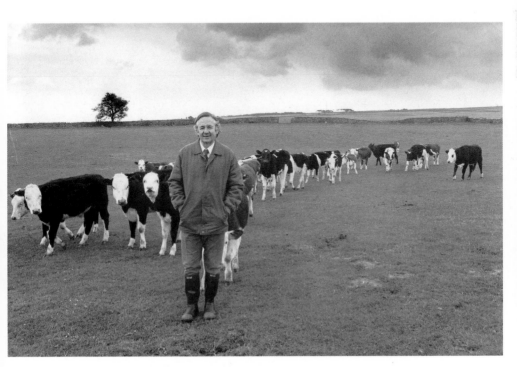

Wethercote Farm at Sutton Bank in North Yorkshire.

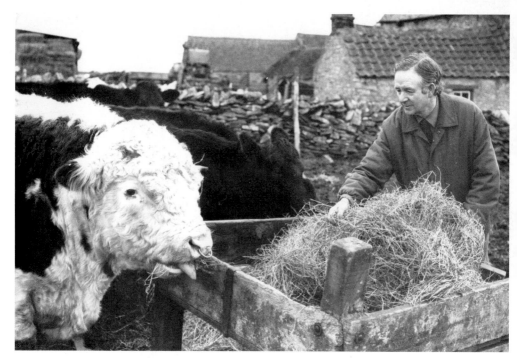

Feeding a young bull at Wethercote Farm.

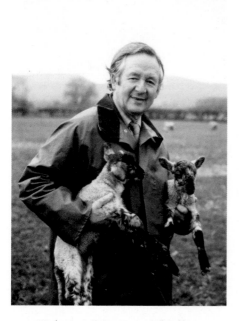

Kelmire Grange in Thirlby.

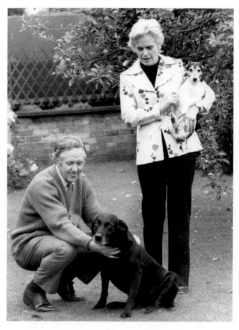

Mum and Dad with Dan and Hector at their home in Thirsk.

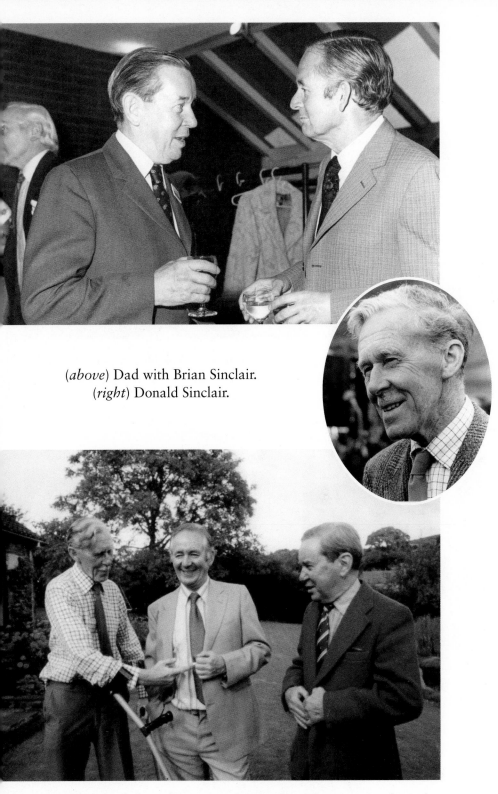

(*above*) Dad with Brian Sinclair.
(*right*) Donald Sinclair.

Dad with Donald (*left*) and Brian (*right*) Sinclair. They remained good friends throughout their lives. Taken at Dad's final home in Thirlby.

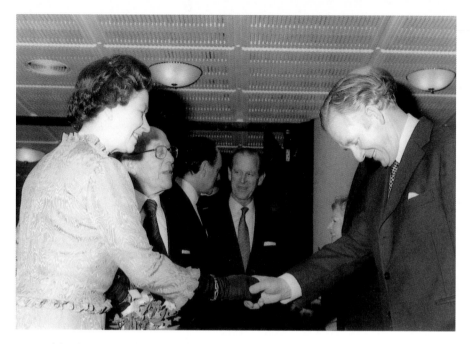

Dad looking very happy to be introduced to the Queen at the annual Hatchards Authors of the Year reception. She was said to be a big fan of the Herriot books.

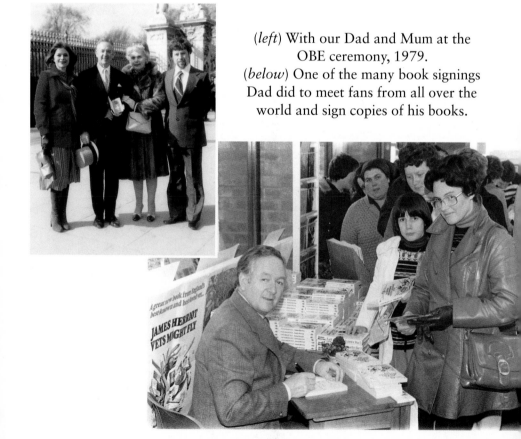

(*left*) With our Dad and Mum at the OBE ceremony, 1979.
(*below*) One of the many book signings Dad did to meet fans from all over the world and sign copies of his books.

fingers. Wordlessly, dry-mouthed, I stitched the gash I had made in the wrong organ. Then the two of us made frantic attempts to swab away the escaped rumenal contents with cotton wool and antiseptic but much of it had run away beyond our reach. The contamination must be massive.

When we had done what we could, I sat back and looked at the student. My voice was a hoarse growl. 'I thought you knew all about these operations.'

He looked at me with frightened eyes. 'They do quite a few of them at the clinic.'

I glared back at him. 'How many caesareans have you seen?'

'Well . . . er . . . one, actually.'

'One! To hear you speak I thought you were an expert! And anyway, even if you'd seen only one you should know a little bit about it.'

'The thing is . . .' Norman shuffled his knees around on the cobbles. 'You see . . . I was right at the back of the class.'

I worked up a sarcastic snarl. 'Oh, I understand. So you couldn't see very well?'

'That's about it.' The young man hung his head.

'Well, you're a stupid young fool!' I said in a vicious whisper. 'Dishing out your confident instructions when you know damn-all. You realize you've killed this good cow? With all that contamination she'll certainly develop peritonitis and die. All we can hope for now is to get the calf out alive.' With an effort I turned my gaze from his stricken face. 'Anyway, let's get on with it.'

Apart from my first shouts of panic the entire interchange had been carried out *pianissimo* and Mr Bushell kept shooting enquiring glances at us.

I gave him what I hoped was a reassuring smile and returned to the attack. Getting the calf out alive was easy to say, but it soon dawned on me that getting the calf out in any way whatsoever was going to be a mammoth task. Plunging my arm deep below what I now knew was the rumen I encountered a smooth and mighty organ lying on the abdominal floor. It contained an enormous bulk with the hardness and immobility of a sack of coal.

I felt my way along the surface and came upon the unmistakable contours of a hock pushing against the slippery wall. That was the calf all right, but it was far far away.

I withdrew my arm and started on Norman again. 'From your position at the back of the class,' I enquired bitingly, 'did you happen to notice what they did next?'

'Next? Ah yes.' He licked his lips and I could see beads of sweat on his brow. 'You are supposed to exteriorize the uterus.'

'Exteriorize it? Bring it up to the wound, you mean?'

'That's right.'

'Good God!' I said. 'King Kong couldn't lift up that bloody uterus. In fact I can't move it an inch. Have a feel.'

The student, who was stripped and soaped like myself, introduced his arm and for a few moments I watched his eyes pop and his face redden. Then he withdrew and nodded sheepishly. 'You're right. It won't move.'

'Only one thing to do.' I picked up a scalpel. 'I'll have to cut into the uterus and grab that hock. There's nothing else to get hold of.'

It was very nasty fiddling about away out of sight down in the dark unknown, my arm buried to the shoulder in the cow, my tongue hanging out with anxiety. I was terrified I might slash into something vital but in fact it was my own fingers that I cut, several times, before I was able to draw the scalpel edge across the bulge made by the hock. A second later I had my hand round the hairy leg. Now I was getting somewhere.

Gingerly I enlarged the incision, inch by inch. I hoped fervently I had made it big enough, but working blind is a terrible thing and it was difficult to be sure.

At any rate I couldn't wait to deliver that calf. I laid aside my knife, seized the leg and tried to lift it, and immediately I knew that another little nightmare lay ahead. The thing was a tremendous weight and it was going to take great strength to bring it up into the light of day. Nowadays when I do a caesar I take care to have a big strong farm lad stripped off ready to help me with this lifting job, but today I had only Norman.

'Come on,' I panted. 'Give me a hand.'

James manages to bring the foot of the calf round and grasp the other hind leg, and then, both men pulling with every vestige of their strength, the tail appears, then a huge ribcage and, finally, with a rush, the shoulders and head. As the calf snorts, the farmer exclaims, 'By gaw, he's a big 'un.' It is indeed a massive bull who would have never come out the usual way.

My attention was whisked back to the cow. Where was the uterus? It had vanished. Again I started my frantic groping inside. My hand became entangled with yards of placenta. Oh hell, that wouldn't do any good floating around among the guts. I pulled it out and dropped it on the floor but I still couldn't find the uterus. For a palpitating moment I wondered what would happen if I never did locate it, then my fingers came upon the ragged edge of my incision.

I pulled as much as possible of the organ up to the light and I noticed with sinking disquiet that my original opening had been enlarged by the passage of that enormous calf and there was a long tear disappearing out of sight towards the cervix.

'Sutures.' I held my hand out and Norman gave me a fresh

needle. 'Hold the lips of the wound,' I said and began to stitch.

I worked as quickly as I could and was doing fine until the tear ran out of sight. The rest was a kind of martyrdom. Norman hung on grimly while I stabbed around at the invisible tissue far below. At times I pricked the young man's fingers, at others my own. And to my dismay a further complication had arisen.

The calf was now on his feet, blundering unsteadily around. The speed with which newly born animals get on to their legs has always fascinated me but at this moment it was an un-mitigated nuisance.

The calf, looking for the udder with that instinct which nobody can explain, kept pushing his nose at the cow's flank and at times toppling head first into the gaping hole in her side.

'Reckon 'e wants back in again,' Mr Bushell said with a grin. 'By 'eck, he is a wick 'un.'

'Wick' is Yorkshire for lively and the word was never more aptly applied. As I worked, eyes half closed, jaws rigid, I had to keep nudging the wet muzzle away with my elbow, but as fast as I pushed him back the calf charged in again and with sick resignation I saw that every time he nosed his way into the cavity he brought particles of straw and dirt from the floor and spread them over the abdominal contents.

'Look at that,' I moaned. 'As if there wasn't enough muck in there.'

Norman didn't reply. His mouth was hanging open and the sweat ran down his blood-streaked face as he grappled with that unseen wound. And in his fixed stare I seemed to read a growing doubt as to his wisdom in deciding to be a veterinary surgeon.

I would rather not go into any more details. The memory is too painful. Sufficient to say that after an eternity I got as far down the uterine tear as I could, then we cleared away a lot of rubbish from the cow's abdomen and covered everything with antiseptic dusting powder. I stitched up the muscle and skin layers with the calf trying all the time to get in on the act and at last the thing was finished.

Norman and I got to our feet very slowly, like two old, old men. It took me a long time to straighten my back and I saw the young man rubbing tenderly at his lumbar region. Then, since we were both plastered with caked blood and filth, we began the slow process of scrubbing and scraping ourselves clean.

Mr Bushell left his position by the head and looked at the row of skin stitches. 'Nice neat job,' he said. 'And a grand calf, too.'

Yes, that was something. The little creature had dried off now and he was a beauty, his body swaying on unsteady legs, his wideset eyes filled with gentle curiosity. But that 'neat job' hid things I didn't dare think about.

Antibiotics were still not in general use but in any case I knew there was no hope for the cow. More as a gesture than anything else I left the farmer some sulpha powders to give her three times a day. Then I got off the farm as quickly as I could.

We drove away in silence. I rounded a couple of corners, then stopped the car under a tree and sank my head against the steering wheel.

'Oh hell,' I groaned. 'What a bloody balls-up.'

Norman replied only with a long sigh and I continued. 'Did you ever see such a performance? All that straw and dirt and rumenal muck in among that poor cow's bowels. Do you know what I was thinking about towards the end? I was remembering the story of that human surgeon of olden times who left his hat inside his patient. It was as bad as that.'

They leave convinced that they will never see Bella alive again, that she probably has a good-sized hole in her uterus and peritonitis (caused by infection) is inevitable. The next morning, however, James phones Mr Bushell to see if Bella has survived the night, only to discover that she is up and eating and 'bright as a cricket'. James is utterly astonished and Bella recovers fully without showing any symptoms from the ordeal.

> That was the way it was at my first caesarean. Over the years Bella went on to have eight more calves normally and unaided, a miracle which I can still hardly believe.
>
> But Norman and I were not to know that. All we felt then was an elation which was all the sweeter for being unexpected. As we drove away I looked at the young man's smiling face.
>
> 'Well, Norman,' I said. 'That's veterinary practice for you. You get a lot of nasty shocks but some lovely surprises too. I've often heard of the wonderful resistance of the bovine peritoneum and thank heavens it's true.'

While cattle can be remarkably resistant to infection, as Bella the cow shows, there are a myriad of complications that can ensue after giving birth. Uterus inversion, when the cow continues to push out the entire uterus, presents veterinary surgeons with one of their most difficult and physically demanding challenges. Returning a uterus, an enormous pink mass, through the relatively small opening of the vagina is both awkward and exhausting work.

> It happens when the cow, after calving, continues to strain until it pushes the entire uterus out and it hangs down as far as the animal's hocks. It is a vast organ and desperately difficult to replace, mainly because the cow, having once got rid of it,

doesn't want it back. And in a straightforward contest between man and beast the odds were very much on the cow.

The old practitioners, in an effort to even things up a bit, used to sling the cow up by its hind limbs and the more inventive among them came up with all sorts of contraptions like the uterine valise which was supposed to squeeze the organ into a smaller bulk. But the result was usually the same — hours of back-breaking work.

The introduction of the epidural anaesthetic made everything easier by removing sensation from the uterus and preventing the cow from straining but, for all that, the words 'calf bed out' coming over the line were guaranteed to wipe the smile off any vet's face.

I decided to take Tristan in case I needed a few pounds of extra push. He came along but showed little enthusiasm for the idea. He showed still less when he saw the patient, a very fat shorthorn lying, quite unconcerned, in her stall. Behind her, a bloody mass of uterus, afterbirth, muck and straw spilled over into the channel.

She wasn't at all keen to get up, but after we had done a bit of shouting and pushing at her shoulder she rose to her feet, looking bored.

The epidural space was difficult to find among the rolls of fat and I wasn't sure if I had injected all the anaesthetic into the right place. I removed the afterbirth, cleaned the uterus and placed it on a clean sheet held by the farmer and his brother. They were frail men and it was all they could do to keep the sheet level. I wouldn't be able to count on them to help much.

I nodded to Tristan; we stripped off our shirts, tied clean sacks round our waists and gathered the uterus in our arms.

It was badly engorged and swollen and it took us just an

hour to get it back. There was a long spell at the beginning when we made no progress at all and the whole idea of pushing the enormous organ through a small hole seemed ludicrous, like trying to thread a needle with a sausage. Then there were a few minutes when we thought we were doing famously only to find we were feeding the thing down through a tear in the sheet (Siegfried once told me he had spent half a morning trying to stuff a uterus up a cow's rectum. What really worried him, he said, was that he nearly succeeded) and at the end, when hope was fading, there was the blissful moment when the whole thing began to slip inside and incredibly disappeared from sight.

Somewhere halfway through we both took a breather at the same time and stood panting, our faces almost touching. Tristan's cheeks were prettily patterned where a spouting artery had sprayed him; I was able to look deep into his eyes and I read there a deep distaste for the whole business.

Lathering myself in the bucket and feeling the ache in my shoulders and back, I looked over at Tristan. He was pulling his shirt over his head as though it cost him the last of his strength. The cow, chewing contentedly at a mouthful of hay, had come best out of the affair.

Out in the car, Tristan groaned. 'I'm sure that sort of thing isn't good for me. I feel as though I've been run over by a steamroller. Hell, what a life this is at times.'

In *It Shouldn't Happen to a Vet* James is called to Dick Rudd's farm to take a look at his prized dairy shorthorn cow, Strawberry. Shorthorns, their red, white and dark roan colours once a common sight in Yorkshire, could be bred for milk or beef. At one point most of the Wensleydale cheese, originally made in the Yorkshire Dales, was made from the milk of shorthorns.

Dick's cows had been scratched together over the years and they were a motley lot. Many of them were old animals discarded by more prosperous farmers because of their pendulous udders or because they were 'three titted 'uns'. Others had been reared by Dick from calves and tended to be rough haired and scruffy. But halfway down the byre, contrasting almost violently with her neighbours, was what seemed to me a perfect dairy shorthorn cow.

In these days when the Friesian has surged over England in a black and white flood and inundated even the Dales which were the very home of the shorthorn, such cows as I looked at that day at Dick Rudd's are no longer to be seen, but she represented all the glory and pride of her breed. The wide pelvis tapering to fine shoulders and a delicate head, the level udder thrusting back between the hind legs, and the glorious colour — dark roan. That was what they used to call a 'good colour' and whenever I delivered a dark roan calf the farmer would say 'It's a good-coloured 'un', and it would be more valuable accordingly. The geneticists are perfectly right, of course: the dark roaned cows gave no more milk than the reds or the whites, but we loved them and they were beautiful.

'Where did she come from, Dick?' I said, still staring.

Dick's voice was elaborately casual. 'Oh, ah went over to Weldon's of Cranby and picked her out. D'you like her?'

'She's a picture — a show cow. I've never seen one better.' Weldon's were the biggest pedigree breeders in the northern Dales and I didn't ask whether Dick had cajoled his bank manager or had been saving up for years just for this.

'Aye, she's a seven-galloner when she gets goin' and top butter fat, too. Reckon she'll be as good as two of my other cows and a calf out of her'll be worth a bit.' He stepped forward and ran his hand along the perfectly level, smoothly fleshed back. 'She's got a great fancy pedigree name but missus 'as called her Strawberry.'

I knew as I stood there in the primitive, cobbled byre with its wooden partitions and rough stone walls that I was looking not just at a cow but at the foundation of the new herd, at Dick Rudd's hopes for the future.

It was about a month later that he phoned me. 'I want you to come and look at Strawberry for me,' he said. 'She's been doing grand, tipplin' the milk out, but there's summat amiss with her this morning.'

The cow didn't really look ill and, in fact, she was eating when I examined her; but I noticed that she gulped slightly when she swallowed. Her temperature was normal and her lungs clear but when I stood up by her head I could just hear a faint snorting sound.

'It's her throat, Dick,' I said. 'It may be just a bit of inflammation but there's a chance that she's starting a little abscess in there.' I spoke lightly but I wasn't happy. Postpharyngeal abscesses were, in my limited experience, nasty things. They were situated in an inaccessible place, right away behind the back of the throat and if they got very large could interfere seriously with the breathing. I had been lucky with the few I had seen; they had either been small and regressed or had ruptured spontaneously.

I gave an injection of Prontosil and turned to Dick. 'I want you to foment this area behind the angle of the jaw with hot water and rub this salve well in afterwards. You may manage to burst it that way. Do this at least three times a day.'

I kept looking in at her over the next ten days and the picture was one of steady development of the abscess. The cow was still not acutely ill but she was eating a lot less, she was thinner and was going off her milk. Most of the time I felt rather helpless as I knew that only the rupture of the abscess would bring relief and the various injections I was giving her were largely irrelevant. But the infernal thing was taking a long time to burst.

After three days, Dick calls James back in and he's shocked to see Strawberry in a terrible way, rasping and little more than a skeleton. James hopes that her abscess will burst that night but when it doesn't, he decides to operate on Strawberry, cutting into and draining the abscess in a procedure he has never done before. The following day, she looks worse than ever and they fear she'll end up at the knacker's yard. Then, thankfully, she turns a corner and thereon starts to recover: 'I saw her three weeks later and her bones were magically clothed with flesh, her skin shone and, most important, the magnificent udder bulged turgid beneath her, a neat little teat proudly erect at each corner.'

It Shouldn't Happen to a Vet opens with James visiting Mr Handshaw's cow, which, despite being treated for milk fever, is unable to get up. Milk fever is a condition that can come on soon after calving, resulting in a cow becoming extremely weak and unable to get on its feet. By the 1930s it was established that a very low level of calcium in the blood caused the symptoms, although in this case James suspects there's another reason why Mr Handshaw's cow won't stand.

I could see that Mr Handshaw didn't believe a word I was saying. He looked down at his cow and his mouth tightened into a stubborn line.

'Broken pelvis? You're trying to tell me she'll never get up n'more? Why, look at her chewing her cud! I'll tell you this, young man – me dad would've soon got her up if he'd been alive today.'

I had been a veterinary surgeon for a year now and I had learned a few things. One of them was that farmers weren't easy men to convince – especially Yorkshire Dalesmen.

And that bit about his dad. Mr Handshaw was in his fifties and I suppose there was something touching about his faith in his late father's skill and judgement. But I could have done very nicely without it.

It had acted as an additional irritant in a case in which I felt I had troubles enough. Because there are few things which get more deeply under a vet's skin than a cow which won't get up. To the layman it may seem strange that an animal can be apparently cured of its original ailment and yet be unable to rise from the floor, but it happens. And it can be appreciated that a completely recumbent milk cow has no future.

The case had started when my boss, Siegfried Farnon, who owned the practice in the little Dales market town of Darrowby, sent me to a milk fever. This suddenly occurring calcium deficiency attacks high-yielding animals just after calving and causes collapse and progressive coma. When I first saw Mr Handshaw's cow she was stretched out motionless on her side, and I had to look carefully to make sure she wasn't dead.

But I got out my bottles of calcium with an airy confidence because I had been lucky enough to qualify just about the time when the profession had finally got on top of this hitherto fatal condition. The breakthrough had come many years earlier with inflation of the udder and I still carried a little blowing-up outfit around with me (the farmers used bicycle pumps), but with the advent of calcium therapy one could bask in a cheap glory by jerking an animal back from imminent death within minutes.

212

The skill required was minimal but it looked very very good.

By the time I had injected the two bottles — one into the vein, the other under the skin — and Mr Handshaw had helped me roll the cow onto her chest the improvement was already obvious; she was looking about her and shaking her head as if wondering where she had been for the last few hours. I felt sure that if I had had the time to hang about for a bit I could see her on her feet. But other jobs were waiting.

When the cow still isn't up the next day, James returns to inject another bottle of calcium, still confident that she'll get back on her feet. After forty-eight hours, however, there's still no change and James is increasingly worried about her condition. Mr Handshaw, now on the offensive, suggests a couple of home-spun remedies popular with farmers, including cutting off the cow's tail to force her to get up. James refuses to resort to that, as it's painful for the cow, but he does try bellowing in the cow's ear, which serves only to stop the cow chewing for a moment.

The next day, James returns to find Mr Handshaw's neighbours assembled around the still-recumbent cow. Putting sacks under her, they heave the cow up onto her feet, but she just hangs there placidly with her legs dangling until, with a lot of puffing and grunting, they lower the inert body back down. Mr Handshaw then suggests dogs might get the cow up and the assembled farmers immediately rush off to get their dogs but the cow just ignores their snapping and snarling, even when the dogs break into a vicious fight. Somehow, despite the din all around, James hears a creaking sound coming from the cow's pelvis and he decides to examine the animal again.

I stripped off my jacket, soaped my arms and pushed a hand into the cow's rectum until I felt the hard bone of the pubis.

Gripping it through the wall of the rectum I looked up at my audience. 'Will two of you get hold of the hook bones and rock the cow gently from side to side.'

Yes, there it was again, no mistake about it. I could both hear and feel it — a looseness, a faint creaking, almost a grating.

I got up and washed my arm. 'Well, I know why your cow won't get up — she has a broken pelvis. Probably did it during the first night when she was staggering about with the milk fever. I should think the nerves are damaged, too. It's hopeless, I'm afraid.' Even though I was dispensing bad news it was a relief to come up with something rational.

Mr Handshaw stared at me. 'Hopeless? How's that?'

'I'm sorry,' I said, 'but that's how it is. The only thing you can do is get her off to the butcher. She has no power in her hind legs. She'll never get up again.'

On hearing the dire prognosis, Mr Handshaw blows his top, points out all of James's shortcomings and the vet has no option but to leave. The whole thing is an unhappy episode for James although he feels certain of his diagnosis until he receives a phone call from Mr Handshaw the next day.

'Is that Mr Herriot? Aye, well, good mornin' to you. I'm just ringing to tell you that me cow's up on her legs and doing fine.'

I gripped the receiver tightly with both hands.

'What? What's that you say?'

'I said me cow's up. Found her walking about byre this morning, fit as a fiddle. You'd think there'd never been owt the matter with her.' He paused for a few moments then spoke with grave deliberation like a disapproving schoolmaster. 'And you stood there and looked at me and said she'd never get up n'more.'

'But . . . but . . .'

'Ah, you're wondering how I did it? Well, I just happened to remember another old trick of me dad's. I went round to t'butcher and got a fresh-killed sheep skin and put it on her back. Had her up in no time — you'll 'ave to come round and see her. Wonderful man was me dad.'

Blindly I made my way into the dining room. I had to consult my boss about this. Siegfried's sleep had been broken by a 3 a.m. calving and he looked a lot older than his thirty-odd years. He listened in silence as he finished his breakfast then pushed away his plate and poured a last cup of coffee. 'Hard luck, James. The old sheep skin, eh? Funny thing — you've been in the Dales over a year now and never come across that one. Suppose it must be going out of fashion a bit now but you know it has a grain of sense behind it like a lot of these old remedies. You can imagine there's a lot of heat generated under a fresh sheep skin and it acts like a great hot poultice on the back — really tickles them up after a while, and if a cow is lying there out of sheer cussedness she'll often get up just to get rid of it.'

'But damn it, how about the broken pelvis? I tell you it was creaking and wobbling all over the place!'

'Well, James, you're not the first to have been caught that way. Sometimes the pelvic ligaments don't tighten up for a few days after calving and you get this effect.'

'Oh God,' I moaned, staring down at the tablecloth. 'What a bloody mess I've made of the whole thing.'

'Oh, you haven't really.' Siegfried lit a cigarette and leaned back in his chair. 'That old cow was probably toying with the idea of getting up for a walk just when old Handshaw dumped the skin on her back. She could just as easily have done it after one of your injections and then you'd have got

215

the credit. Don't you remember what I told you when you first came here? There's a very fine dividing line between looking a real smart vet on the one hand and an immortal fool on the other.'

The story with Mr Handshaw was inspired by a visit that Alf Wight made to a cow belonging to a local farmer, Billy Goodyear. Having been told by Alf that his cow would never get up, Billy ignored his advice, kept her alive and she eventually got to her feet. Billy never forgot the incident and five decades later, when an assistant from the Thirsk practice visited his farm, he was still bragging about it! 'Downer' cows are something all veterinary surgeons come up against, even today. When working at the Thirsk practice, Jim Wight was frequently called out to attend to cows that wouldn't get up – they would usually end up at the knacker's yard after a week or so, but there was always the odd cow that would defy all scientific knowledge and suddenly get up after two or three weeks. Alf was happy to try the age-old methods and remedies of the farmers, sometimes to humour his clients or because he had nothing more scientific to offer.

Alf was also called out frequently to treat cows with mastitis, which can cause an udder to swell, redden or harden and in some cases emit a stinking serum-like liquid instead of milk. Expected to produce three or four gallons of milk a day, dairy cows are prone to the condition, which is caused by getting dirt on the end of a teat, perhaps by lying down in muck or when they are milked. In *It Shouldn't Happen to a Vet*, James pays a visit to a cow with acute mastitis, a condition vets often saw in the summer months when a cow had stopped milking and flies got onto the end of its teat. Modern vets can now administer antibiotics as soon as a cow dries off but in the

1930s and 1940s there was little vets could do other than cutting the teat off or drawing any liquid out by hand.

I got back into the car and looked at my list of visits; it was good to be back and the day passed quickly. It was about seven o'clock in the evening, when I thought I had finished, that I had a call from Terry Watson, a young farm worker who kept two cows of his own. One of them, he said, had summer mastitis. Mid-July was a bit early for this but in the later summer months we saw literally hundreds of these cases; in fact a lot of the farmers called it 'August bag'. It was an unpleasant condition because it was just about incurable and usually resulted in the cow losing a quarter (the area of the udder which supplies each teat with milk) and sometimes even her life.

Terry Watson's cow looked very sick. She had limped in from the field at milking time, swinging her right hind leg wide to keep it away from the painful udder, and now she stood trembling in her stall, her eyes staring anxiously in front of her. I drew gently at the affected teat and, instead of milk, a stream of dark, foul-smelling serum spurted into the tin can I was holding.

'No mistaking that stink, Terry,' I said. 'It's the real summer type all right.' I felt my way over the hot, swollen quarter and the cow lifted her leg quickly as I touched the tender tissue. 'Pretty hard, too. It looks bad, I'm afraid.'

The poor outlook for the cow comes as a blow to Terry Watson, a young man with a wife and baby, whose smallholding of two cows, a few pigs and hens provides him with a little extra income on top of a day's labouring. James injects the cow and tells Terry to strip the teat out, by working away at the udder every half-hour to draw out the stinking liquid, and then to bathe and massage it in warm water. Terry immediately grabs a milking stool and bucket and starts to massage straight away. The following morning, James drops in and sees Terry in the same position and, amazingly, the cow looks far more comfortable.

I bent down by the udder, feeling carefully for the painful swelling of last night, but my hand came up against a smooth, yielding surface and in disbelief, I kneaded the tissue between my fingers. The animal showed no sign of discomfort. With a feeling of bewilderment I drew on the teat with thumb and forefinger; the quarter was nearly empty but I did manage to squeeze a single jet of pure white milk onto my palm.

'What's going on here, Terry? You must have switched cows on me. You're having me on, aren't you?'

'Nay, guvnor,' the young man said with his slow smile. 'It's same cow all right – she's better, that's all.'

'But it's impossible! What the devil have you done to her?'

'Just what you told me to do. Rub and strip.'

I scratched my head. 'But she's back to normal. I've never seen anything like it.'

'Aye, I know you haven't.' It was a woman's voice and I turned and saw young Mrs Watson standing at the door holding her baby. 'You've never seen a man that would rub and strip a cow right round the clock, have you?'

'Round the clock?' I said.

She looked at her husband with a mixture of concern and exasperation. 'Yes, he's been there on that stool since you left last night. Never been to bed, never been in for a meal. I've been bringing him bits and pieces and cups of tea. Great fool – it's enough to kill anybody.'

I looked at Terry and my eyes moved from the pallid face

over the thin, slightly swaying body to the nearly empty bowl of goose grease at his feet. 'Good Lord, man,' I said. 'You've done the impossible but you must be about all in. Anyway, your cow is as good as new – you don't need to do another thing to her, so you can go in and have a bit of a rest.'

'Nay, I can't do that.' He shook his head and straightened his shoulders. 'I've got me work to go to and I'm late as it is.'

As Siegfried frequently tells James, veterinary work provides countless opportunities for practitioners to look like fools, and bovine care is no exception. The Sidlow family, as described in Chapter 6, already consider vets to be 'useless creatures . . . expensive layabouts who really know nothing about animals or their diseases'. As a result, they only send for a vet when their animals are on the brink of death, often as a result of the black magic remedies they have tried first. James has the misfortune to be called to the Sidlow farm several times, where invariably something goes wrong or he has to assign a poor beast to the knacker's yard, which only confirms their conviction that vets are a menace to the animal population. When Mr Sidlow calls him in again to see a cow, James is yet again forced to leave the farm in disgrace.

A numbness filled me as we went into the byre. It continued as Mr Sidlow described how he had battled against this cow's recurring bouts of diarrhoea for several months; how he had started quietly with ground eggshells in gruel and worked up to his most powerful remedy, blue vitriol and dandelion tea, but all to no avail. I hardly heard him because it was fairly obvious at a glance that the cow had Jöhne's disease.

Nobody could be quite sure, of course, but the animal's advanced emaciation, especially in the hind end, and the stream of bubbly, foetid scour which she had ejected as I walked in were almost diagnostic. Instinctively I grasped her tail and thrust my thermometer into the rectum: I wasn't much interested in her temperature but it gave me a couple of minutes to think.

However, in this instance I got only about five seconds because, without warning, the thermometer disappeared from my fingers. Some sudden suction had drawn it inside the cow. I ran my fingers round just inside the rectum – nothing; I pushed my hand inside without success; with a feeling of rising panic I rolled up my sleeve and groped about in vain.

There was nothing else for it – I had to ask for a bucket of hot water, soap and a towel and strip off as though preparing for some large undertaking. Over my thirty-odd years in practice I can recall many occasions when I looked a complete fool, but there is a peculiarly piercing quality about the memory of myself, bare to the waist, the centre of a ring of hostile stares, guddling frantically inside that cow. At the time, all I could think of was that this was the Sidlow place; anything could happen here. In my mental turmoil I had discarded all my knowledge of pathology and anatomy and could visualize the little glass tube working its way rapidly along the intestinal tract until it finally pierced some vital organ. There was another hideous image of myself carrying out a major operation, a full-scale laparotomy on the cow to recover my thermometer.

It is difficult to describe the glorious relief which flooded through me when at last I felt the thing between my fingers; I pulled it out, filthy and dripping, and stared down stupidly at the graduations on the tube.

Mr Sidlow cleared his throat. 'Well, wot does it say? Has she got a temperature?'

I whipped round and gave him a piercing look. Was it possible that this man could be making a joke? But the dark, tight-shut face was expressionless.

'No,' I mumbled in reply. 'No temperature.'

The farming industry saw many changes in the years that James worked as a veterinary surgeon, particularly in the small dairy farms in the area. When Alf first worked in Thirsk, the practice had around seventy to eighty dairy farms but after the war, small farms struggled to survive and were gradually subsumed into industrial-size farms where large herds of cows were milked by machines in modern milking parlours. Today there are just two dairy farms in the Thirsk practice. In *Vet in a Spin* James is called to Mr Blackburn's new big dairy farm to take a look at one of their cows in labour, and he finds the concrete surroundings less than welcoming.

I think it was the early-morning calls in the winter which were the worst. It was a fairly common experience to be walking sleepy-eyed into a cow byre at 6 a.m. for a calving but at Mr Blackburn's farm there was a difference. In fact several differences.

Firstly, there was usually an anxious-faced farmer to greet me with news of how the calf was coming, when labour had started, but today I was like an unwelcome stranger. Secondly, I had grown accustomed to the sight of a few cows tied up in a cobbled byre with wooden partitions and an oil lamp, and now I was gazing down a long avenue of concrete under blazing electric light with a seemingly endless succession of bovine backsides protruding from tubular metal standings. Thirdly, instead of the early-morning peace there was a clattering of buckets, the rhythmic pulsing of a milking machine and the blaring of a radio loudspeaker. There was also a frantic scurrying of white-coated, white-capped men, but none of them paid the slightest attention to me.

This was one of the new big dairy farms. In place of a solitary figure on a milk stool, head buried in the cow's side, pulling forth the milk with a gentle 'hiss-hiss' there was this impersonal hustle and bustle.

James catches Mr Blackburn, who is hurrying past, and asks him to point him in the direction of the calving cow. He discovers that no one has had time to check on the cow as the staff have been too busy milking the other cows, ready for the collection of the churns by the big dairy companies. James therefore must examine the cow alone, treat it for milk fever, and then birth its calf without any help.

I filled a bucket, found a piece of soap and threw a towel over my shoulder. When I reached my patient I looked in vain for some sign of a name. So many of the cows of those days had their names printed above their stalls but there were no Marigolds, Alices or Snowdrops here, just numbers.

Before taking off my jacket I looked casually in the ear where the tattoo marks stood out plainly against the creamy white surface. She was number eighty-seven.

Alf similarly preferred working on the small farms, where he could build up relationships with the farmers and their animals. In the first years after the war, there were still plenty of small farmsteads that retained the old traditions, including giving names to their livestock. Some farmers, however, such as the Rowney brothers in *The Lord God Made Them All*, come up with some unusual names for their herd of cows.

I recall a visit I made to test the herd of Rupe and Will Rowney. Rupe and Will just didn't get on. They were bachelor brothers who had run a dairy farm for many years together but they didn't seem to be able to agree about anything.

Visits there could be embarrassing as the brothers argued continually and criticized each other's every move, but on this particular day I found they had forgotten to keep the cows in for me.

I stood to one side as they castigated each other.

'Ah told ye the postcard said today.'

'Naw, ye didn't, ye said Tuesday. It was me as said today.'

'Well, fetch the bloody card from t'house and let's 'ave another look at it.'

'How can I? Ye burned it, ye daft bugger!'

I let the debate go on for a few minutes, then intervened tactfully.

'It's all right,' I said. 'There's no harm done. The cows are just there in the field. It shouldn't take long to get them in.'

Rupe gave his brother a final glare and turned to me. 'Nay, it won't take long, Mr Herriot. The byre door's open. Ah'll soon call 'em in.'

He inflated his lungs and began a series of shrill cries. 'Come on, Spotty Nose, come on, Big Lugs, come on, Mucky Tail, come on, Fat Tits, come on, Fuzzy Top!'

Will, nettled at being upstaged, broke in with his own shout. 'Come on, Long Legs! Come on, Slow Coach!'

Rupe froze him with a stare then bent towards me. 'Ye'll have to excuse me brother, Mr Herriot,' he said in a confidential whisper. 'Ah've tried to tell 'im many a time, but he will call the cows them daft names.'

Alongside the many cows James treats, bulls are also regular patients. In *Vet in Harness*, the young vet heads to Mr Dacre's farm to conduct a tuberculin test on his bull, Bill. The test consists of injecting tuberculin into the animal's skin and then measuring any swelling around the injection site after seventy-two hours – and any infected animal must be slaughtered. James has no concerns about Mr Dacre's bull on this front – instead, he is more concerned about his own safety.

'Move over, Bill!' Mr Dacre cried some time later as he tweaked the big bull's tail.

Nearly every farmer kept a bull in those days and they were all called Billy or Bill. I suppose it was because this was a very mature animal that he received the adult version. Being a docile beast he responded to the touch on his tail by shuffling his great bulk to one side, leaving me enough space to push in between him and the wooden partition against which he was tied by a chain.

I was reading a tuberculin test and all I wanted to do was to measure the intradermal reaction. I had to open my calipers very wide to take in the thickness of the skin on the enormous neck.

'Thirty,' I called out to the farmer.

He wrote the figure down on the testing book and laughed.

'By heck, he's got some pelt on 'im.'

'Yes,' I said, beginning to squeeze my way out. 'But he's a big fellow, isn't he?'

Just how big he was was brought home to me immediately because the bull suddenly swung round, pinning me against the partition. Cows did this regularly and I moved them by bracing my back against whatever was behind me and pushing them away. But it was different with Bill.

Gasping, I pushed with all my strength against the rolls of fat which covered the vast roan-coloured flank, but I might as well have tried to shift a house.

The farmer dropped his book and seized the tail again but this time the bull showed no response. There was no malice in his behaviour — he was simply having a comfortable lean against the boards and I don't suppose he even noticed the morsel of puny humanity wriggling frantically against his ribcage.

Still, whether he meant it or not, the end result was the same; I was having the life crushed out of me. Pop-eyed, groaning, scarcely able to breathe, I struggled with everything I had, but I couldn't move an inch. And just when I thought things couldn't get any worse, Bill started to rub himself up and down against the partition. So that was what he had come round for; he had an itch and he just wanted to scratch it.

The effect on me was catastrophic. I was certain my internal organs were being steadily ground to pulp and as I thrashed about in complete panic the huge animal leaned even more heavily.

I don't like to think what would have happened if the wood behind me had not been old and rotten, but just as I felt my senses leaving me there was a cracking and splintering and I fell through into the next stall. Lying there like a stranded fish on a bed of shattered timbers I looked up at Mr Dacre, waiting till my lungs started to work again.

The farmer, having got over his first alarm, was rubbing his upper lip vigorously in a polite attempt to stop himself laughing. His little girl who had watched the whole thing from her vantage point in one of the hay racks had no such inhibitions. Screaming with delight, she pointed at me.

'Ooo, Dad, Dad, look at that man! Did you see him, Dad, did you see him? Ooo what a funny man!' She went into

THE WONDERFUL WORLD of JAMES HERRIOT

helpless convulsions. She was only about five but I had a feeling she would remember my performance all her life.

At length I picked myself up and managed to brush the matter off lightly, but after I had driven a mile or so from the farm I stopped the car and looked myself over. My ribs ached pretty uniformly as though a light road roller had passed over them and there was a tender area on my left buttock where I had landed on my calipers but otherwise I seemed to have escaped damage. I removed a few spicules of wood from my trousers, got back into the car and consulted my list of visits.

On cattle farms, the main job of a bull is to breed with cows and any innovations brought in to help with this were greeted enthusiastically by veterinary surgeons and farmers alike. Artificial insemination revolutionized the breeding of cattle although the vets' first experience with an artificial vagina – as related in *The Lord God Made Them All* – doesn't quite go to plan.

The bull with the bowler hat.

That was one of the irreverent terms for artificial insemination when it first arrived on the post-war scene. Of course AI was a wonderful advance. Up till the official licensing of bulls the farmers had used any available male bovine to get their cows in calf. A cow had to produce a calf before it would give milk and it was milk that was the goal of the dairy farmers, but unfortunately the progeny of these 'scrub' bulls were often low grade and weakly.

But AI was a great improvement on licensing. To use a high-class, pedigree, proven bull to inseminate large numbers of cows for farmers who could never afford to own such an animal was and is a splendid idea. Over the years I have seen countless thousands of superior young heifers, bullocks and bulls populate the farms of Britain and I have rejoiced.

I am speaking theoretically, however. My own practical experience of artificial insemination was brief and unhappy.

When the thing first began, most practitioners thought they would be rushing about, doing a lot of insemination on their own account, and Siegfried and I could hardly wait to get started. We purchased an artificial vagina, which was a tube of hard vulcanized rubber about eighteen inches long with a lining of latex. There was a little tap on the tube and warm water was run into this to simulate the temperature of a genuine bovine vagina. On one end of the AV was a latex cone secured by rubber bands and this cone terminated in a glass tube in which the semen was collected.

Apart from its use in insemination this instrument provided an excellent means of testing the farmers' own bulls for fertility. It was in this context that I had my first experience.

Wally Hartley had brought a young Ayrshire bull from one of the big dairy farmers and he wanted the animal's fertility tested by the new method. He rang me to ask if I would do the job and I was elated at the chance to try out our new acquisition.

At the farm I filled the liner with water just nicely at blood heat and fastened on the cone and glass tube. I was ready and eager for action.

The required cow in oestrus was in a large loose box off the yard and the farmer led the bull towards it.

'He's nobbut a little 'un,' Mr Hartley said, 'but I wouldn't trust 'im. He's a cheeky young bugger. Never served a cow yet, but keen as mustard.'

I eyed the bull. Certainly he wasn't large, but he had mean eyes and the sharp curving horns of the typical Ayrshire.

Anyway, this job shouldn't be much trouble. I had never seen it done but had flipped through a pamphlet on the subject and it seemed simple enough.

All you did was wait till the bull started to mount, then you directed the protruded penis into the AV. Apparently then, the bull, with surprising gullibility, thrust happily into the water-filled cylinder and ejaculated into the tube. I had been told repeatedly that there was nothing to it.

I went into the box. 'Let him in, Wally,' I said, and the farmer opened the half door.

The bull trotted inside, and the cow, fastened by a halter to a ring on the wall, submitted calmly as he sniffed around her. He seemed to like what he saw because he finally stationed himself behind her with eager anticipation.

This was the moment. Take up position on the right side of the bull, the pamphlet had said, and the rest would be easy.

With surprising speed the young animal threw his forelegs on the cow's rump and surged forward. I had to move quickly and as the penis emerged from the sheath I grabbed it and poised the AV for action.

But I didn't get the chance. The bull dismounted immediately and swung round on me with an affronted glare. He looked me carefully up and down as though he didn't quite believe what he saw and there was not an ounce of friendliness in his expression. Then he appeared to remember the rather pressing business on hand and turned his attention to the cow again.

He leaped up, I grabbed, and once more he suspended his activities abruptly and brought his forefeet thudding to the ground. This time there was more than outraged dignity in his eyes, there was anger. He snorted, shook the needle-sharp horns in my direction and dragged a little straw along the floor with a hoof before fixing me with a long appraising stare. He didn't have to speak, his message was unequivocal. Just try that once more, chum, and you've had it.

As his eyes lingered on me everything seemed to become silent and motionless as though I were part of a picture. The cow standing patiently, the churned straw beneath the animals, and beyond them the farmer out in the yard, leaning over the half door, waiting for the next move.

I wasn't particularly looking forward to that next move. I felt a little breathless and my tongue pressed against the roof of my mouth.

At length the bull, with a final warning glance at me, decided to resume his business and reared up on the cow once more. I gulped, bent quickly and as his slim red organ shot forth I grasped it and tried to bring the AV down on it.

This time the bull didn't mess about. He sprang away from the cow, put his head down and came at me like a bullet.

In that fleeting instant I realized what a fool I had been to stand with the animals between me and the door. Behind me was the dark corner of the box. I was trapped.

Fortunately the AV was dangling from my right hand and as the bull charged I was able to catch him an upward blow on the snout. If I had hit him on the top of the head he would never have felt it and one or both of those nasty horns would inevitably have started to explore my interior. But as it was, the hard rubber cylinder thumping against his nose brought him to a slithering halt, and while he was blinking and making up his mind about having a second go I rained blows on him with a frenzy born of terror.

I have often wondered since that day if I am the only veterinary surgeon to have used an artificial vagina as a defensive weapon. It certainly was not built for the purpose because it soon began to disintegrate under my onslaught. First the glass tube hurtled past the ear of the startled farmer who was watching, wide-eyed, from the doorway, then the cone spun away against the flank of the cow, who had started to chew her cud placidly, oblivious of the drama being enacted by her side.

I alternated my swipes with thrusts and lunges worthy of a fencing master but I still couldn't jockey my way out of that corner. However, although my puny cylinder couldn't hurt the bull I obviously had him puzzled. Apart from a lot of weaving and prodding with his horns he made no sign of repeating his first headlong charge and seemed content to keep me penned in the few feet of space.

But I knew it was only a matter of time. He was out to get me and I was wondering how it felt to receive a cornada when he took a step back and came in again full tilt, head down.

I met him with a back-handed slash, and that was what saved me because the elastic holding the latex lining came off and the warm water from within fountained into the bull's eyes.

He stopped suddenly and it was then I think he just decided to give up. In his experience of humans I was something new to him. I had taken intimate liberties with him in the pursuit of his lawful duty, I had belaboured him with a rubber instrument and finally squirted water in his face. He had plainly had enough of me.

During his pause for thought I dodged past him, threw open the door and escaped into the yard.

Chapter 8

SHEEP, PIGS *and* OTHER CREATURES

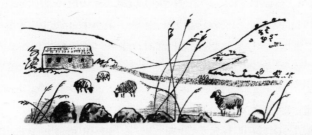

This was my third spring in the Dales but it was like the two before — and all the springs after. The kind of spring, that is, that a country vet knows; the din of the lambing pens, the bass rumble of the ewes and the high, insistent bawling of the lambs. This, for me, has always heralded the end of winter and the beginning of something new. This and the piercing Yorkshire wind and the hard, bright sunshine flooding the bare hillsides.

At the top of the grassy slope the pens, built of straw bales, formed a long row of square cubicles each holding a ewe with her lambs and I could see Rob Benson coming round the far end carrying two feeding buckets. Rob was hard at it; at this time of the year he didn't go to bed for about six weeks; he would maybe take off his boots and doze by the kitchen fire at night but he was his own shepherd and never very far from the scene of action.

'Ah've got a couple of cases for you today, Jim.' His face, cracked and purpled by the weather, broke into a grin. 'It's not really you ah need, it's that little lady's hand of yours and right sharpish, too.'

Lambing time marks not only the end of a long harsh winter but the start of the busiest period in the year for a veterinary surgeon. Just as sheep farmers like Rob Benson can hardly sleep during the weeks of lambing, so too are veterinary surgeons dragged from their beds on a nightly basis to attend to the tidal wave of lambing. For ten months of the year, sheep hardly figure in a vet's calendar: they are, as James Herriot puts it, just 'woolly things on the hills', but for the other two months, from around March to May, they're almost all vets can think about.

To add to their busy schedule, other animals are also at a low ebb in spring: cattle have been confined in their byres all winter and their calves have little resistance to disease. Despite the relentless work, Alf Wight enjoyed this time of year and often said lambing ewes was easily his favourite job as 'it had all the thrill and interest of calving without the hard labour'. He became very adept at it – once lambing sixteen ewes in just one afternoon – his small hands enabling him gently to ease out lambs. It's for this reason that Rob Benson calls for the services of James, knowing that only he can help his distressed ewe.

He led the way to a bigger enclosure, holding several sheep. There was a scurry as we went in but he caught expertly at the fleece of a darting ewe. 'This is the first one. You can see we haven't a deal o' time.'

I lifted the woolly tail and gasped. The lamb's head was protruding from the vagina, the lips of the vulva clamped tightly behind the ears, and it had swollen enormously to more than twice its size. The eyes were mere puffed slits in the great oedematous ball and the tongue, blue and engorged, lolled from the mouth.

'Well I've seen a few big heads, Rob, but I think this takes the prize.'

'Aye, the little beggar came with his legs back. Just beat me to it. Ah was only away for an hour but he was up like a football. By hell it doesn't take long. I know he wants his legs bringin' round but what can I do with bloody great mitts like mine.' He held out his huge hands, rough and swollen with the years of work.

While he spoke I was stripping off my jacket and as I rolled my shirtsleeves high the wind struck like a knife at my shrinking flesh. I soaped my fingers quickly and began to feel for a space round the lamb's neck. For a moment the little eyes opened and regarded me disconsolately.

'He's alive, anyway,' I said. 'But he must feel terrible and he can't do a thing about it.'

Easing my way round, I found a space down by the throat where I thought I might get through. This was where my 'lady's hand' came in useful and I blessed it every spring; I could work inside the ewes with the minimum of discomfort to them and this was all-important because sheep, despite their outdoor hardiness, just won't stand rough treatment.

With the utmost care I inched my way along the curly wool of the neck to the shoulder. Another push forward and I was able to hook a finger round the leg and draw it forward until I could feel the flexure of the knee; a little more twiddling and I had hold of the tiny cloven foot and drew it gently out into the light of day.

With farm animals, vets are usually called in to deal with problem births – those that farmers cannot handle themselves.

Lambs are often born in twos or threes, which can result in a jumble of heads and legs which a vet must untangle and ease out as gently as possible. A large, single lamb can also prove challenging if it gets stuck in its mother's pelvis, and there's no extra room for a vet's hand – in which case some vets would put a bit of string around the lamb's head and ease the lamb out by pulling on the string. Alf Wight, as the subsequent story shows, had a different method.

Dealing with various complications meant that lambing could take time, although it was invariably undertaken in the open fields, often with just the aid of cold water and a meagre bit of soap, exposed to the biting Yorkshire wind and rain. For Alf Wight the rewards, however, outweighed the hardships and years later in the late 1970s he wrote: 'Delivering these uniquely appealing little creatures is an unfailing joy and the charm of seeing them struggling to their feet while the mother "talks" to them has never grown dim for me.'

In *Every Living Thing* James must attend to a difficult lambing on a particularly bitter day, where there is snow still on the ground.

I wondered if there was any chance of the ewe being under cover. In the early fifties, it didn't seem to occur to many of the farmers to bring their lambing ewes into the buildings and I attended to the great majority out in the open fields. There were happy times when I almost chuckled in relief at the sight of a row of hurdles in a warm fold yard or sometimes the farmers would build pens from stacked-up straw bales, but on this occasion my spirits plummeted when I drew up at the farm and met Mr Walton who came out of the house carrying a bucket of water and headed for the gate. 'Outside, is she?' I asked, trying to sound airy.

'Aye, just ower there.' He pointed over the long, bracken-splashed pasture to a prone woolly form in the distance which looked a hell of a long way 'ower there'. As I trailed across the frosty grass, my medical bag and obstetric overall dangling, a merciless wind tore at me, picking up an extra Siberian cold from the long drifts of snow which still lay behind the walls in this late Yorkshire spring.

As I stripped off and knelt behind the ewe I looked around. We were right on top of the world and the panorama of hills and valleys with grey farmhouses and pebbled rivers in their depths was beautiful but would have been more inviting if it had been a warm summer afternoon and me preparing for a picnic with my family.

I held out my hand and the farmer deposited a tiny sliver of soap on my palm. I always felt that farmers kept special pieces of soap for the vet — minute portions of scrubbing soap which were too small and hard to be of any use. I rubbed this piece frantically with my hands, dipping frequently into the water, but I could work up only the most meagre film of lather. Not enough to protect my tender arm as I inserted it into the ewe, and the farmer looked at me enquiringly as I softly ooh'd and aah'd my way towards the cervix.

I found just what I didn't want to find. A big single lamb, jammed tight. Two lambs are the norm and three quite common, but a big single lamb often spells trouble. It was one of my joys in practice to sort out the tangles of twins and triplets but with the singles it was a case of not enough room and the big lamb had to be eased and pulled out as gently as possible — a long and tedious business. Also, often the single lamb was dead through pressure and had to be removed by embryotomy or a caesarean operation.

Resigning myself to the fact that I was going to spend a long

235

time crouched on that windy hilltop, I reached as far as possible and poked a finger into the lamb's mouth, feeling a surge of relief as the little tongue stirred against my hand. He was alive, anyway, and with a lifting of my spirits I began the familiar ritual of introducing lubricating jelly, locating the tiny legs and fastening them with snares and, finally, as I sat back on my heels for a breather I knew that all I had to do now was to bring the head through the pelvis. That was the tricky bit. If it came through I was home and dry; if it didn't I was in trouble. Mr Walton, holding back the wool from the vulva, watched me in silence. Despite his lifetime experience with sheep he was helpless in a case like this because, like most farmers, he had huge, work-roughened hands with fingers like bananas and could not possibly have got inside a ewe. My small 'lady's hand' as they called it was a blessing.

I hooked my forefinger into the eye socket — my favourite trick, there was nothing else to get hold of except the lower jaw which was dangerously fragile — and began to pull with infinite care. The ewe strained, crushing my hand against the pelvic bones — not as bad as in a cow but painful, and my mouth opened wide as I eased and twisted and pulled until, with a blessed surge, the head slipped through the bony pelvic opening.

It wasn't long, then, until feet, legs and nose appeared at the vulva and I brought the little creature out onto the grass. He lay still for a moment, snuffling at the cold world he had entered, then he shook his head vigorously. I smiled. That was the best sign of all.

I had another wrestle with the morsel of soap, then the farmer wordlessly handed me a piece of sacking to dry my arms. This was quite common in those days. Towels were scarce commodities on the farms and I couldn't blame the farmers' wives for hesitating to send out a clean towel to a man who had just had his arms up the back end of an animal. An old soiled one was the usual and, if not, the hessian sack was always at hand. I couldn't rub my painful arms with the coarse material and contented myself with a careful patting, before pushing them, still damp, into the sleeves of my jacket.

The ewe, hearing a high-pitched call from her lamb, began to talk back with the soft deep baa I knew so well, and as she got up and began an intensive licking of the little creature I stood there, forgetful of the cold, listening to their conversation, enthralled as ever by the miracle of birth. When the lamb, apparently feeling he was wasting time, struggled to his feet and tottered unsteadily round to the milk bar I grinned in satisfaction and made my way back to the car.

~

While for much of the year, sheep can be left to their own devices, pigs represent year-round work for James and Siegfried. In the 1930s and 1940s nearly all working people in Yorkshire kept a pig or two, so they'd be self-sufficient in the local staple of ham and fatty bacon. Many farms kept dairy cattle and sheep along with pigs, hens and perhaps a few goats, while townsfolk would keep pigs in gardens or yards often in ramshackle tin sheds.

In *If Only They Could Talk*, Siegfried decides they too must keep a few pigs, alongside the mare he already stables in the yard, with some hens at the bottom of the garden. Not only would they save a bit of money – always an attractive proposition to Siegfried – but the scheme would also give his work-shy younger brother Tristan something to do.

He put down his cup with a clatter. 'You know, there's no reason why we should have to go to the grocer for our bacon and eggs. There's a perfectly good henhouse at the bottom of the garden and a pigsty in the yard with a boiler for the swill. All our household waste could go towards feeding a pig. We'd probably do it quite cheaply.'

He rounded on Tristan who had just lit a Woodbine and was shaking out his *Mirror* with the air of ineffable pleasure which was peculiar to him. 'And it would be a useful job for you. You're not producing much sitting around here on your arse all day. A bit of stock keeping would do you good.'

Once Siegfried decides to do something he doesn't muck about and within forty-eight hours ten little pigs have taken up residence in the yard and twelve light Sussex pullet hens are pecking about in the henhouse. Tristan, however, does not share his brother's enthusiasm for the scheme and, under his half-hearted care, the hens fail to produce any eggs over the subsequent weeks and frequently escape in search of substance. Eventually, much to Siegfried's irritation, he accepts the hens must go, ranting at Tristan: 'I must have been mad to think that any hens under your care would ever lay eggs . . . Not one solitary egg have we seen. The bloody hens are flying about the countryside like pigeons.' He gives them away to Mrs Dale, a pensioner down the road, who just a fortnight later informs Siegfried she's getting ten eggs a day from them, as he bellows at Tristan: 'Ten eggs, do you hear, ten eggs!'

Fortunately, Tristan finds the piglets more interesting and is frequently found resting his elbows on the sty door watching them gobbling their swill or conducting conferences with old Boardman who considers himself something of expert in pig husbandry. Before long the piglets grow into ten solid, no-nonsense porkers and in the process lose much of their charm. At the rattle of the swill bucket, they squeal loudly, and Tristan has to brandish a heavy stick before he dares enter the sty, plunging himself among the grunting, jostling animals. On one fateful day, however, they too, like the hens, make a break for liberty.

It was on a market day when the pigs had almost reached bacon weight that I came upon Tristan sprawled in his favourite chair. But there was something unusual about him; he wasn't asleep, no medicine bottle, no Woodbines, no *Daily Mirror*. His arms hung limply over the sides of the chair, his eyes were half closed and sweat glistened on his forehead.

'Jim,' he whispered. 'I've had the most hellish afternoon I've ever had in my life.'

I was alarmed at his appearance. 'What's happened?'

'The pigs,' he croaked. 'They escaped today.'

'Escaped! How the devil could they do that?'

Tristan tugged at his hair. 'It was when I was feeding the mare. I gave her her hay and thought I might as well feed the pigs at the same time. You know what they've been like lately — well, today they went berserk. Soon as I opened the door they charged out in a solid block. Sent me up in the air, bucket and all, then ran over the top of me.' He shuddered and looked up at me wide-eyed. 'I'll tell you this, Jim, when I was lying there on the cobbles, covered with swill and that lot trampling on me, I thought it was all over. But they didn't savage me. They belted out through the yard door at full gallop.'

'The yard door was open then?'

'Too true it was. I would just choose this day to leave it open.'

Tristan sat up and wrung his hands. 'Well, you know, I

239

thought it was all right at first. You see, they slowed down when they got into the lane and trotted quietly round into the front street with Boardman and me hard on their heels. They formed a group there. Didn't seem to know where to go next. I was sure we were going to be able to head them off, but just then one of them caught sight of itself in Robson's shop window.'

He gave a remarkable impression of a pig staring at its reflection for a few moments then leaping back with a startled grunt.

'Well, that did it, Jim. The bloody animal panicked and shot off into the market place at about fifty miles an hour with the rest after it.'

I gasped. Ten large pigs loose among the packed stalls and market-day crowds was difficult even to imagine.

'Oh God, you should have seen it.' Tristan fell back wearily into his chair. 'Women and kids screaming. The stallholders, police and everybody else cursing me. There was a terrific traffic jam too — miles of cars tooting like hell while the policeman on point duty concentrated on browbeating me.' He wiped his brow. 'You know that fast-talking merchant on the china stall — well, today I saw him at a loss for words. He was balancing a cup on his palm and in full cry when one of the pigs got its forefeet on his stall and stared him straight in the face. He stopped as if he'd been shot. Any other time it would have been funny but I thought the perishing animal was going to wreck the stall. The counter was beginning to rock when the pig changed its mind and made off.'

'What's the position now?' I asked. 'Have you got them back?'

'I've got nine of them back,' Tristan replied, leaning back and closing his eyes. 'With the help of almost the entire male population of the district I've got nine of them back. The tenth was last seen heading north at a good pace. God knows where it is now. Oh, I didn't tell you — one of them got into the post office. Spent quite some time in there.' He put his hands over his face. 'I'm for it this time, Jim. I'll be in the hands of the law after this lot. There's no doubt about it.'

I leaned over and slapped his leg. 'Oh, I shouldn't worry. I don't suppose there's been any serious damage done.'

Tristan replied with a groan. 'But there's something else. When I finally closed the door after getting the pigs back in their sty I was on the verge of collapse. I was leaning against the wall gasping for breath when I saw the mare had gone. Yes, gone. I'd gone straight out after the pigs and forgot to close her box. I don't know where she is. Boardman said he'd look around — I haven't the strength.'

Tristan lit a trembling Woodbine. 'This is the end, Jim. Siegfried will have no mercy this time.'

As he spoke, the door flew open and his brother rushed in. 'What the hell is going on?' he roared. 'I've just been speaking to the vicar and he says my mare is in his garden eating his wallflowers. He's hopping mad and I don't blame him. Go on, you lazy young scoundrel. Don't lie there, get over to the vicarage this instant and bring her back!'

Tristan did not stir. He lay inert, looking up at his brother. His lips moved feebly.

'No,' he said.

'What's that?' Siegfried shouted incredulously. 'Get out of that chair immediately. Go and get that mare!'

'No,' replied Tristan.

I felt a chill of horror. This sort of mutiny was unprecedented. Siegfried had gone very red in the face and I steeled myself for an eruption; but it was Tristan who spoke. 'If you want your mare you can get her yourself.' His voice was quiet with no note of defiance. He had the air of a man to whom the future is of no account.

Even Siegfried could see that this was one time when Tristan had had enough. After glaring down at his brother for a few seconds he turned and walked out. He got the mare himself.

Nothing more was said about the incident but the pigs were moved hurriedly to the bacon factory and were never replaced. The stock-keeping project was at an end.

Tristan is not alone being wary of pigs – sows can grow into enormous, formidable beasts, and can become especially aggressive when their piglets require treatment. Alf Wight's son Jim frequently joined his father on visits to treat pigs and keenly remembers the cacophony of squealing piglets and the terror of a huge sow roaring towards him. It's no surprise that smallholders were frequently injured by their pigs and Jim soon learned to seek out an escape route whenever he entered a pen. Alf, however, showed little fear, although often he armed himself with a board or an old broom if he needed to inject a sow. In *If Only They Could Talk*, Tristan has another run-in with a pig, this time an enormous sow with a swollen ear which Siegfried sends him to treat.

'All right,' he said suddenly. 'It's maybe just as well you are staying. I want you to do a job for me. You can open that haematoma on Charlie Dent's pig's ear.'

This was a bombshell. Charlie Dent's pig's ear was something we didn't talk about.

A few weeks earlier, Siegfried himself had gone to the smallholding halfway along a street on the outskirts of the town to see a pig with a swollen ear. It was an aural haematoma and the only treatment was to lance it, but, for some reason, Siegfried had not done the job but had sent me the following day.

I had wondered about it, but not for long. When I climbed into the sty, the biggest sow I had ever seen rose from the straw, gave an explosive bark and rushed at me with its huge mouth gaping. I didn't stop to argue. I made the wall about six inches ahead of the pig and vaulted over into the passage. I stood there, considering the position, looking thoughtfully at the mean little red eyes, the slavering mouth with its long, yellow teeth.

Usually, I paid no attention when pigs barked and grumbled at me but this one really seemed to mean it. As I wondered what the next step would be, the pig gave an angry roar, reared up on its hind legs and tried to get over the wall at me. I made up my mind quickly.

'I'm afraid I haven't got the right instrument with me, Mr Dent. I'll pop back another day and open the ear for you. It's nothing serious – only a small job. Goodbye.'

There the matter had rested, with nobody caring to mention it till now.

Tristan is aghast but Siegfried insists the job must be done before the younger brother heads off to a village dance that evening. Like Siegfried and James, Tristan comes up with endless excuses to get out of the dreaded task, returning to the house and claiming he can't find the address, then the family are out, and finally that it's too dark in the sty. Siegfried is having none of it – 'Don't give me any more of your bloody excuses . . . Now get the hell out of here and don't come back until it's done!' Tristan has no choice but to face the terrifying beast and James waits with anticipation for his return.

243

A moment later, the man of destiny entered but the penetrating smell of pig got into the room just ahead of him, and as he walked over to the fire, pungent waves seemed to billow round him. Pig muck was splattered freely over his nice suit, and on his clean collar, his face and hair. There was a great smear of the stuff on the seat of his trousers but despite his ravaged appearance he still maintained his poise.

Siegfried pushed his chair back hurriedly but did not change expression.

'Have you got that ear opened?' he asked quietly.

'Yes.'

Siegfried returned to his book without comment. It seemed that the matter was closed and Tristan, after staring briefly at his brother's bent head, turned and marched from the room. But even after he had gone, the odour of the pigsty hung in the room like a cloud.

Later, in the Drovers', I watched Tristan draining his third pint. He had changed, and if he didn't look as impressive as when he started the evening, at least he was clean and hardly smelled at all. I had said nothing yet, but the old light was returning to his eye. I went over to the bar and ordered my second half and Tristan's fourth pint and, as I set the glasses on the table, I thought that perhaps it was time.

'Well, what happened?'

Tristan took a long, contented pull at his glass and lit a Woodbine. 'Well now, all in all, Jim, it was rather a smooth operation, but I'll start at the beginning. You can imagine me standing all alone outside the sty in the pitch darkness with that bloody great pig grunting and growling on the other side of the wall. I didn't feel so good, I can tell you.

'I shone my torch on the thing's face and it jumped up and ran at me, making a noise like a lion and showing all those dirty yellow teeth. I nearly wrapped it up and came home there and then, but I got to thinking about the dance and all and, on the spur of the moment, I hopped over the wall.

'Two seconds later, I was on my back. It must have charged me but couldn't see enough to get a bite in. I just heard a bark, then a terrific weight against my legs and I was down.

'Well, it's a funny thing, Jim. You know I'm not a violent chap, but as I lay there, all my fears vanished and all I felt was a cold hatred of that bloody animal. I saw it as the cause of all my troubles and before I knew what I was doing I was up on my feet and booting its arse round and round the sty. And, do you know, it showed no fight at all. That pig was a coward at heart.'

I was still puzzled. 'But the ear — how did you manage to open the haematoma?'

'No problem, Jim. That was done for me.'

'You don't mean to say . . .'

'Yes,' Tristan said, holding his pint up to the light and studying a small foreign body floating in the depths. 'Yes, it was really very fortunate. In the scuffle in the dark, the pig ran up against the wall and burst the thing itself. Made a beautiful job.'

In *It Shouldn't Happen to a Vet*, James visits hotel landlord Mr Worley who keeps Tamworth pigs, including a huge sow Queenie and her litter of piglets. As Mr Worley gently croons in Queenie's ear, James applies ointment to an overgrown claw and sensitive foot. Once that's done, Mr Worley thanks James profusely, almost as if he has saved the animal's life, and James sets out to leave.

We went out into what was really the back yard of an inn. Because Mr Worley wasn't a regular farmer, he was the

245

landlord of the Langthorpe Falls Hotel and his precious live-stock were crammed into what had once been the stables and coach houses of the inn. They were all Tamworths and which-ever door you opened you found yourself staring into the eyes of ginger-haired pigs; there were a few porkers and the odd one being fattened for bacon but Mr Worley's pride was his sows. He had six of them — Queenie, Princess, Ruby, Marigold, Delilah and Primrose.

For years expert farmers had been assuring Mr Worley that he'd never do any good with his sows. If you were going in for breeding, they said, you had to have proper premises; it wasn't a bit of use shoving sows into converted buildings like this. And for years Mr Worley's sows had responded by producing litters of unprecedented size and raising them with tender care. They were all good mothers and didn't savage their families or crush them clumsily under their bodies so it turned out with uncanny regularity that at the end of eight weeks Mr Worley had around twelve chunky weaners to take to market.

It must have spoiled the farmers' beer — none of them could equal that, and the pill was all the more bitter because the landlord had come from the industrial West Riding — Halifax, I think it was — a frail, short-sighted little retired newsagent with no agricultural background. By all the laws he just didn't have a chance.

Mr Worley makes his living from running a hotel but it's clear his pigs are his number one priority. He delights in welcoming James into the bar of the hotel, bringing up a tall jug from the cellar, before exclaiming: 'Well now, let's have a piggy talk!' and they go on to discuss swine fever, brine poisoning and various aspects of pig husbandry, while pictures of his sows with show rosettes look down at them from the walls.

His devotion resulted in my being called out frequently for very trivial things and I swore freely under my breath when I heard his voice on the other end of the line at one o'clock one morning.

'Marigold pigged this afternoon, Mr Herriot, and I don't think she's got much milk. Little pigs look very hungry to me. Will you come?'

I groaned my way out of bed and downstairs and through the long garden to the yard. By the time I had got the car out into the lane I had begun to wake up and when I rolled up to the inn was able to greet Mr Worley fairly cheerfully.

But the poor man did not respond. In the light from the oil lamp his face was haggard with worry.

'I hope you can do something quick. I'm real upset about her — she's just laid there doing nothin' and it's such a lovely litter. Fourteen she's had.'

I could understand his concern as I looked into the pen. Marigold was stretched motionless on her side while the tiny piglets swarmed around her udder; they were rushing from teat to teat, squealing and falling over each other in their desperate quest for nourishment. And the little bodies had the narrow, empty look which meant they had nothing in their stomachs. I hated to see a litter die off from sheer starvation but it could happen so easily. There came a time when they stopped trying to suck and began to lie about the pen. After that it was hopeless.

Crouching behind the sow with my thermometer in her rectum I looked along the swelling flank, the hair a rich copper red in the light from the lamp. 'Did she eat anything tonight?'

'Aye, cleaned up just as usual.'

The thermometer reading was normal. I began to run my hands along the udder, pulling in turn at the teats. The ravenous

247

piglets caught at my fingers with their sharp teeth as I pushed them to one side but my efforts failed to produce a drop of milk. The udder seemed full, even engorged, but I was unable to get even a bead down to the end of the teat.

'There's nowt there, is there?' Mr Worley whispered anxiously.

I straightened up and turned to him 'This is simply agalactia. There's no mastitis and Marigold isn't really ill, but there's something interfering with the let-down mechanism of the milk. She's got plenty of milk and there's an injection which ought to bring it down.'

I tried to keep the triumphant look off my face as I spoke, because this was one of my favourite party tricks. There is a flavour of magic in the injection of pituitrin in these cases; it works within a minute and though no skill is required the effect is spectacular.

Marigold didn't complain as I plunged in the needle and administered three cc deep into the muscle of her thigh. She was too busy conversing with her owner — they were almost nose to nose, exchanging soft pig noises.

After I had put away my syringe and listened for a few moments to the cooing sounds from the front end I thought it might be time. Mr Worley looked up in surprise as I reached down again to the udder.

'What are you doing now?'

'Having a feel to see if the milk's come down yet.'

'Why damn, it can't be! You've only just given t'stuff and she's bone dry!'

Oh, this was going to be good. A roll of drums would be appropriate at this moment. With finger and thumb I took hold of one of the teats at the turgid back end of the udder. I suppose it is a streak of exhibitionism in me which always makes me send the jet of milk spraying against the opposite wall in these circumstances; this time I thought it would be more impressive if I directed my shot past the innkeeper's left ear, but I got my trajectory wrong and sprinkled his spectacles instead.

He took them off and wiped them slowly as if he couldn't believe what he had seen. Then he bent over and tried for himself.

'It's a miracle!' he cried as the milk spouted eagerly over his hand. 'I've never seen owt like it!'

It didn't take the little pigs long to catch on. Within a few seconds they had stopped their fighting and squealing and settled down in a long, silent row. Their utterly rapt expressions all told the same story — they were going to make up for lost time.

Mr Worley was in reality based on pig-owner Mrs Bush who ran a country inn at Byland Abbey near Thirsk, exemplifying how Alf sometimes changed the gender of the odd book character. Mrs Bush kept some formidable saddleback pigs in her yard at the back of the inn and she was equally devoted to them and convinced that Alf loved them too. After *If Only They Could Talk* was published, Alf was at the inn one day having a drink, when he saw Mrs Bush making a beeline for him. Alf's daughter Rosie remembered him freezing as he never liked people recognizing themselves in his books, but Mrs Bush went on to say how much she liked the chapter about the man and the pigs and how she could understand *just* how he felt! Alf simply smiled politely and said he was pleased, no doubt relieved by her response.

∾

When you work with an array of farm animals, even Christmas Day can be busy. James's hopes for a restful day are dashed when he's called early, first to see to a cow with milk fever and then to a choking goat. Dorothy the goat belongs to old Mr Kirby, a retired farmer who has a cottage and a mixture of animals on his land, including a cow, a few pigs and some goats, although he's always been particularly fond of the latter.

The cottage was in a village high up the Dale. Mr Kirby met me at the gate.

'Ee, lad,' he said. 'I'm right sorry to be bothering you this early in the morning and Christmas an' all, but I didn't have no choice. Dorothy's real bad.'

He led the way to a stone shed which had been converted into a row of pens. Behind the wire of one of them a large white Saanen goat peered out at us anxiously and as I watched her she gulped, gave a series of retching coughs, then stood trembling, saliva drooling from her mouth.

The farmer turned to me, wide-eyed. 'You see, I had to get you out, didn't I? If I left her till tomorrow she'd be a goner.'

'You're right, Mr Kirby,' I replied. 'You couldn't leave her. There's something in her throat.'

We went into the pen and as the old man held the goat against the wall I tried to open her mouth. She didn't like it very much and as I prised her jaws apart she startled me with a loud, long-drawn, human-sounding cry. It wasn't a big mouth but I have a small hand and, as the sharp back teeth tried to nibble me, I poked a finger deep into the pharynx.

There was something there all right. I could just touch it but I couldn't get hold of it. Then the animal began to throw her head about and I had to come out; I stood there, saliva dripping from my hand, looking thoughtfully at Dorothy.

After a few moments I turned to the farmer. 'You know, this is a bit baffling. I can feel something in the back of her throat, but it's soft — like cloth. I'd been expecting to find a bit of twig, or something sharp sticking in there — it's funny what a goat will pick up when she's pottering around outside. But if it's cloth, what the heck is holding it there? Why hasn't she swallowed it down?'

James is mystified – what on earth has Dorothy swallowed? As the goat descends into a paroxysm of coughs, he heads to his car to retrieve a torch.

The old man held the torch as I once more pulled the goat's mouth open and again heard the curious child-like wailing. It was when the animal was in full cry that I noticed something under the tongue — a thin, dark band.

'I can see what's holding the thing now,' I cried. 'It's hooked round the tongue with string or something.' Carefully I pushed my forefinger under the band and began to pull.

It wasn't string. It began to stretch as I pulled carefully at it . . . like elastic. Then it stopped stretching and I felt a real resistance . . . whatever was in the throat was beginning to move. I kept up a gentle traction and very slowly the mysterious obstruction came sliding up over the back of the tongue and into the mouth, and when it came within reach I let go the elastic, grabbed the sodden mass and hauled it forth. It seemed as if there was no end to it — a long snake of dripping material nearly two feet long — but at last I had it out onto the straw of the pen.

Mr Kirby seized it and held it up and as he unravelled the mass wonderingly he gave a sudden cry.

'God 'elp us, it's me summer drawers!'

'Your what?'

'Me summer drawers. Ah don't like them long johns when weather gets warmer and I allus change into these little short 'uns. Missus was havin' a clear-out afore the end of t'year and she didn't know whether to wash 'em or mek them into dusters. She washed them at t'finish and Dorothy must have got 'em off the line.' He held up the tattered shorts and regarded them ruefully. 'By gaw, they've seen better days, but I reckon Dorothy's fettled them this time.'

The goat, after belching, is immediately better and Mr Kirby, unlike the farmer on James's previous case who doesn't greet James with so much as a Merry Christmas, invites the vet into his cottage. There, in a tiny living room by a blazing fire, James is treated to Christmas cake and an enormous wedge of Wensleydale cheese – a traditional Yorkshire combination – washed down with a large glass of whisky. After listening to the carols on the wireless, the young vet returns to Skeldale House feeling decidedly more festive than when he arrived.

In *Vet in Harness*, after having been almost crushed by Mr Dacre's bull, as we've seen in Chapter 7, James returns to the practice and is relieved to read that his next call is: 'Mrs Tompkin, 14, Jasmine Terrace. Clip budgie's beak.' Veterinary practice can be enormously varied and a call-out to a budgie feels like a welcome break from the care of hefty farm animals. James arrives at the little terrace of old Mrs Tompkin and is greeted by her neighbour Mrs Dodd who keeps an eye out for the octogenarian.

She led me into the cramped little room. 'Here y'are, love,' she said to the old woman who sat in a corner. She put the pension book and money on the mantelpiece. 'And here's Mr Herriot come to see Peter for you.'

Mrs Tompkin nodded and smiled. 'Oh that's good. Poor little feller can't hardly eat with 'is long beak and I'm worried about him. He's me only companion, you know.'

'Yes, I understand, Mrs Tompkin.' I looked at the cage by the window with the green budgie perched inside. 'These little birds can be wonderful company when they start chattering.'

She laughed. 'Aye, but it's a funny thing. Peter never has said owt much. I think he's lazy! But I just like havin' him with me.'

'Of course you do,' I said. 'But he certainly needs attention now.'

The beak was greatly overgrown, curving away down till it touched the feathers of the breast. I would be able to revolutionize his life with one quick snip from my clippers.

The way I was feeling, this job was right up my street.

I opened the cage door and slowly inserted my hand.

'Come on, Peter,' I wheedled as the bird fluttered away from me. And I soon cornered him and enclosed him gently in my fingers. As I lifted him out I felt in my pocket with the other hand for the clippers, but as I poised them I stopped.

The tiny head was no longer poking cheekily from my fingers but had fallen loosely to one side. The eyes were closed. I stared at the bird uncomprehendingly for a moment then opened my hand. He lay quite motionless on my palm. He was dead.

Dry-mouthed, I continued to stare; at the beautiful iridescence of the plumage, the long beak which I didn't have to cut now, but mostly at the head dropping down over my forefinger. I hadn't squeezed him or been rough with him in any way but he was dead. It must have been sheer fright.

James and Mrs Dodd are aghast at the turn of events although Mrs Tompkin, who has poor hearing and sight, has not noticed the calamity. Agreeing that the shock of losing the bird would be terrible for the old lady, James rushes out to see if he can find a replacement. Hurriedly purchasing a green budgie, he races back to Jasmine Terrace and hangs the cage containing the new bird up at the window: 'I think you'll find all is well now.' Months later, James strikes up the courage to go back to Mrs Tompkin's and tentatively enquires after the bird.

> His mistress reached up, tapped the metal and looked lovingly at him.
>
> 'You know, you wouldn't believe it,' she said. 'He's like a different bird.'
>
> I swallowed. 'Is that so? In what way?'
>
> 'Well he's so active now. Lively as can be. You know 'e chatters to me all day long. It's wonderful what cuttin' a beak can do.'

Turkey and geese are also found on the odd farm or small-holding and in *The Lord Made Them All* dairy farmer Mr Bogg keeps a few turkeys and chickens alongside his main herd of Ayrshire cows. He is a regular client at the Darrowby practice, and James and Siegfried have grown accustomed to his penny-pinching ways, which, even by Yorkshire standards, are impressive.

> Then there was Mr Bogg, whose tight-fistedness was a byword in a community where thrift was the norm. I had heard many tales of his parsimony but I have a few experiences of my own which I cherish.

He owned a herd of good Ayrshire cows and ran a few turkeys and chickens on the side. He certainly would not be short of money.

His turkeys were frequently afflicted with blackhead and he used to come to us for Stovarsol tablets which were the popular treatment at that time.

One afternoon he approached me in the surgery.

'Look,' he said. 'Ah keep comin' here for fifty or a hundred of them little tablets and it's a flippin' nuisance. I'd rather buy a whole tinful — it 'ud save a lot of journeys.'

'Yes, Mr Bogg, you're right,' I replied. 'It would be a much better idea. I'll get you some now.'

When I returned from the dispensary I held up the tin. 'This contains a thousand tablets and as it happens it's the only one we have in stock. It has been opened and a few have been taken out but it is virtually a new tin.'

'A few . . . taken out . . .?' I could read the alarm in his eyes at the idea of paying for the full thousand when he was getting less than that.

'Oh, don't worry,' I said. 'There's maybe something like a dozen tablets short — no more.'

My words failed to reassure him and as he left the surgery he looked gloomy and preoccupied.

He was back again that same evening. He rang the bell at about eight o'clock and I faced him on the front doorstep.

'I've just come in to tell ye,' he said. 'I've been counting them tablets and there's nine hundred and eighty-seven.'

On another occasion I went to buy some eggs from Mr Bogg. I got a dozen from him most weeks because his farm was on the outskirts of the town. When I returned home with this particular batch I found that there were only eleven eggs in the bag, so when I saw him a week later I mentioned the fact.

'Mr Bogg,' I said. 'There were only eleven eggs in last week's lot.'

'Aye, ah knaw,' he replied, fixing me with a steady eye. 'But one of 'em was a double-yolked 'un.'

Chapter 9

DOGS *and* CATS

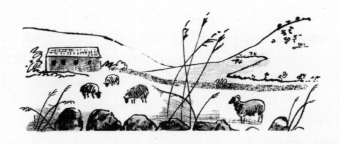

There was one marvellous thing about the set-up in Darrowby. I had the inestimable advantage of being a *large animal practitioner with a passion for dogs and cats.* So that although I spent most of my time in the wide outdoors of Yorkshire there was always the captivating background of the household pets to make a contrast.

I treated some of them every day and it made an extra interest in my life; interest of a different kind, based on sentiment instead of commerce and because of the way things were it was something I could linger over and enjoy. I suppose with a very intensive small animal practice it would be easy to regard the thing as a huge sausage machine, an endless procession of hairy forms to prod with hypodermic needles. But in Darrowby we got to know them all as individual entities.

Driving through the town I was able to identify my ex-patients without difficulty; Rover Johnson, recovered from his ear canker, coming out of the ironmonger's with his mistress, Patch Walker whose broken leg had healed beautifully, balanced happily on the back of his owner's coal wagon, or Spot Briggs who was a bit of a rake anyway and would soon be tearing himself again on barbed wire, ambling all alone across the market place cobbles in search of adventure.

I got quite a kick out of recalling their ailments and mulling over their characteristics. Because they all had their own personalities and they were manifested in different ways.

Like James, Alf saw plenty of family pets at the Thirsk practice and the James Herriot books are full of memorable stories about cats and dogs. As a teenager, Alf Wight ranged the hills and parks of Glasgow with his dog Don, a glossy and beautiful Irish setter with whom he developed a close bond. Thereon he set upon pursuing a veterinary career and, while he loved working with all animals over the subsequent decades, whenever he was asked what his favourite animal was, he invariably answered, 'most definitely dogs'.

His veterinary training, however, focused mainly on horses and large farm animals, dogs were still deemed more of a sideline concern for vets, and cats were hardly covered at all. Despite this, Alf was able to set up a small animal surgery at the Thirsk practice – Donald was happy to focus on their equine patients and Alf, with the help of Brian and various assistants, could attend to dogs and cats in between farm visits. The surgery wasn't the gleaming operating room he'd envisaged during student days, but simply the consulting room of 23 Kirkgate or a dark corner of a cow byre or farmyard kitchen, but Alf nonetheless found the treatment of dogs and cats rewarding work.

The fascination and love that Alf had for dogs – the huge range of breeds, their various personalities, quirks, ailments and devotion to humans – shines through in the James Herriot books.

Dogs and Cats

Cedric the boxer, who features in *Vets Might Fly*, is just one of the many memorable dogs we are introduced to after James receives a telephone call from Cedric's owner, Mrs Rumney.

'Mr Herriot . . . I should be grateful if you would come and see my dog.' It was a woman, obviously upper class.

'Certainly. What's the trouble?'

'Well . . . he . . . er . . . he seems to suffer from . . . a certain amount of flatus.'

'I beg your pardon?'

There was a long pause. 'He has . . . excessive flatus.'

'In what way, exactly?'

'Well . . . I suppose you'd describe it as . . . windiness.' The voice had begun to tremble.

I thought I could see a gleam of light. 'You mean his stomach . . .?'

'No, not his stomach. He passes . . . er . . . a considerable quantity of . . . wind from his . . . his . . .' A note of desperation had crept in.

'Ah, yes!' All became suddenly clear. 'I quite understand. But that doesn't sound very serious. Is he ill?'

'No, he's very fit in other ways.'

'Well then, do you think it's necessary for me to see him?'

'Oh yes, indeed, Mr Herriot. I wish you would come as soon as possible. It has become quite . . . quite a problem.'

'All right,' I said. 'I'll look in this morning. Can I have your name and address, please?'

'It's Mrs Rumney, The Laurels.'

The Laurels was a very nice house on the edge of the town standing back from the road in a large garden. Mrs Rumney herself let me in and I felt a shock of surprise at my first sight of her. It wasn't just that she was strikingly beautiful; there was

259

an unworldly air about her. She would be around forty but had the appearance of a heroine in a Victorian novel – tall, willowy, ethereal. And I could understand immediately her hesitation on the phone. Everything about her suggested fastidiousness and delicacy.

'Cedric is in the kitchen,' she said. 'I'll take you through.'

I had another surprise when I saw Cedric. An enormous boxer hurled himself on me in delight, clawing at my chest with the biggest, horniest feet I had seen for a long time. I tried to fight him off but he kept at me, panting ecstatically into my face and wagging his entire rear end.

'Sit down, boy!' the lady said sharply, then, as Cedric took absolutely no notice, she turned to me nervously. 'He's so friendly.'

'Yes,' I said breathlessly, 'I can see that.' I finally managed to push the huge animal away and backed into a corner for safety. 'How often does this . . . excessive flatus occur?'

As if in reply an almost palpable sulphurous wave arose from the dog and eddied around me. It appeared that the excitement of seeing me had activated Cedric's weakness. I was up against the wall and unable to obey my first instinct to run for cover so I held my hand over my face for a few moments before speaking.

'Is that what you meant?'

Mrs Rumney waved a lace handkerchief under her nose and the faintest flush crept into the pallor of her cheeks. 'Yes,' she replied almost inaudibly. 'Yes . . . that is it.'

'Oh well,' I said briskly. 'There's nothing to worry about. Let's go into the other room and we'll have a word about his diet and a few other things.'

It turned out that Cedric was getting rather a lot of meat and I drew up a little chart cutting down the protein and adding extra carbohydrates. I prescribed a kaolin antacid mixture to be given night and morning and left the house in a confident frame of mind.

Cedric's flatulence, however, does not improve. James goes on to try various powders, remedies and vast quantities of charcoal biscuits, as recommended by Siegfried, all of which make not the slightest difference to his condition. At the end of a long day, James decides to pay Mrs Rumney a visit, just as she is holding an elegant drinks party where James is mortified to see Cedric bound enthusiastically into the room and leap upon the guests, almost tearing off one lady's dress. To make matters worse, the room then fills with 'an unmistakable effluvium' of which Cedric is clearly the guilty party.

James finally comes to the conclusion that Cedric is simply not the dog for Mrs Rumney. Con Fenton, however, a retired farm worker who helps out in the garden of Laurel House, has taken a liking to the dog, so James suggests he take Cedric and that Mrs Rumney find herself a more suitable pet. She agrees and acquires a poodle, while Con Fenton takes in Cedric and they become devoted to each other. When James visits the pair, however, he notices a familiar pungency rising from Cedric, although Con is entirely oblivious to it. It soon becomes clear why, as the two men chat and James takes in the fragrance of some carnation flowers in a vase.

Con watched me approvingly. 'Aye, they're lovely flowers, aren't they? T'missus at Laurels lets me bring 'ome what I want and I reckon them carnations is me favourite.'

'Yes, they're a credit to you.' I still kept my nose among the blooms.

'There's only one thing,' the old man said pensively. 'Ah don't get t'full benefit of 'em.'

'How's that, Con?'

He pulled at his pipe a couple of times. 'Well, you can hear ah speak a bit funny, like?'

'No . . . no . . . not really.'

'Oh aye, ye know ah do. I've been like it since I were a lad. I 'ad a operation for adenoids and summat went wrong.'

'Oh, I'm sorry to hear that,' I said.

'Well, it's nowt serious, but it's left me lackin' in one way.'

'You mean . . .?' A light was beginning to dawn in my mind, an elucidation of how man and dog had found each other, of why their relationship was so perfect, of the certainty of their happy future together. It seemed like fate.

'Aye,' the old man went on sadly. 'I 'ave no sense of smell.'

Just as the people of the Dales have different personalities, so too do their dogs. Judy the sheepdog, who features in *Vet in a Spin*, has a particularly caring nature and instinctively looks after other animals around her. While treating a bullock on the farm of Eric Abbot, James notices the big dog sitting nearby.

I inserted the needle into the jugular and tipped up the bottle of clear fluid. Two drachms of the iodide I used to use, in eight ounces of distilled water and it didn't take long to flow in. In fact the bottle was nearly empty before I noticed Judy.

I had been aware of a big dog sitting near me all the time, but as I neared the end of the injection a black nose moved ever closer till it was almost touching the needle. Then the nose moved along the rubber tube up to the bottle and back again, sniffing with the utmost concentration. When I removed the needle the nose began a careful inspection of the injection site.

Then a tongue appeared and began to lick the bullock's neck methodically.

I squatted back on my heels and watched. This was something more than mere curiosity; everything in the dog's attitude suggested intense interest and concern.

'You know, Eric,' I said. 'I have the impression that this dog isn't just watching me. She's supervising the whole job.'

The farmer laughed. 'You're right there. She's a funny old bitch is Judy — sort of a nurse. If there's anything amiss she's on duty. You can't keep her away.'

Judy looked up quickly at the sound of her name. She was a handsome animal; not the usual colour, but a variegated brindle with waving lines of brown and grey mingling with the normal black and white of the farm collie. Maybe there was a cross somewhere but the result was very attractive and the effect was heightened by her bright-eyed, laughing-mouthed friendliness.

I reached out and tickled the backs of her ears and she wagged mightily — not just her tail but her entire rear end. 'I suppose she's just good-natured.'

'Oh aye, she is,' the farmer said. 'But it's not only that. It sounds daft but I think Judy feels a sense of responsibility to all the stock on t'farm.'

Judy sniffs the rug covering the bullock, then gives its shaggy forehead a lick and stations herself facing the patient. The farmer Eric assures James that 'nothing'll shift her till he's dead or better'. Five days later, James discovers Judy is still with the bullock, which is much better. The farmer tells James how she gives every new-born calf a good lick over as soon as it comes into the world, as she does with any kittens, and always sleeps with the farm animals every night. A week later James returns to see the bullock which is galloping around his box like a racehorse. Enquiring after Judy, Eric points her out.

I looked through the doorway. Judy was stalking importantly across the yard. She had something in her mouth — a yellow, fluffy object.

I craned out further. 'What is she carrying?'

'It's a chicken.'

'A chicken?'

'Aye, there's a brood of them runnin' around just now. They're only a month old and t'awd bitch seems to think they'd be better off in the stable. She's made a bed for them in there and she keeps tryin' to curl herself round them. But the little things won't 'ave it.'

I watched Judy disappear into the stable. Very soon she came out, trotted after a group of tiny chicks which were pecking happily among the cobbles and gently scooped one up. Busily she made her way back to the stable but as she entered the previous chick reappeared in the doorway and pottered over to rejoin his friends.

She was having a frustrating time but I knew she would keep at it because that was the way she was. Judy the nurse dog was still on duty.

In Thirsk, Alf Wight continued to keep his own dogs, all of them becoming cherished companions. They invariably accompanied him on rounds and, as a break between visits, Alf liked nothing more than getting out of the car and escaping for walks with his dog, where he often revelled in the beauty and solitude of the Dales. In the books, James describes walking with his dog Sam, a composite beagle dog based on his real dogs Danny and Dinah. Danny originally belonged to Alf's wife Joan and after their marriage he went on to accompany Alf everywhere. He had a look of a West Highland white terrier but was probably a mix of breeds and went on to live to a ripe old age of fourteen, when he was sadly killed on the main road outside their house. Dinah was the successor to Danny, one of a pack of beagle hunting dogs bred by Donald Sinclair which he gave to Alf and his family in 1953 as a successor to Danny.

This was the real Yorkshire with the clean limestone wall riding the hill's edge and the path cutting brilliant green through the crowding heather. And, walking face-on to the scented breeze I felt the old tingle of wonder at being alone on the wide moorland where nothing stirred and the spreading miles of purple blossom and green turf reached away till it met the hazy blue of the sky.

But I wasn't really alone. There was Sam, and he made all the difference. Helen had brought a lot of things into my life and Sam was one of the most precious; he was a beagle and her own personal pet. He would be about two years old when I first saw him and I had no way of knowing that he was to be my faithful companion, my car dog, my friend who sat by my side through the lonely hours of driving till his life ended at the age of fourteen. He was the first of a series of cherished dogs whose comradeship have warmed and lightened my working life.

Sam adopted me on sight. It was as though he had read the Faithful Hound Manual because he was always near me; paws on the dash as he gazed eagerly through the windscreen on my rounds, head resting on my foot in our bed-sitting room, trotting just behind me wherever I moved. If I had a beer in a pub he would be under my chair and even when I was having a haircut you only had to lift the white sheet to see Sam crouching beneath my legs. The only place I didn't dare take him was the cinema and on these occasions he crawled under the bed and sulked.

Most dogs love car-riding but to Sam it was a passion which never waned — even in the night hours; he would gladly leave his basket when the world was asleep, stretch a couple of times and follow me out into the cold. He would be on to the seat before I got the car door fully open and this action became so much a part of my life that for a long time after his death I still held the door open unthinkingly, waiting for him. And I still remember the pain I felt when he did not bound inside.

And having him with me added so much to the intermissions I granted myself on my daily rounds. Whereas in offices and factories they had tea breaks I just stopped the car and stepped out into the splendour which was always at hand and walked for a spell down hidden lanes, through woods, or as today, along one of the grassy tracks which ran over the high tops.

This thing which I had always done had a new meaning now. Anybody who has ever walked a dog knows the abiding satisfaction which comes from giving pleasure to a loved animal, and the sight of the little form trotting ahead of me lent a depth which had been missing before.

By the time of *Every Living Thing*, James has a new dog Dinah, based on Alf's real dog Dinah, who also grew fat. The beagle loved her food and few could resist her liquid brown eyes when she was after a morsel of something tasty. The family never could and the dog grew very large, despite going out with Alf for regular walks. Practice assistant Calum, who has a way with all animals, is not shy in pointing out Dinah's portliness.

Everything was going with a bang when Dinah, our second beagle and successor to Sam, ran in from the garden.

'This is Dinah,' I said.

'Oh-ho, oh-ho, little fat Dinah,' said Calum in a rumbling bass. It was not a complimentary remark, because my little dog was undoubtedly too fat, and an embarrassment to a vet who was constantly adjuring people to keep their dogs slim, but Dinah didn't seem to mind. She wagged her whole back end until I thought she would tie herself in a knot. Her response was remarkable and she clearly found this new voice immensely attractive. Calum bent down and she rolled on her back in ecstasy as he rubbed her tummy.

Helen laughed. 'Gosh, she really likes you!'

The real Dinah died in 1963 at the age of eleven, having unwittingly consumed some rat-poison, much to the distress of the family. As a dog-lover, James can empathize with the sadness or heartbreak owners experience when their dogs die or suffer an injury. As Alf Wight put it: 'I am as soppy over my dogs as any old lady and it is a trait which has always stood me in good stead in my dealing with clients.' That sensitivity also resulted in some very poignant stories about dogs in his books, including that of Bob the Labrador who features in *If Only They Could Talk*.

'I've come to see your dog,' I said, and the old man smiled.

'Oh, I'm glad you've come, sir,' he said. 'I'm getting a bit worried about the old chap. Come inside, please.'

He led me into the tiny living room. 'I'm alone now, sir. Lost my missus over a year ago. She used to think the world of the old dog.'

The grim evidence of poverty was everywhere. In the

worn-out lino, the fireless hearth, the dank, musty smell of the place. The wallpaper hung away from the damp patches and on the table the old man's solitary dinner was laid; a fragment of bacon, a few fried potatoes and a cup of tea. This was life on the old-age pension.

In the corner, on a blanket, lay my patient, a cross-bred Labrador. He must have been a big, powerful dog in his time, but the signs of age showed in the white hairs round his muzzle and the pale opacity in the depth of his eyes. He lay quietly and looked at me without hostility.

'Getting on a bit, isn't he, Mr Dean?'

'Aye he is that. Nearly fourteen, but he's been like a pup galloping about until these last few weeks. Wonderful dog for his age is old Bob and he's never offered to bite anybody in his life. Children can do anything with him. He's my only friend now — I hope you'll soon be able to put him right.'

'Is he off his food, Mr Dean?'

'Yes, clean off, and that's a strange thing because, by gum, he could eat. He always sat by me and put his head on my knee at meal times, but he hasn't been doing it lately.'

I looked at the dog with growing uneasiness. The abdomen was grossly distended and I could read the tell-tale symptoms of pain; the catch in the respirations, the retracted commissures of the lips, the anxious, preoccupied expression in the eyes.

When his master spoke, the tail thumped twice on the blankets and a momentary interest showed in the white old eyes; but it quickly disappeared and the blank, inward look returned.

I passed my hand carefully over the dog's abdomen. Ascites was pronounced and the dropsical fluid had gathered till the pressure was intense. 'Come on, old chap,' I said, 'let's see if we can roll you over.' The dog made no resistance as I eased him slowly onto his other side, but, just as the movement was completed, he whimpered and looked round. The cause of the trouble was now only too easy to find.

I palpated gently. Through the thin muscle of the flank I could feel a hard, corrugated mass; certainly a splenic or hepatic carcinoma, enormous and completely inoperable. I stroked the old dog's head as I tried to collect my thoughts. This wasn't going to be easy.

'Is he going to be ill for long?' the old man asked, and again came the thump, thump of the tail at the sound of the loved voice. 'It's miserable when Bob isn't following me round the house when I'm doing my little jobs.'

'I'm sorry, Mr Dean, but I'm afraid this is something very serious. You see this large swelling. It is caused by an internal growth.'

'You mean . . . cancer?' the little man said faintly.

'I'm afraid so, and it has progressed too far for anything to be done. I wish there was something I could do to help him, but there isn't.'

The old man looked bewildered and his lips trembled. 'Then he's going to die?'

I swallowed hard. 'We really can't just leave him to die, can we? He's in some distress now, but it will soon be an awful lot worse. Don't you think it would be kindest to put him to sleep? After all, he's had a good, long innings.' I always aimed at a brisk, matter-of-fact approach, but the old clichés had an empty ring.

The old man was silent, then he said, 'Just a minute,' and slowly and painfully knelt down by the side of the dog. He did not speak, but ran his hand again and again over the grey old muzzle and the ears, while the tail thump, thump, thumped on the floor.

He knelt there a long time while I stood in the cheerless

269

room, my eyes taking in the faded pictures on the walls, the frayed, grimy curtains, the broken-springed armchair.

At length the old man struggled to his feet and gulped once or twice. Without looking at me, he said huskily, 'All right, will you do it now?'

I filled the syringe and said the things I always said. 'You needn't worry, this is absolutely painless. Just an overdose of an anaesthetic. It is really an easy way out for the old fellow.'

The dog did not move as the needle was inserted, and, as the barbiturate began to flow into the vein, the anxious expression left his face and the muscles began to relax. By the time the injection was finished, the breathing had stopped.

'Is that it?' the old man whispered.

'Yes, that's it,' I said. 'He is out of his pain now.'

The old man stood motionless except for the clasping and unclasping of his hands. When he turned to face me his eyes were bright. 'That's right, we couldn't let him suffer, and I'm grateful for what you've done. And now, what do I owe you for your services, sir?'

'Oh, that's all right, Mr Dean,' I said quickly. 'It's nothing – nothing at all. I was passing right by here – it was no trouble.'

The old man was astonished. 'But you can't do that for nothing.'

'Now please say no more about it, Mr Dean. As I told you, I was passing right by your door.' I said goodbye and went out of the house, through the passage and into the street. In the bustle of people and the bright sunshine, I could still see only the stark, little room, the old man and his dead dog.

As I walked towards my car, I heard a shout behind me. The old man was shuffling excitedly towards me in his slippers. His cheeks were streaked and wet, but he was smiling. In his hand he held a small, brown object.

'You've been very kind, sir. I've got something for you.' He held out the object and I looked at it. It was tattered but just recognizable as a precious relic of a bygone celebration.

'Go on, it's for you,' said the old man. 'Have a cigar.'

Providing services for free or at a much-reduced rate to clients living in poverty was an all-too-common occurrence at the Darrowby practice. While vets' bills are a stretch for some animal owners, there is one client who can easily meet the cost of calling out a vet – as she does regularly. Mrs Pumphrey, whom we meet in *If Only They Could Talk*, calls in James to attend to her Pekinese dog Tricki Woo and his reoccurring 'flop-bott'.

Mrs Pumphrey was an elderly widow. Her late husband, a beer baron whose breweries and pubs were scattered widely over the broad bosom of Yorkshire, had left her a vast fortune and a beautiful house on the outskirts of Darrowby. Here she lived with a large staff of servants, a gardener, a chauffeur and Tricki Woo. Tricki Woo was a Pekinese and the apple of his mistress's eye.

Standing now in the magnificent doorway, I furtively rubbed the toes of my shoes on the backs of my trousers and blew on my cold hands. I could almost see the deep armchair drawn close to the leaping flames, the tray of cocktail biscuits, the bottle of excellent sherry. Because of the sherry, I was always careful to time my visits for half an hour before lunch.

A maid answered my ring, beaming on me as an honoured guest, and led me to the room, crammed with expensive furniture and littered with glossy magazines and the latest novels. Mrs Pumphrey, in the high-backed chair by the fire, put down her book with a cry of delight. 'Tricki! Tricki! Here is your Uncle Herriot.' I had been made an uncle very early and, sensing the advantages of the relationship, had made no objection.

Tricki, as always, bounded from his cushion, leaped onto the back of a sofa and put his paws on my shoulders. He then licked my face thoroughly before retiring, exhausted. He was soon exhausted because he was given roughly twice the amount of food needed for a dog of his size. And it was the wrong kind of food.

'Oh, Mr Herriot,' Mrs Pumphrey said, looking at her pet anxiously. 'I'm so glad you've come. Tricki has gone flop-bott again.'

This ailment, not to be found in any textbook, was her way of describing the symptoms of Tricki's impacted anal glands. When the glands filled up, he showed discomfort by sitting down suddenly in mid-walk and his mistress would rush to the phone in great agitation.

'Mr Herriot! Please come, he's going flop-bott again!'

I hoisted the little dog on to a table and, by pressure on the anus with a pad of cotton wool, I evacuated the glands.

It baffled me that the Peke was always so pleased to see me. Any dog who could still like a man who grabbed him and squeezed his bottom hard every time they met had to have an incredibly forgiving nature. But Tricki never showed any resentment; in fact he was an outstandingly equable little animal, bursting with intelligence, and I was genuinely attached to him. It was a pleasure to be his personal physician.

The squeezing over, I lifted my patient from the table, noticing the increased weight, the padding of extra flesh over the ribs. 'You know, Mrs Pumphrey, you're overfeeding him again. Didn't I tell you to cut out all those pieces of cake and give him more protein?'

'Oh yes, Mr Herriot,' Mrs Pumphrey wailed. 'But what can I do? He's so tired of chicken.'

I shrugged; it was hopeless. I allowed the maid to lead me to the palatial bathroom where I always performed a ritual handwashing after the operation. It was a huge room with a fully stocked dressing-table, massive green ware and rows of glass shelves laden with toilet preparations. My private guest towel was laid out next to the slab of expensive soap.

Then I returned to the drawing room, my sherry glass was filled and I settled down by the fire to listen to Mrs Pumphrey. It couldn't be called a conversation because she did all the talking, but I always found it rewarding.

Mrs Pumphrey launches into a variety of charming but entirely fanciful stories about the wonders of Tricki Woo, who apparently studies the horse racing columns so he can tell his owner which horse to place a bet on. Mrs Pumphrey also tells James how frightened she was when Tricki Woo went 'completely crackerdog' the previous week, suddenly running about in circles, barking and yelping and then falling over on his side 'like a little dead thing' before getting up and walking away as if nothing has happened.

Hysteria, I thought, brought on by wrong feeding and over-excitement. I put down my glass and fixed Mrs Pumphrey with a severe glare. 'Now look, this is just what I was talking about. If you persist in feeding all that fancy rubbish to Tricki you are going to ruin his health. You really must get him on to a sensible dog diet of one or, at the most, two small meals a day of meat and brown bread or a little biscuit. And nothing in between.'

Mrs Pumphrey shrank into her chair, a picture of abject guilt. 'Oh, please don't speak to me like that. I do try to give him

273

the right things, but it is so difficult. When he begs for his little titbits, I can't refuse him.' She dabbed her eyes with a handkerchief.

But I was unrelenting. 'All right, Mrs Pumphrey, it's up to you, but I warn you that if you go on as you are doing, Tricki will go crackerdog more and more often.'

I left the cosy haven with reluctance, pausing on the gravelled drive to look back at Mrs Pumphrey waving and Tricki, as always, standing against the window, his wide-mouthed face apparently in the middle of a hearty laugh.

Driving home, I mused on the many advantages of being Tricki's uncle. When he went to the seaside he sent me boxes of oak-smoked kippers; and when the tomatoes ripened in his greenhouse, he sent a pound or two every week. Tins of tobacco arrived regularly, sometimes with a photograph carrying a loving inscription.

But it was when the Christmas hamper arrived from Fortnum and Mason's that I decided that I was on a really good thing which should be helped along a bit. Hitherto, I had merely rung up and thanked Mrs Pumphrey for the gifts, and she had been rather cool, pointing out that it was Tricki who had sent the things and he was the one who should be thanked.

With the arrival of the hamper it came to me, blindingly, that I had been guilty of a grave error of tactics. I set myself to compose a letter to Tricki. Avoiding Siegfried's sardonic eye, I thanked my doggy nephew for his Christmas gifts and for all his generosity in the past. I expressed my sincere hopes that the festive fare had not upset his delicate digestion and suggested that if he did experience any discomfort he should have recourse to the black powder his uncle always prescribed. A vague feeling of professional shame was easily swamped by floating visions of kippers, tomatoes and hampers. I addressed the envelope to Master Tricki Pumphrey, Barlby Grange and slipped it into the post box with only a slight feeling of guilt.

On my next visit, Mrs Pumphrey drew me to one side. 'Mr Herriot,' she whispered, 'Tricki adored your charming letter and he will keep it always, but he was very put out about one thing — you addressed it to Master Tricki and he does insist upon Mister. He was dreadfully affronted at first, quite beside himself, but when he saw it was from you he soon recovered his good temper. I can't think why he should have these little prejudices. Perhaps it is because he is an only dog — I do think an only dog develops more prejudices than one from a large family.'

Alf Wight and his family were similarly fond of Bambi – another little Pekinese dog and the real 'Tricki Woo'. Bambi was the much-loved and very indulged pet of Miss Marjorie Warner who lived in a large house in Sowerby. Alf saw a lot of Bambi and developed a genuine liking for the little dog and his owner. As children Rosie and Jim remember the exciting gifts addressed to 'Uncle Wight' that would arrive on the doorstep of 23 Kirkgate whenever Bambi went on holiday, from Whitby kippers (a favourite of Alf's) to hampers filled with caviar, hams and an array of exotic foods. Alf also got himself into trouble when he addressed a thank you letter to Miss Warner and not to Bambi himself, and the correct terminology – 'Bambi Warner Esq' and not 'Master Bambi Warner' – was a must. Miss Warner didn't throw parties like her fictional personification, that was another well-to-do client of the Thirsk practice who invited Alf to one of her balls. Miss Warner nonetheless recognized herself in the books and was happy to be featured in what was an affectionate and memorable portrayal.

Another client who devotes her life to the care of dogs,

which, unlike Tricki Woo, are without home or owners, is Sister Rose. She runs a shelter for abandoned dogs and in *The Lord God Made Them All* asks James to pay her a visit to take a look at one of her dogs, Amber.

I looked at the pale, almost honey-coloured shading of the hair on the dog's ears and flanks. 'I can see why you've given her that name. I bet she'd really glow in the sunshine.'

The nurse laughed. 'Yes, funnily enough it was sunny when I first saw her and the name just jumped into my mind.' She gave me a sideways glance. 'I'm good at names, as you know.'

'Oh yes, without a doubt,' I said, smiling. It was a little joke between us. Sister Rose had to be good at christening the endless stream of unwanted animals which passed through the little dog sanctuary which lay behind her house and which she ran and maintained by organizing small shows, jumble sales, etc., and by spending her own money.

And she didn't only give her money, she also gave her precious time, because as a nursing sister she led a full life of service to the human race. I often asked myself how she found the time to fight for the animals, too. It was a mystery to me, but I admired her.

'Where did this one come from?' I asked.

Sister Rose shrugged. 'Oh, found wandering in the streets of Hebbleton. Nobody knows her and there have been no enquiries to the police. Obviously abandoned.'

James examines Amber, who has some bare patches around her toes, eyes and cheek. He prescribes some ointment for Sister Rose to rub in morning and night. Two weeks later, however, she phones to say the patches are spreading, and James takes another look at Amber who's now in a worse state. James is sorry to diagnose a very serious case of demodectic mange, which is often incurable but he tells Sister Rose to try rubbing a lotion in every day just in case that works. A week later, though, Amber's condition has worsened, she has lost even more hair but is still wagging her tail. Further treatment also fails and the situation starts to look increasingly desperate until James decides to take Amber back to the surgery with him.

Veterinary surgeons would never last in their profession if they became too involved with their patients. I knew from experience that most of my colleagues were just as sentimental over animals as the owners, but before I knew what was happening I became involved with Amber.

I fed her myself, changed her bedding and carried out the treatment. I saw her as often as possible during the day, but when I think of her now it is always night. It was late November when darkness came in soon after four o'clock and the last few visits were a dim-sighted fumbling in cow byres, and when I came home I always drove round to the yard at the back of Skeldale House and trained my headlights on the stable.

When I threw open the door Amber was always there, waiting to welcome me, her forefeet resting on the plywood sheet, her long yellow ears gleaming in the bright beam. That is my picture of her to this day. Her temperament never altered and her tail swished the straw unceasingly as I did all the uncomfortable things to her; rubbing the tender skin with the lotion, injecting her with the staph toxoid, taking further skin scrapings to check progress.

As the days and the weeks went by and I saw no improvement I became a little desperate. I gave her sulphur baths, and derris baths, although I had done no good with such things in the past, and I also began to go through all the proprietary things on the market. In veterinary practice every resistant disease spawns a multitude of quack 'cures' and I lost count of the shampoos and washes I swilled over the young animal in the hope that there might be some magic element in them despite my misgivings.

These nightly sessions under the headlights became part of my life and I think I might have gone on blindly for an indefinite period until one very dark evening with the rain beating on the cobbles of the yard I seemed to see the young dog for the first time.

The condition had spread over the entire body, leaving only tufts and straggling wisps of hair. The long ears were golden no longer. They were almost bald, as was the rest of her face and head. Everywhere her skin was thickened and wrinkled and had assumed a bluish tinge. And when I squeezed it a slow ooze of pus and serum came up around my fingers.

I flopped back and sat down in the straw while Amber leaped around me, licking and wagging. Despite her terrible state, her nature was unchanged.

James eventually realizes that he can do no more for Amber, who is clearly now uncomfortable and soon to be in a lot of pain. He drives into the practice yard and opens the garage door.

And it was like all the other times. Amber was there in the beam, paws on the plywood, body swinging with her wagging, mouth open and panting with delight, welcoming me.

I put the barbiturate and syringe into my pocket before climbing into the pen. For a long time I made a fuss of her, patting her and talking to her as she leaped up at me. Then I filled the syringe.

278

'Sit, girl,' I said, and she flopped obediently onto her hindquarters. I gripped her right leg above the elbow to raise the radial vein. There was no need for clipping — all the hair had gone. Amber looked at me interestedly, wondering what new game this might be as I slipped the needle into the vein. I realized that there was no need to say the things I always said. 'She won't know a thing.' 'This is just an overdose of anaesthetic.' 'It's an easy way out for her.' There was no sorrowing owner to hear me. There were just the two of us.

And as I murmured, 'Good girl, Amber, good lass,' as she sank down on the straw, I had the conviction that if I had said those things they would have been true. She didn't know a thing between her playfulness and oblivion and it was indeed an easy way out from that prison which would soon become a torture chamber.

I stepped from the pen and switched off the car lights and in the cold darkness the yard had never seemed so empty. After the weeks of struggle the sense of loss and of failure was overpowering, but at the end I was at least able to spare Amber the ultimate miseries: the internal abscesses and septicaemia which await a dog suffering from a progressive and incurable demodectic mange.

For a long time I carried a weight around with me, and I feel some of it now after all these years. Because the tragedy of Amber was that she was born too soon. At the present time we can cure most cases of demodectic mange by a long course of organo-phosphates and antibiotics, but neither of these things were available then when I needed them.

It is still a dread condition, but we have fought patiently with our modern weapons and won most of the battles over the past few years. I know several fine dogs in Darrowby who have survived, and when I see them in the streets, healthy and

glossy-coated, the picture of Amber comes back into my mind.
It is always dark and she is always in the headlights' beam.

Sister Rose was based on another Sister, Ann Lilley, who ran
several small animal sanctuaries in North Yorkshire and who
dedicated her life to caring for homeless animals. She also helped
to set up the Jerry Green Centre for cats and dogs at Catton
near Thirsk. There, Alf had become very attached to a golden
retriever cared for by Sister Ann Lilley but which sadly died.

James sees other dogs who come from happy homes but
who repeatedly get themselves into trouble, usually by eating
something they shouldn't. Brandy is a golden Labrador who
likes nothing more than to root through dustbins only to emerge
with a tin can wedged on his face.

In the semi-darkness of the surgery passage I thought it was a
hideous growth dangling from the side of the dog's face but
as he came closer I saw that it was only a condensed milk can.
Not that condensed milk cans are commonly found sprouting
from dogs' cheeks, but I was relieved because I knew I was
dealing with Brandy again.

I hoisted him onto the table. 'Brandy, you've been at the
dustbin again.'

The big golden Labrador gave me an apologetic grin and
did his best to lick my face. He couldn't manage it since his
tongue was jammed inside the can, but he made up for it by a
furious wagging of tail and rear end.

'Oh, Mr Herriot, I am sorry to trouble you again.' Mrs Westby,
his attractive young mistress, smiled ruefully. 'He just won't
keep out of that dustbin. Sometimes the children and I can get
the cans off ourselves but this one is stuck fast. His tongue is
trapped under the lid.'

'Yes . . . yes . . .' I eased my finger along the jagged edge of the metal. 'It's a bit tricky, isn't it? We don't want to cut his mouth.'

As I reached for a pair of forceps I thought of the many other occasions when I had done something like this for Brandy. He was one of my patients, a huge, lolloping, slightly goofy animal, but this dustbin raiding was becoming an obsession.

He liked to fish out a can and lick out the tasty remnants, but his licking was carried out with such sudden dedication that he burrowed deeper and deeper until he got stuck. Again and again he had been freed by his family or myself from fruit salad cans, corned beef cans, baked bean cans, soup cans. There didn't seem to be any kind of can he didn't like.

I gripped the edge of the lid with my forceps and gently bent it back along its length till I was able to lift it away from the tongue. An instant later, that tongue was slobbering all over my cheek as Brandy expressed his delight and thanks.

'Get back, you daft dog!' I said, laughing, as I held the panting face away from me.

'Yes, come down, Brandy.' Mrs Westby hauled him from the table and spoke sharply. 'It's all very fine making a fuss now, but you're becoming a nuisance with this business. It will have to stop.'

The scolding had no effect on the lashing tail and I saw that his mistress was smiling. You just couldn't help liking Brandy, because he was a great ball of affection and tolerance without an ounce of malice in him.

Along with his fondness for dustbins, Brandy has other peculiar traits. While walking his dog in Darrowby, James often sees him playing in the fields and one day witnesses something extraordinary.

There is a little children's playground in one corner — a few swings, a roundabout and a slide. Brandy was disporting himself on the slide.

For this activity he had assumed an uncharacteristic gravity of expression and stood calmly in the queue of children. When his turn came he mounted the steps, slid down the metal slope, all dignity and importance, then took a staid walk round to rejoin the queue.

The little boys and girls who were his companions seemed to take him for granted, but I found it difficult to tear myself away. I could have watched him all day.

The character of Brandy is a composite of a few dogs Alf knew, including a golden retriever called Moses who also loved to go down the slides in playgrounds. The dog belonged to locals John and Sue Garside, who are still close friends with the Wight family and John worked with Alf's daughter Rosie as a GP in Thirsk. Jim also remembers one particular dog coming into the practice with a tin can firmly stuck on his face, although he seemed entirely unfazed by it as he was still rooting about, sniffing and cocking his leg as if nothing had happened. There was another troublesome dog who, living in a pub, constantly ate bar cloths, so much so that Jim and his dad had to operate on him four times to remove the offending articles. Some dogs never learn!

In *Let Sleeping Vets Lie* old Mrs Barker brings her twelve-year-old spaniel into the practice. The dog has a bad infection in her womb and requires an operation. Although James is gradually doing more small animal surgery, the dog is in a bad way, panting and trembling with the signs of a weak heart, and he decides to send her to Granville Bennett, a small animal specialist based in Hartington.

By the end of the 1950s Alf was similarly performing the odd hysterectomy on cats and bitches but he had to send more complex cases to a small animal surgeon, Denton Pette, in Darlington, on whom Granville Bennett is based. Like Granville Bennett, Pette was an immensely skilled surgeon, operating on his small animal patients with great speed and finesse, despite his large, solid bulk. He and his wife Eve were also generous with their hospitality and Alf often ended evenings with them slightly worse for wear, unable to keep up with Pette who had a seemingly indestructible constitution. Alf's son Jim also worked at Pette's practice as a student in 1964 and 1965 and, even as a young man, he could never match the older vet's ability to drink. Despite his fondness for alcohol, Pette was always immaculately dressed and charming with clients, and his focus on family pets rather than farm animals would become increasingly common across veterinary practice from the 1960s onwards.

There was no doubt Granville Bennett had become something of a legend in northern England. In those days when specialization was almost unknown he had gone all out for small animal work – never looked at farm stock – and had set a new standard by the modern procedures in his animal hospital which was run as nearly as possible on human lines. It was, in fact, fashionable for veterinary surgeons of that era to belittle dog and cat work; a lot of the older men who had spent their lives among the teeming thousands of draught horses in city and agriculture would sneer 'Oh I've no time to bother with those damn things.' Bennett had gone dead in the opposite direction.

I had never met him but I knew he was a young man in his early thirties. I had heard a lot about his skill, his business acumen, and about his reputation as a bon viveur. He was, they said, a dedicated devotee of the work-hard-play-hard school.

The Veterinary Hospital was a long low building near the top of a busy street. I drove into a yard and knocked at a door in the corner. I was looking with some awe at a gleaming Bentley dwarfing my own battered little Austin when the door was opened by a pretty receptionist.

'Good evening,' she murmured with a dazzling smile which I thought must be worth another half-crown on the bill for a start. 'Do come in, Mr Bennett is expecting you.'

I was shown into a waiting room with magazines and flowers on a corner table and many impressive photographs of dogs and cats on the walls — taken, I learned later, by the principal himself. I was looking closely at a superb study of two white poodles when I heard a footstep behind me. I turned and had my first view of Granville Bennett.

He seemed to fill the room. Not over tall but of tremendous bulk. Fat, I thought at first, but as he came nearer it seemed to me that the tissue of which he was composed wasn't distributed like fat. He wasn't flabby, he didn't stick out in any particular place, he was just a big wide, solid, hard-looking man. From the middle of a pleasant blunt featured face the most magnificent pipe I had ever seen stuck forth shining and glorious, giving out delicious wisps of expensive smoke. It was an enormous pipe, in fact it would have looked downright silly with a smaller man but on him it was a thing of beauty. I had a final impression of a beautifully cut dark suit and sparkling shirt cuffs as he held out a hand.

'James Herriot!' He said it as somebody else might have said 'Winston Churchill'.

Bennett proceeds to operate on Dinah the spaniel – who is no relation to Alf's real dog Dinah who appears in a later book – expertly removing a mass around her womb within minutes. James watches on, taking in the white-tiled walls and rows of gleaming instruments, and is suddenly reminded that this was the kind of work he had envisaged for himself when he first started training in veterinary practice, and yet here he is, a 'shaggy cow doctor'. But he then realizes that the life he has is one of magical fulfilment: 'I would rather spend my days driving over the unfenced roads of the high country than stooping over that operating table.'

While they wait for the spaniel to wake up from the anaesthetic, the two vets pop into the 'old boys' club' across the road from the practice. Bennett orders pints for them, and drains his with amazing speed, while James desperately tries to keep up, downing four pints in total. They then head to Bennett's house, Granville pushes James towards a leather armchair and disappears off to the kitchen to sort out some grub for them.

Immensely gratified, Granville hurried through to the kitchen again. This time when he came back he bore a tray with an enormous cold roast, a loaf of bread, butter and mustard.

'I think a beef sandwich would go down rather nicely, Jim,' he murmured as he stropped his carving knife on a steel. Then he noticed my glass of whisky still half full.

'C'mon, c'mon, c'mon!' he said with some asperity. 'You're not touching your drink.' He watched me benevolently as I drained the glass then he refilled it to its old level. 'That's better. And have another onion.'

I stretched my legs out and rested my head on the back of the chair in an attempt to ease my internal turmoil. My stomach was a lake of volcanic lava bubbling and popping fiercely in its crater with each additional piece of onion, every sip of whisky setting up a fresh violent reaction. Watching Granville at work, a great wave of nausea swept over me. He was sawing busily at the roast, carving off slices which looked to be an inch thick, slapping mustard on them and enclosing them in the bread. He hummed with contentment as the pile grew. Every now and then he had another onion.

'Now then, laddie,' he cried at length, putting a heaped plate at my elbow. 'Get yourself round that lot.' He took his own supply and collapsed with a sigh into another chair.

He took a gargantuan bite and spoke as he chewed. 'You know Jim, this is something I enjoy — a nice little snack. Zoe always leaves me plenty to go at when she pops out.' He engulfed a further few inches of sandwich. 'And I'll tell you something, though I say it myself, these are bloody good, don't you think so?'

'Yes indeed.' Squaring my shoulders I bit, swallowed and held my breath as another unwanted foreign body slid down to the ferment below.

Just then I heard the front door open.

'Ah, that'll be Zoe,' Granville said and was about to rise when a disgracefully fat Staffordshire bull terrier burst into the room, waddled across the carpet and leaped into his lap.

'Phoebles, my dear, come to daddykins!' he shouted. 'Have you had nice walkies with Mummy?'

The Staffordshire was closely followed by a Yorkshire terrier which was also enthusiastically greeted by Granville.

'Yoo-hoo, Victoria, yoo-hoo!'

The Yorkie, an obvious smiler, did not jump up but contented herself with sitting at her master's feet, baring her teeth ingratiatingly every few seconds.

I smiled through my pain. Another myth exploded; the one about these specialist small animal vets not being fond of dogs themselves. The big man crooned over the two little animals. The fact that he called Phoebe 'Phoebles' was symptomatic.

Alf and Denton Pette became good friends and Alf trusted Pette so much that he asked him to put down one of his much-loved dogs, Hector. A Jack Russell terrier, Hector replaced Alf's previous dog Dinah who had died in 1963. Hector was an immensely energetic dog, who accompanied Alf on his daily rounds, barking as they drove around, and, despite becoming virtually blind aged five or six, he always had a zest for life. Of all the dogs Alf shared his life with, Hector was his favourite and appeared in many photographs with the vet when he became a famous author. With suspected cancer of the oe-sophagus, fourteen-year-old Hector was put to sleep by Denton Pette, who also agreed to bury him in his garden in Aldborough St John.

Cats also feature in the James Herriot books – most farms keep a cat or two, as do the villagers and townsfolk of Darrowby. Alf was used to having cats around and his friend and colleague Brian Sinclair, the real Tristan, had something of a soft spot for the creatures and the pair frequently treated feline patients when they were brought in. Cats can be difficult to catch or handle and Alf took great pride in his technique of 'wrapping' cats so he could examine them, as he did with the stray cat Alfred in *Vet in Harness*.

I had heard of the Bonds, of course. They were Londoners who for some obscure reason had picked on North Yorkshire for their retirement. People said they had a 'bit o' brass' and they had bought an old house on the outskirts of Darrowby where they kept themselves to themselves — and the cats. I had heard that Mrs Bond was in the habit of taking in strays and feeding them and giving them a home if they wanted it and this had predisposed me in her favour, because in my experience the unfortunate feline species seemed to be fair game for every kind of cruelty and neglect. They shot cats, threw things at them, starved them and set their dogs on them for fun. It was good to see somebody taking their side.

My patient on this first visit was no more than a big kitten, a terrified little blob of black and white crouching in a corner.

'He's one of the outside cats,' Mrs Bond boomed.

'Outside cats?'

'Yes. All these you see here are the inside cats. The others are the really wild ones who simply refuse to enter the house. I feed them of course but the only time they come indoors is when they are ill.'

'I see.'

'I've had frightful trouble catching this one. I'm worried about his eyes — there seemed to be a skin growing over them, and I do hope you can do something for him. His name, by the way, is Alfred.'

'Alfred? Ah yes, quite.' I advanced cautiously on the little half-grown animal and was greeted by a waving set of claws and a series of open-mouthed spittings. He was trapped in his corner or he would have been off with the speed of light.

Examining him was going to be a problem. I turned to Mrs Bond. 'Could you let me have a sheet of some kind? An old ironing sheet would do. I'm going to have to wrap him up.'

'Wrap him up?' Mrs Bond looked very doubtful but she

disappeared into another room and returned with a tattered sheet of cotton which looked just right.

I cleared the table of an amazing variety of cat feeding dishes, cat books, cat medicines and spread out the sheet, then I approached my patient again. You can't be in a hurry in a situation like this and it took me perhaps five minutes of wheedling and 'Puss-pussing' while I brought my hand nearer and nearer. When I got as far as being able to stroke his cheek I made a quick grab at the scruff of his neck and finally bore Alfred, protesting bitterly and lashing out in all directions, over to the table. There, still holding tightly to his scruff, I laid him on the sheet and started the wrapping operation.

This is something which has to be done quite often with obstreperous felines and, although I say it, I am rather good at it. The idea is to make a neat, tight roll, leaving the relevant piece of cat exposed; it may be an injured paw, perhaps the tail, and in this case of course the head. I think it was the beginning of Mrs Bond's unquestioning faith in me when she saw me quickly enveloping that cat till all you could see of him was a small black and white head protruding from an immovable cocoon of cloth. He and I were now facing each other, more or less eyeball to eyeball, and Alfred couldn't do a thing about it.

As I say, I rather pride myself on this little expertise and even today my veterinary colleagues have been known to remark: 'Old Herriot may be limited in many respects but by God he can wrap a cat.'

As it turned out, there wasn't a skin growing over Alfred's eyes. There never is.

'He's got a paralysis of the third eyelid, Mrs Bond. Animals have this membrane which flicks across the eye to protect it. In this case it hasn't gone back, probably because the cat is in low condition — maybe had a touch of cat flu or something else which has weakened him. I'll give him an injection of vitamins and leave you some powder to put in his food if you could keep him in for a few days. I think he'll be all right in a week or two.'

James visits Mrs Bond many more times, as she adds more stray cats to her collection, naming many of the toms after Arsenal players. James is adept at coaxing nervous cats out of their hiding places, knowing that it's mainly fear that makes them lash out. Boris, however, is particularly ferocious.

Boris was an enormous blue-black member of the outside cats and my bête noire in more senses than one. I always cherished a private conviction that he had escaped from a zoo; I had never seen a domestic cat with such sleek, writhing muscles, such dedicated ferocity. I'm sure there was a bit of puma in Boris somewhere.

It had been a sad day for the cat colony when he turned up. I have always found it difficult to dislike any animal; most of the ones which try to do us a mischief are activated by fear, but Boris was different; he was a malevolent bully and after his arrival the frequency of my visits increased because of his habit of regularly beating up his colleagues. I was forever stitching up tattered ears, dressing gnawed limbs.

We had one trial of strength fairly early. Mrs Bond wanted me to give him a worm dose and I had the little tablet all ready held in forceps. How I ever got hold of him I don't quite know, but I hustled him onto the table and did my wrapping act at lightning speed, swathing him in roll upon roll of stout material. Just for a few seconds I thought I had him as he stared up at me, his great brilliant eyes full of hate. But as I pushed my loaded forceps into his mouth he clamped his teeth viciously down on them and I could feel claws of amazing power tearing inside the sheet. It was all over in moments. A long leg shot out and ripped its way down my wrist, I let go my tight hold of the neck and in a flash Boris sank his teeth through the gauntlet into the ball of my thumb and was away. I was left standing there stupidly, holding the fragmented worm tablet in a bleeding hand and looking at the bunch of ribbons which had once been my wrapping sheet. From then on Boris loathed the very sight of me and the feeling was mutual.

In *Vet in a Spin* a teenage girl brings in a badly injured tabby cat. As it appears to be a stray, no one is sure how it has been injured. It may have been hit by a car or even struck or kicked by a person – such acts of cruelty a sad and all-too-common occurrence with cats. Alf and Donald, like most veterinary practices, saw their fair share of strays brought in by the public – including injured cats, birds, and even hedgehogs, which they would have to treat for free unless someone claimed them.

'It's a cat,' Tristan said. He pulled back a fold of the blanket and I looked down at a large, deeply striped tabby. At least he would have been large if he had had any flesh on his bones, but ribs and pelvis stood out painfully through the fur and as I passed my hand over the motionless body I could feel only a thin covering of skin.

Tristan cleared his throat. 'There's something else, Jim.'

I looked at him curiously. For once he didn't seem to have a joke in him. I watched as he gently lifted one of the cat's hind legs and rolled the abdomen into view. There was a gash on the ventral surface through which a coiled cluster of intestines spilled grotesquely onto the cloth. I was still shocked and staring when the girl spoke.

'I saw this cat sittin' in the dark, down Brown's yard. I thought 'e looked skinny, like, and a bit quiet and I bent down to give 'im a pat. Then I saw 'e was badly hurt and I went home for a blanket and brought 'im round to you.'

'That was kind of you,' I said. 'Have you any idea who he belongs to?'

The girl shook her head. 'No, he looks like a stray to me.'

The cat is so badly injured, with its intestines spilling out and covered in dirt, that the kindest plan is to put the poor thing out of its misery. But when Tristan gently strokes the cheek of the cat, he and James are astonished to hear it purr. Tristan insists they do what they can to clean and stitch up the perforated intestines, aware that they're probably fighting a lost cause.

Two hours and yards of catgut later, we dusted the patched-up peritoneal surface with sulphonamide and pushed the entire mass back into the abdomen. When I had sutured muscle layers and skin everything looked tidy but I had a nasty feeling of sweeping undesirable things under the carpet. The extensive damage, all that contamination — peritonitis was inevitable.

'He's alive, anyway, Triss,' I said as we began to wash the instruments. 'We'll put him on to sulphapyridine and keep our fingers crossed.' There were still no antibiotics at that time but the new drug was a big advance.

The door opened and Helen came in. 'You've been a long time, Jim.' She walked over to the table and looked down at the sleeping cat. 'What a poor skinny little thing. He's all bones.'

'You should have seen him when he came in.' Tristan

switched off the sterilizer and screwed shut the valve on the anaesthetic machine. 'He looks a lot better now.'

She stroked the little animal for a moment. 'Is he badly injured?'

'I'm afraid so, Helen,' I said. 'We've done our best for him but I honestly don't think he has much chance.'

'What a shame. And he's pretty, too. Four white feet and all those unusual colours.' With her finger she traced the faint bands of auburn and copper-gold among the grey and black.

Tristan laughed. 'Yes, I think that chap has a ginger tom somewhere in his ancestry.'

Helen smiled, too, but absently, and I noticed a broody look about her. She hurried out to the stock room and returned with an empty box.

'Yes . . . yes . . .' she said thoughtfully. 'I can make a bed in this box for him and he'll sleep in our room, Jim.'

'He will?'

'Yes, he must be warm, mustn't he?'

'Of course.'

Later, in the darkness of our bed-sitter, I looked from my pillow at a cosy scene; Sam in his basket on one side of the flickering fire and the cat cushioned and blanketed in his box on the other.

As I floated off into sleep it was good to know that my patient was so comfortable, but I wondered if he would be alive in the morning . . .

Over the next few days, Helen assiduously tends to the weak cat, spooning in milk, baby foods and various liquids. The cat remains entirely still, day after day, but still purrs, until eventually he gets up and gradually grows into the handsome cat he once was. Helen decides she wants to keep him and to call him Oscar and from that day 'his purr became part of our lives'. He becomes firm friends with their dog Sam, but they constantly worry when he keeps disappearing. They then realize that when he goes missing, he is in fact visiting the pub, the church house and various places around town – he is simply a sociable cat, known to many in town, and always returns to Skeldale House.

From that night our delight in him increased. There was endless joy in watching this facet of his character unfolding.

He did the social round meticulously, taking in most of the activities of the town. He became a familiar figure at whist drives, jumble sales, school concerts and scout bazaars. Most of the time he was made welcome, but was twice ejected from meetings of the Rural District Council who did not seem to relish the idea of a cat sitting in on their deliberations.

At first I was apprehensive about his making his way through the streets but I watched him once or twice and saw that he looked both ways before tripping daintily across. Clearly he had excellent traffic sense and this made me feel that his original injury had not been caused by a car.

Taking it all in all, Helen and I felt that it was a kind stroke of fortune which had brought Oscar to us. He was a warm and cherished part of our home life. He added to our happiness.

When the blow fell it was totally unexpected.

I was finishing the evening surgery. I looked round the door and saw only a man and two little boys.

'Next, please,' I said.

The man stood up. He had no animal with him. He was middle-aged, with the rough weathered face of a farm worker.

He twirled a cloth cap nervously in his hands.

'Mr Herriot?' he said.

'Yes, what can I do for you?'

He swallowed and looked me straight in the eyes. 'Ah think you've got ma cat.'

'What?'

'Ah lost ma cat a bit since.' He cleared his throat. 'We used to live at Missdon but ah got a job as ploughman to Mr Horne of Wederly. It was after we moved to Wederly that t'cat went missin'. Ah reckon he was tryin' to find 'is way back to his old home.'

'Wederly? That's on the other side of Brawton — over thirty miles away.'

'Aye, ah knaw, but cats is funny things.'

'But what makes you think I've got him?'

He twisted the cap around a bit more. 'There's a cousin o' mine lives in Darrowby and ah heard tell from 'im about this cat that goes around to meetin's. I 'ad to come. We've been huntin' everywhere.'

'Tell me,' I said. 'This cat you lost. What did he look like?'

'Grey and black and sort o' gingery. Right bonny 'e was. And 'e was allus goin' out to gatherin's.'

A cold hand clutched at my heart. 'You'd better come upstairs. Bring the boys with you.'

Helen was putting some coal on the fire of the bed-sitter.

'Helen,' I said. 'This is Mr — er — I'm sorry, I don't know your name.'

'Gibbons, Sep Gibbons. They called me Septimus because ah was the seventh in family and it looks like ah'm goin' t'same way 'cause we've got six already. These are our two youngest.' The two boys, obvious twins of about eight, looked up at us solemnly.

I wished my heart would stop hammering. 'Mr Gibbons thinks Oscar is his. He lost his cat some time ago.'

My wife put down her little shovel. 'Oh . . . oh . . . I see.' She stood very still for a moment then smiled faintly. 'Do sit down. Oscar's in the kitchen, I'll bring him through.'

She went out and reappeared with the cat in her arms. She hadn't got through the door before the little boys gave tongue. 'Tiger!' they cried. 'Oh, Tiger, Tiger!'

The man's face seemed lit from within. He walked quickly across the floor and ran his big work-roughened hand along the fur.

'Hullo, awd lad,' he said, and turned to me with a radiant smile. 'It's 'im, Mr Herriot. It's 'im awright, and don't 'e look well!'

With heavy hearts, Helen and James return Oscar to his original owners but Helen is particularly upset about having to let him go. The story was inspired by a real stray cat, also named Oscar, which turned up at Alf and Joan's house. He stayed for a few weeks but sadly disappeared, never to be seen again.

After Oscar left their lives, no more cats would live with Alf until he and Joan were visited by two strays, which made themselves at home in a log shed in the garden of their house in Thirlby. This feline pair, Olly and Ginny, star in *Every Living Thing*.

During the next few weeks they came close to Helen as she fed them but fled immediately at the sight of me. All my attempts to catch Ginny to remove the single little stitch in her spay incision were fruitless. That stitch remained for ever and I realized that Herriot had been cast firmly as the villain of the piece, the character who would grab you and bundle you into a wire cage if you gave him half a chance.

It soon became clear that things were going to stay that way because, as the months passed and Helen plied them with all manner of titbits and they grew into truly handsome, sleek cats, they would come arching along the wall top when she appeared at the back door, but I had only to poke my head from the door to send them streaking away out of sight. I was the chap to be avoided at all times and this rankled with me because I have always been fond of cats and I had become particularly attached to these two. The day finally arrived when Helen was able to stroke them gently as they ate and my chagrin deepened at the sight.

Usually they slept in the log shed but occasionally they disappeared to somewhere unknown and stayed away for a few days and we used to wonder if they had abandoned us or if something had happened to them. When they reappeared, Helen would shout to me in great relief, 'They're back, Jim, they're back!' They had become part of our lives.

Summer lengthened into autumn and when the bitter Yorkshire winter set in we marvelled at their hardiness. We used to feel terrible, looking at them from our warm kitchen as they sat out in the frost and snow, but no matter how harsh the weather, nothing would induce either of them to set foot inside the house. Warmth and comfort had no appeal for them.

When the weather was fine we had a lot of fun just watching them. We could see right up into the log shed from our kitchen, and it was fascinating to observe their happy relationship. They were such friends. Totally inseparable, they spent hours licking each other and rolling about together in gentle play and they never pushed each other out of the way when they were given their food. At nights we could see the two furry little forms curled close together in the straw.

Months pass without any thawing of relations between James and the two stray cats. The vet then notices that Olly's fur is becoming knotted and tangled and resolves to catch him so he can take the cat down to the surgery. He leaves his favourite food, raw haddock, on the wall, and an open cage nearby. As the cat eats it, Helen strokes him and then James manages to grab him by the scruff of the neck and somehow thrust him into the cage 'amid a flurry of flailing black limbs'. At the surgery, under anaesthetic, they snip, trim and clip, and he emerges with lustrous smooth fur. Olly, however, distrusts James even more, scurrying away whenever he opens the back door. James, nonetheless, gradually and very cautiously starts feeding the cats, until Olly eventually allows James to stroke him.

Tragedy strikes when Olly is discovered in the garden having suffered some kind of stroke or seizure, from which he never recovers. It's a huge blow, particularly for Ginny who is now entirely alone, and James and Helen are distressed to see her looking for Olly for weeks afterwards. James resolves to make friends with Ginny, but he knows he's taking on a long and maybe hopeless challenge.

For a long time, although she accepted the food from me, she would not let me near her. Then, maybe because she needed companionship so desperately that she felt she might as well even resort to me, the day came when she did not back away but allowed me to touch her cheek with my finger as I had done with Olly.

After that, progress was slow but steady. From touching I moved week by week to stroking her cheek then to gently rubbing her ears, until finally I could run my hand the length of her body and tickle the root of her tail. From then on, undreamed-of familiarities gradually unfolded until she would not look at her food until she had paced up and down the wall top, again and again, arching herself in delight against my hand

and brushing my shoulders with her body. Among these daily courtesies one of her favourite ploys was to press her nose against mine and stand there for several moments looking into my eyes.

It was one morning several months later that Ginny and I were in this posture — she on the wall, touching noses with me, gazing into my eyes, drinking me in as though she thought I was rather wonderful and couldn't quite get enough of me — when I heard a sound from behind me.

'I was just watching the veterinary surgeon at work,' Helen said softly.

'Happy work, too,' I said, not moving from my position, looking deeply into the green eyes, alight with friendship, fixed on mine a few inches away. 'I'll have you know that this is one of my greatest triumphs.'

Chapter 10

NEVER FAILS *to* GIVE RELIEF

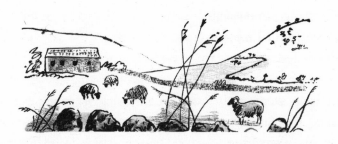

Farnon led me to the first of several doors which opened off a passage where the smell of ether and carbolic hung on the air. 'This,' he said, with a secret gleam in his eye as though he were about to unveil the mysteries of Aladdin's cave, 'is the dispensary.'

The dispensary was an important place in the days before penicillin and the sulphonamides. Rows of gleaming Winchester bottles lined the white walls from floor to ceiling. I savoured the familiar names: Sweet Spirits of Nitre, Tincture of Camphor, Chlorodyne, Formalin, Salammoniac, Hexamine, Sugar of Lead, Linimentum Album, Perchloride of Mercury, Red Blister. The lines of labels were comforting.

I was an initiate among old friends. I had painfully accumulated their lore, ferreting out their secrets over the years. I knew their origins, actions and uses, and their maddeningly varied dosage. The examiner's voice — 'And what is the dose for the horse? — and the cow? — and the sheep? — and the pig? — and the dog? — and the cat?'

These shelves held the vet's entire armoury against disease and, on a bench under the window, I could see the instruments for compounding them; the graduated vessels and beakers, the mortars and pestles. And underneath, in an open cupboard, the medicine bottles, piles of corks of all sizes, pill boxes, powder papers.

The dispensary that Siegfried proudly shows to James in *If Only They Could Talk* belongs to a bygone era, when veterinary surgeons relied upon a variety of age-old remedies to treat their animals, with varying success. Antibiotics, vaccines and modern drugs were on the horizon but were yet to revolutionize veterinary treatment and in the pre-war years veterinary surgeons were working much as they had for decades. Instead of injecting drugs, vets often dispensed liquids that they or a farmer would pour down the throat of an animal – known as drenching – with the use of bottles or drenching horns. For skin conditions, they might slaver on tar or diesel oil or apply mustard plasters to an animal's chest if it had pneumonia. The James Herriot books provide a fascinating insight into this former world and chronicle the huge impact the introduction of new drugs and methods had on veterinary practice in the 1930s and post-war years.

As we moved around, Farnon's manner became more and more animated. His eyes glittered and he talked rapidly. Often, he reached up and caressed a Winchester on its shelf; or he would lift out a horse ball or an electuary from its box, give it a friendly pat and replace it with tenderness.

'Look at this stuff, Herriot,' he shouted without warning. 'Adrevan! This is the remedy, par excellence, for red worms in horses. A bit expensive, mind you — ten bob a packet. And these gentian violet pessaries. If you shove one of these into a cow's uterus after a dirty cleansing, it turns the discharges a very pretty colour. Really looks as though it's doing something. And have you seen this trick?'

He placed a few crystals of resublimated iodine on a glass dish and added a drop of turpentine. Nothing happened for a second, then a dense cloud of purple smoke rolled heavily to the ceiling. He gave a great bellow of laughter at my startled face.

'Like witchcraft, isn't it? I use it for wounds in horses' feet. The chemical reaction drives the iodine deep into the tissues.'

'It does?'

'Well, I don't know, but that's the theory, and anyway, you must admit it looks wonderful. Impresses the toughest client.'

Some of the bottles on the shelves fell short of the ethical standards I had learned in college. Like the one labelled 'Colic Drench' and featuring a floridly drawn picture of a horse rolling in agony. The animal's face was turned outwards and wore an expression of very human anguish. Another bore the legend 'Universal Cattle Medicine' in ornate script — 'A sovereign Remedy for coughs, chills, scours, pneumonia, milk fever, gargett and all forms of indigestion.' At the bottom of the label, in flaring black capitals, was the assurance, 'Never Fails to Give Relief'.

Farnon had something to say about most of the drugs. Each one had its place in his five years' experience of practice; they all had their fascination, their individual mystique. Many of the bottles were beautifully shaped, with heavy glass stoppers and their Latin names cut deeply into their sides; names familiar to physicians for centuries, gathering fables through the years.

The two of us stood gazing at the gleaming rows without any idea that it was nearly all useless and that the days of the old medicines were nearly over. Soon they would be hustled into oblivion by the headlong rush of the new discoveries and they would never return.

'This is where we keep the instruments.' Farnon showed me into another little room. The small animal equipment lay on green baize shelves, very neat and impressively clean. Hypodermic syringes, whelping forceps, tooth scalers, probes, searchers and, in a place of prominence, an ophthalmoscope.

Farnon lifted it lovingly from its black box. 'My latest purchase,' he murmured, stroking its smooth shaft. 'Wonderful thing. Here, have a peep at my retina.'

I switched on the bulb and gazed with interest at the glistening, coloured tapestry in the depths of his eye. 'Very pretty. I could write you a certificate of soundness.'

He laughed and thumped my shoulder. 'Good, I'm glad to hear it. I always fancied I had a touch of cataract in that one.'

He began to show me the large animal instruments which hung from hooks on the walls. Docking and firing irons, bloodless castrators, emasculators, casting ropes and hobbles, calving ropes and hooks. A new, silvery embryotome hung in the place of honour, but many of the instruments, like the drugs, were museum pieces. Particularly the blood stick and fleam, a relic of medieval times, but still used to bring the rich blood spouting into a bucket.

In the early days of veterinary practice, vets were also required to mix up potions and powders to their own recipes. 'Materia medica', as it was called at veterinary college (today known as pharmacology), formed a key part of the curriculum in the 1930s and 1940s, and required students to learn the different medicines, liquids and relevant doses. When he was a student, it was Alf Wight's least favourite subject, partly because he hadn't taken science as a Higher at school and he had a poor grasp of maths, which was critical when working out the doses of medicines that might contain arsenic, turpentine and a variety of toxic substances.

The job of grinding, weighing and mixing up potions often fell to the more junior members of the practice, as is the case at Skeldale House, where James and Tristan are frequently found blending up concoctions in the dispensary.

Looking back, I can scarcely believe we used to spend all those hours in making up medicines. But our drugs didn't come to us in proprietary packages and before we could get out on the road we had to fill our cars with a wide variety of carefully compounded and largely useless remedies.

When Siegfried came upon me that morning I was holding a twelve-ounce bottle at eye level while I poured syrup of coccilana into it. Tristan was moodily mixing stomach powders with a mortar and pestle and he stepped up his speed of stroke when he saw his brother's eye on him. He was surrounded by packets of the powder and, further along the bench, were orderly piles of pessaries which he had made by filling cellophane cylinders with boric acid.

Armed with their various pills and potions, James and Siegfried then administer them to the farm animals of the Dales, exactly as Alf and Donald did in the late 1930s. Dispensary staples included stomach powders and bloat drenches which they gave cattle to reduce the potentially lethal build-up of gases in their digestive tracts which caused them to bloat up (a condition less frequently seen today as much more is known about cattle nutrition). For horses and cattle that had 'stoppages' in their bowels, they would pour liquid paraffin or castor oil down their throats in order to get things moving again.

In the early days, Alf used great quantities of the antiseptic Acriflavine to wash out stomachs and to clean wounds or various orifices. Jim also remembers that his dad had one glass syringe – rather than the hundreds of disposable syringes used by vets today – which was stored in a black plastic cylindrical container filled with surgical spirit along with a supply of metal needles. Stimulant medicines were also a staple of the dispensary, including 'Universal Cattle Medicine', a rich red fluid that consti- tuted the last line of defence in the battle with animal disease.

> It was a pity it didn't do any good because there was something compelling about its ruby depths when you held it up to the light and about the solid camphor-ammonia jolt when you sniffed at it and which made the farmers blink and shake their heads and say 'By gaw, that's powerful stuff,' with deep respect. But our specific remedies were so few and the possibilities of error so plentiful that it was comforting in cases of doubt to be able to hand over a bottle of the old standby. Whenever an entry of Siegfried's or mine appeared in the day book stating 'Visit attend cow, advice, 1 UCM' it was a pretty fair bet we didn't know what was wrong with the animal.

Alf Wight and Donald Sinclair regularly resorted to using Universal Cattle Medicine for a variety of bovine complaints. Cows might splutter after being drenched with the stuff – unsurprising as it consisted, amongst other things, of ammonia and arsenic – but its stimulant properties often helped. Its powerful odour meant that just sniffing it was enough for most people but there was one raucous night at the Thirsk practice when Donald, after a few too many drinks, decided to take a few swigs from the bottle of UCM as a form of self-medication. Clutching his throat, he then staggered out into the garden and collapsed in the flowerbed. Thankfully, Donald survived the incident but it didn't stop his younger brother Brian recreating the whole event in the pub afterwards. Lying on the floor, twitching and convulsing, the theatrics soon became a regular party piece of Brian's, as entertaining as his 'mad conductor'.

The arrival of James Herriot comes with a certain amount of expectation by the farmers in the region, not least that the newly qualified vet will be acquainted with some of the modern drugs they've heard about. Dairy farmer Phin Calvert – who was based on the real farmer Fred Thompson, known by everyone as Atom Thompson – is hoping the young vet will come up with 'summat real and scientific like' when James visits to look at his sickly calves. But sometimes the old remedies work just as well and, having diagnosed lead poisoning, James prescribes Epsom salts, which work as an effective antidote to the poisoning, and the calves soon recover. James is then called in again to Mr Calvert's, this time to see his prized pedigree shorthorn bull who's 'puffin' like a bellows'.

The bull was standing as though rooted to the middle of the pen. His great ribcage rose and fell with the most laboured respirations I had ever seen. His mouth gaped wide, a bubbling foam hung round his lips and his flaring nostrils; his eyes, almost starting from his head in terror, stared at the wall in front of him. This wasn't pneumonia, it was a frantic battle for breath; and it looked like a losing one.

He didn't move when I inserted my thermometer and though my mind was racing I suspected the half-minute wasn't going to be long enough this time. I had expected accelerated breathing, but nothing like this.

'Poor aud beggar,' Phin muttered. 'He's bred me the finest calves I've ever had and he's as quiet as a sheep, too. I've seen me little grandchildren walk under 'is belly and he's took no notice. I hate to see him sufferin' like this. If you can't do no good, just tell me and I'll get the gun out.'

I took the thermometer out and read it. One hundred and ten degrees Fahrenheit. This was ridiculous; I shook it vigorously and pushed it back into the rectum.

I gave it nearly a minute this time so that I could get in some extra thinking. The second reading said a hundred and ten again and I had an unpleasant conviction that if the thermometer had been a foot long the mercury would still have been jammed against the top.

What in the name of God was this? Could be anthrax . . . must be . . . and yet . . . I looked over at the row of heads above the half door; they were waiting for me to say something and their silence accentuated the agonized groaning and panting. I looked above the heads to the square of deep blue and a tufted cloud moving across the sun. As it passed, a single dazzling ray made me close my eyes and a faint bell rang in my mind.

'Has he been out today?' I asked.

'Aye, he's been out on the grass on his tether all morning. It was that grand and warm.'

The bell became a triumphant gong. 'Get a hosepipe in here quick. You can rig it to that tap in the yard.'

'A hosepipe? What the 'ell . . .?'

'Yes, quick as you can — he's got sunstroke.'

They had the hose fixed in less than a minute. I turned it full on and began to play the jet of cold water all over the huge form — his face and neck, along the ribs, up and down the legs. I kept this up for about five minutes but it seemed a lot longer as I waited for some sign of improvement. I was beginning to think I was on the wrong track when the bull gulped just once.

It was something – he had been unable to swallow his saliva before in his desperate efforts to get the air into his lungs; and I really began to notice a change in the big animal. Surely he was looking just a little less distressed and wasn't the breathing slowing down a bit?

Then the bull shook himself, turned his head and looked at us. There was an awed whisper from one of the young men: 'By gaw, it's working!'

I enjoyed myself after that. I can't think of anything in my working life that has given me more pleasure than standing in that pen directing the life-saving jet and watching the bull savouring it. He liked it on his face best and as I worked my way up from the tail and along the steaming back he would turn his nose full into the water, rocking his head from side to side and blinking blissfully.

Within half an hour he looked almost normal. His chest was still heaving a little but he was in no discomfort. I tried the temperature again. Down to a hundred and five.

'He'll be all right now,' I said. 'But I think one of the lads should keep the water on him for another twenty minutes or so. I'll have to go now.'

Phin Calvert offers James a drink before he goes and, sitting in the farm kitchen, he is a little lost for words over the miraculous recovery of his bull. However, he soon finds his voice again at the next meeting of the farmers' discussion group, where various gentlemen are discussing the latest advances in veterinary medicine. It's all too much for Phin and he jumps up and cries: 'Ah think you're talking a lot of rubbish. There's a young feller in Darrowby not long out of college and it doesn't matter what you call 'im out for he uses nowt but Epsom salts and cold water.'

Much of Siegfried's and James's work is undertaken in stables, cow byres or fields, with owners helping to hold their animals or looking on, meaning they must also witness various medical procedures and the gore that goes with it. Most farmers are able to cope with the more visceral aspects of animal husbandry but there are some – and it's often the big, burly types – who grow weak at the knees at the sight of a needle or blood.

So this morning I looked with satisfaction at the two men holding the cow. It wasn't a difficult job — just an intravenous injection of magnesium lactate — but still it was reassuring to have two such sturdy fellows to help me. Maurice Bennison, medium-sized but as tough as one of his own hill beasts, had a horn in his right hand while the fingers of his left gripped the nose; I had the comfortable impression that the cow wouldn't jump very far when I pushed the needle in. His brother George, whose job it was to raise the vein, held the choke rope limply in enormous hands like bunches of carrots. He grinned down at me amiably from his six feet four inches.

'Right, George,' I said. 'Tighten up that rope and lean against the cow to stop her coming round on me.' I pushed my way between the cow and her neighbour, past George's unyielding bulk and bent over the jugular vein. It was standing out very nicely. I poised the needle, feeling the big man's elbow on me as he peered over my shoulder, and thrust quickly into the vein.

'Lovely!' I cried as the dark blood fountained out and spattered thickly on the straw bedding beneath. 'Slacken your rope,

George.' I fumbled in my pocket for the flutter valve. 'And for God's sake, get your weight off me!'

Because George had apparently decided to rest his full fourteen stones on me instead of the cow, and as I tried desperately to connect the tube to the needle I felt my knees giving way. I shouted again, despairingly, but he was inert, his chin resting on my shoulder, his breathing stertorous in my ear.

There could only be one end to it. I fell flat on my face and lay there writhing under the motionless body. My cries went unheeded; George was unconscious.

Mr Bennison, attracted by the commotion, came into the byre just in time to see me crawling out from beneath his eldest son. 'Get him out, quick!' I gasped, 'before the cows trample on him.' Wordlessly, Maurice and his father took an ankle apiece and hauled away in unison. George shot out from under the cows, his head beating a brisk tattoo on the cobbles, traversed the dung channel, then resumed his sleep on the byre floor.

Mr Bennison moved back to the cow and waited for me to continue with my injection but I found the presence of the sprawled body distracting. 'Look, couldn't we sit him up against the wall and put his head between his legs?' I suggested apologetically. The others glanced at each other then, as though deciding to humour me, grabbed George's shoulders and trundled him over the floor with the expertise of men used to throwing around bags of fertilizer and potatoes. But even propped against the rough stones, his head slumped forward and his great long arms hanging loosely, the poor fellow still didn't look so good.

I couldn't help feeling a bit responsible. 'Don't you think we might give him a drink?'

But Mr Bennison had had enough. 'Nay, nay, he'll be right,'

he muttered testily. 'Let's get on with t'job.' Evidently he felt he had pampered George too much already.

The incident started me thinking about this question of people's reactions to the sight of blood and other disturbing realities. Even though it was only my second year of practice I had already formulated rules about this and one was that it was always the biggest men who went down. (I had, by this time, worked out a few other, perhaps unscientific theories, e.g. big dogs were kept by people who lived in little houses and vice versa. Clients who said 'spare no expense' never paid their bills, ever. When I asked my way in the Dales and was told 'you can't miss it', I knew I'd soon be hopelessly lost.)

I had begun to wonder if perhaps country folk, despite their closer contact with fundamental things, were perhaps more susceptible than city people. Ever since Sid Blenkhorn had staggered into Skeldale House one evening. His face was ghastly white and he had obviously passed through a shattering experience. 'Have you got a drop o' whisky handy, Jim?' he quavered, and when I had guided him to a chair and Siegfried had put a glass in his hand he told us he had been at a first aid lecture given by Dr Allinson, a few doors down the street. 'He was talking about veins and arteries and things,' groaned Sid, passing a hand across his forehead. 'God, it was awful!' Apparently Fred Ellison the fishmonger had been carried out unconscious after only ten minutes and Sid himself had only just made it to the door. It had been a shambles.

I was interested because this sort of thing, I had found, was always just round the corner. I suppose we must have more trouble in this way than the doctors because in most cases when our medical colleagues have any cutting or carving to do they send their patients to hospital while the vets just have to get their jackets off and operate on the spot. It means that the owners and attendants of the animals are pulled in as helpers and are subjected to some unusual sights.

A veterinary surgeon must also be paid and this sometimes proved a problem for Alf and Donald at the Thirsk practice. Most clients paid their bills on time but there were the stubborn few who racked up debt with the practice or resented having to pay veterinary bills, particularly when the National Health Service was launched in 1948 and doctors were no longer charging for their services. Bill-paying days were often accompanied with the usual grumbles, that the practice had been 'ower heavy wi' t'pen' or they wanted a 'bit knockin' off'.

Alf loved his work, but neither he nor Donald were businesspeople and often exclaimed: 'Why can't I just drive around, doing the job I love and receive a decent sum of money at the end of the week?' James and Siegfried similarly must deal with the 'ten per cent' or so of clients who avoid paying their bills, as James muses upon in *It Shouldn't Happen to a Vet*.

As time passed and I painfully clothed the bare bones of my theoretical knowledge with practical experience I began to realize there was another side to veterinary practice they didn't mention in the books. It had to do with money. Money has always formed a barrier between the farmer and the vet. I think this is because there is a deeply embedded, maybe subconscious conviction in many farmers' minds that they know more about their stock than any outsider and it is an admission of defeat to pay somebody else to doctor them.

The wall was bad enough in those early days when they had to pay the medical practitioners for treating their own ailments and when there was no free agricultural advisory service. But it is worse now when there is the Health Service and NAAS

[an advisory arm of the Ministry of Agriculture] and the veterinary surgeon stands pitilessly exposed as the only man who
has to be paid.

Most farmers, of course, swallow the pill and get out their
cheque books, but there is a proportion — maybe about ten
per cent — who do their best to opt out of the whole business.

We had our own ten per cent in Darrowby and it was a small
but constant irritation. As an assistant I was not financially
involved and it didn't seem to bother Siegfried unduly except
when the quarterly bills were sent out. Then it really got through
to him.

Siegfried goes through the outstanding bills, muttering and
occasionally raging about the non-payers, some of whom he's
seen betting at the races or driving around in brand-new cars.
There are some debtors, however, that he can't help but admire,
including the very charming and erudite Major Bullivant who
for years has got away without paying his vet bills or those
of most of the tradesmen in Darrowby. He eventually leaves
the area, still without paying what he owes, and yet Siegfried
holds little bitterness towards the major.

Siegfried's attitude to his debtors was remarkably ambivalent.
At times he would fly into a fury at the mention of their names,
at others he would regard them with a kind of wry benevolence.
He often said that if ever he threw a cocktail party for the
clients he'd have to invite the non-payers first because they
were all such charming fellows.

Nevertheless he waged an inexorable war against them by
means of a series of letters graduated according to severity
which he called his PNS system (Polite, Nasty, Solicitor's) and
in which he had great faith. It was a sad fact, however, that the

system seldom worked with the real hard cases who were accustomed to receiving threatening letters with their morning mail. These people yawned over the polite and nasty ones and were unimpressed by the solicitor's because they knew from experience that Siegfried always shrank from following through to the limit of the law.

Some clients resent having to call in a veterinary surgeon because they feel they know, or should know, more about caring for their own livestock than any vet. When examining animals on farms, James must frequently deal with farmers and their neighbours pontificating on the ailments of animals – rural folk are often experts when it comes to other people's livestock – who swear by a range of home-spun remedies. James and veterinary surgeons like him must also contend with an army of unqualified practitioners, many of whom had built up thriving businesses and were trusted by local farmers.

Marmaduke Skelton was an object of interest to me long before our paths crossed. For one thing I hadn't thought people were ever called Marmaduke outside of books and for another he was a particularly well-known member of the honourable profession of unqualified animal doctors.

Before the Veterinary Surgeons' Act of 1948 anybody who fancied his chance at it could dabble in the treatment of animal disease. Veterinary students could quite legally be sent out to cases while they were seeing practice, certain members of the lay public did a bit of veterinary work as a sideline while others did it as a full-time job. These last were usually called 'quacks'.

The disparaging nature of the term was often unjust because, though some of them were a menace to the animal population, others were dedicated men who did their job with responsibility and humanity and after the Act were brought into the profession's fold as Veterinary Practitioners.

But long before all this there were all sorts and types among them. The one I knew best was Arthur Lumley, a charming little ex-plumber who ran a thriving small animal practice in Brawton, much to the chagrin of Mr Angus Grier MRCVS. Arthur used to drive around in a small van. He always wore a white coat and looked very clinical and efficient, and on the side of the van in foot-high letters which would have got a qualified man a severe dressing down from the Royal College was the legend, 'Arthur Lumley MKC, Canine and Feline Specialist'. The lack of 'letters' after their name was the one thing which differentiated these men from qualified vets in the eyes of the general public and I was interested to see that Arthur did have an academic attainment. However the degree of MKC was unfamiliar to me and he was somewhat cagey when I asked him about it; I did find out eventually what it stood for; Member of the Kennel Club.

Marmaduke Skelton was a vastly different breed. I had been working long enough round the Scarburn district to become familiar with some of the local history and it seemed that when Mr and Mrs Skelton were producing a family in the early 1900s they must have thought their offspring were destined for great things; they named their four sons Marmaduke, Sebastian, Cornelius and, incredibly, Alonzo. The two middle brothers drove lorries for the Express Dairy and Alonzo was a small farmer; one of my vivid memories is the shock of surprise when I was filling up the forms after his tuberculin test and asked him for his first name. The exotic appellation pronounced in gruff Yorkshire was so incongruous that I thought he was pulling my leg; in fact I was going to make a light comment but something in his eye prompted me to leave it alone.

315

Marmaduke, or Duke as he was invariably called, was the colourful member of the family. I had heard a lot about him on my visits to the Scarburn farms; he was a 'right good hand' at calving, foaling and lambing, and 'as good as any vitnery' in the diagnosis and treatment of animals' ailments. He was also an expert castrator, docker and pig-killer. He made a nice living at his trade and in Ewan Ross he had the ideal professional opposition; a veterinary surgeon who worked only when he felt like it and who didn't bother to go to a case unless he was in the mood. Much as the farmers liked and in many cases revered Ewan, they were often forced to fall back on Duke's services. Ewan was in his fifties and unable to cope with the growing volume of testing in his Scarburn practice. I used to help him out with it and in consequence saw a lot of Ewan and his wife, Ginny.

The flamboyant names of Marmaduke and his brothers were inspired by one of the Thirsk practice clients, Alonzo Cornforth, whose farm Greendales was just a couple of miles outside the town. Alf couldn't get over the fact that a Yorkshire farmer had the rather splendid, but unusual name of Alonzo, which clearly stayed in his mind when he wrote the James Herriot books.

Alf used to help out the real Ewan Ross, who was based on the nearby veterinary surgeon and later great friend, Frank Bingham. Twenty years Alf's senior, Frank was laidback in his approach but immensely experienced, with veterinary skills that frequently impressed Alf. In *Let Sleeping Vets Lie* Ewan Ross is called to a farm to deal with the prolapsed uterus of a cow and James comes with him. On arrival, the farmer Mr Thwaite guiltily tells them that Marmaduke Skelton is in with the cow and that despite having wrestled with the cow for an hour and a half, he is no further forward and 'about buggered an' all'. Ewan at first refuses to interfere until Mr Thwaite begs him to take over, fearing he'll lose one of his best cows. They head to the byre and find an exhausted Duke Skelton stood next to a huge everted uterus, still dangling behind the cow: 'Blood and filth streaked his face and covered his arms and as he stared at us from under his shaggy brows he looked like something from the jungle.' Duke refuses to let the vet help, so Ewan squats on a milking stool, rests against a wall, rolls a cigarette and watches the sweaty, struggling figure a few feet from him.

Duke had got the uterus about halfway back. Grunting and gasping, legs straddled, he had worked the engorged mass inch by inch inside the vulva till he had just about enough cradled in his arms for one last push; and as he stood there taking a breather with the great muscles of his shoulders and arms rigid his immense strength was formidably displayed. But he wasn't as strong as that cow. No man is as strong as a cow and this cow was one of the biggest I had ever seen with a back like a table top and rolls of fat round her tail-head.

I had been in this position myself and I knew what was coming next. I didn't have to wait long. Duke took a long wheezing breath and made his assault, heaving desperately, pushing with arms and chest, and for a second or two he seemed to be winning as the mass disappeared steadily inside. Then the cow gave an almost casual strain and the whole thing welled out again till it hung down bumping against the animal's hocks.

As Duke almost collapsed against her pelvis in the same attitude as when we first came in I felt pity for the man. I found him uncharming but I felt for him. That could easily be me standing there; my jacket and shirt hanging on that nail, my strength ebbing, my sweat mingling with the blood. No man could do what he was trying to do. You could push back a calf bed with the aid of an epidural anaesthetic to stop the straining or you could sling the animal up to a beam with a block and tackle; you couldn't just stand there and do it from scratch as this chap was trying to do.

I was surprised Duke hadn't learned that with all his experience; but apparently it still hadn't dawned on him even now because he was going through all the motions of having another go. This time he got even further — a few more inches inside before the cow popped it out again. The animal appeared to have a sporting streak because there was something premeditated about the way she played her victim along before timing her thrust at the very last moment. Apart from that she seemed somewhat bored by the whole business; in fact with the possible exception of Ewan she was the calmest among us.

Duke was trying again. As he bent over wearily and picked up the gory organ I wondered how often he had done this since he arrived nearly two hours ago. He had guts, there was no doubt. But the end was near. There was a frantic urgency about his movements as though he knew himself it was his last throw and as he yet again neared his goal his grunts changed to an agonized whimpering, an almost tearful sound as though he were appealing to the recalcitrant mass, beseeching it to go away inside and stay away, just this once.

And when the inevitable happened and the poor fellow, panting and shaking, surveyed once more the ruin of his hopes I had the feeling that somebody had to do something.

Mr Thwaite did it. 'You've had enough, Duke,' he said. 'For God's sake come in the house and get cleaned up. Missus'll give you a bit o' dinner and while you're having it Mr Ross'll see what he can do.'

The big man, arms hanging limp by his sides, chest heaving, stared at the farmer for a few seconds then he turned abruptly and snatched his clothes from the wall.

'Aw right,' he said and began to walk slowly towards the door. He stopped opposite Ewan but didn't look at him. 'But ah'll tell you summat, Maister Thwaite. If ah can't put that calf bed back this awd bugger never will.'

James watches in amazement as Ewan effortlessly replaces the uterus back into the cow, with the use of rope, a pig stool, a pound of sugar, a whisky bottle and a beer tray (complete with 'John Smith's Magnet Pale Ale' emblazoned on the side). He loops the rope around the cow's body and pulls, causing it to collapse on top of the stool with her rear end stuck high in the air. He first dusts sugar over the uterus, which causes it to shrink, and then hoists it onto the beer tray. Then, without even breaking a sweat, he pushes the uterus back in, before carefully passing the whisky bottle into the vagina the length of an arm and moving his shoulder vigorously so he can position the uterus correctly in place.

He was drying his hands when the byre door opened and Duke Skelton slouched in. He was washed and dressed, with his red handkerchief knotted again round his neck and he glared fierce-eyed at the cow which, tidied up and unperturbed, looked now just like all the other cows in the row. His lips moved once or twice before he finally found his voice.

'Aye, it's all right for some people,' he snarled. 'Some people with their bloody fancy injections and instruments! It's bloody easy that way, isn't it!' Then he swung round and was gone.

Alf had similarly seen Frank Bingham perform the difficult procedure with the same rudimentary items and with similar finesse.

∾

To keep their dispensary stocked up, James and Siegfried also
receive visits from various company representatives who carry
weighty catalogues of liquids and remedies, each one peculiar
to their own firm. One such representative is Mr Barge, based
on a real company representative, Mr Collinson, known to the
family as 'Collie', who was a regular visitor to the Thirsk
practice. Mr Barge's dignified presence elicits deference even
from Siegfried.

> Nowadays the young men from the pharmaceutical companies
> who call on veterinary surgeons are referred to as 'reps', but
> nobody would have dreamed of applying such a term to Mr
> Barge. He was definitely a 'representative' of Cargill and Sons,
> Manufacturers of Fine Chemicals since 1850, and he was so
> old that he might have been in on the beginning.

After lunch, Siegfried and James browse though Mr Barge's
catalogue of exotic remedies and Siegfried orders fever drinks,
castration clamps and a variety of now obsolete items, Mr
Barge responding gravely to each order 'I do thank you' or
'Thank you indeed'.

> Finally Siegfried lay back in his chair. 'Well now, Mr Barge, I
> think that's it — unless you have anything new.'
> 'As it happens, my dear Mr Farnon, we have.' The eyes in
> the pink face twinkled. 'I can offer you our latest product,
> "Soothitt", an admirable sedative.'
> In an instant Siegfried and I were all attention. Every animal

doctor is keenly interested in sedatives. Anything which makes our patients more amenable is a blessing. Mr Barge extolled the unique properties of Soothitt and we probed for further information.

'How about unmaternal sows?' I asked. 'You know — the kind which savage their young. I don't suppose it's any good for that?'

'My dear young sir,' Mr Barge gave me the kind of sorrowing smile a bishop might bestow on an erring curate, 'Soothitt is a specific for this condition. A single injection to a farrowing sow and you will have no problems.'

'That's great,' I said. 'And does it have any effect on car sickness in dogs?'

The noble old features lit up with quiet triumph. 'Another classical indication, Mr Herriot. Soothitt comes in tablet form for that very purpose.'

'Splendid.' Siegfried drained his cup and stood up. 'Better send us a good supply then. And if you will excuse us, we must start the afternoon round, Mr Barge. Thank you so much for calling.'

Within a week, the new supplies from Cargill and Sons arrive in a wooden chest – including the much-anticipated Soothitt. That same day James decides to try Soothitt on a spaniel who howls like mad every time he's in the back of a car as well as an aggressive sow who is attacking her piglets. The Soothitt has no effect on Gertrude the pig, who seems, if anything, more fierce after injections of the stuff – it's only after she's given two gallons of strong ale that she allows her piglets to suckle from her. Soothitt similarly proves totally ineffective with Coco the spaniel whose howls can still be heard long after his owner next drives past the practice.

Gradually modern drugs began to make their presence felt in veterinary practice and by the early 1940s, vets like Alf could see for themselves just how effective they are in the treatment of disease. In *Vet in Harness*, James visits some very sickly calves belonging to Mr Clark, whose farm is covered in rusting agricultural implements, derelict cars and a converted railway wagon in which the calves are kept. They are suffering from white scour, diarrhoea caused by a lethal bacterial enteritis that once had a depressingly high mortality rate. He tries the usual age-old treatments which 'whiskered veterinary surgeons in top hats and tail coats' had been using a hundred years before, which include astringent powders of chalk, opium and catechu and wrapping each calf in a big sack to ensure they are warm and sheltered. James returns the next day but finds the calves lying motionless on their sides and looking so close to death that Mr Clark calls in the knacker man Mr Mallock. James, however, has some new drugs and suggests he gives them a try.

I took the tin from my pocket and read the label. 'It's called M and B 693, or sulphapyridine, to give it its scientific name. Just came in the post this morning. It's one of a completely new range of drugs — they're called the sulphonamides and we've never had anything like them before. They're supposed to actually kill certain germs, such as the organisms which cause scour.'

Mr Clark took the tin from me and removed the lid. 'A lot of little blue tablets, eh? Well ah've seen a few wonder cures for this ailment but none of 'em's much good — this'll be another, I'll bet.'

'Could be,' I said. 'But there's been a lot of discussion about these sulphonamides in our veterinary journals. They're not

quack remedies, they're a completely fresh field. I wish I could
have tried them on your calves.'

Almost to humour James, Mr Clark agrees to him trying the
new drug, although he and Mr Mallock are convinced it won't
work. Having pounded the tablets with Mrs Clark's potato
masher in the kitchen, James measures out five doses which
he and Mr Clark trickle into each of the calves' mouths. The
next morning, James is stunned to discover the calves much
recovered, now with normal temperatures and standing
munching hay.

I didn't know it at the time but I had witnessed the beginning
of the revolution. It was my first glimpse of the tremendous
therapeutic breakthrough which was to sweep the old remedies
into oblivion. The long rows of ornate glass bottles with their
carved stoppers and Latin inscriptions would not stand on the
dispensary shelves much longer and their names, dearly familiar
for many generations – Sweet Spirits of Nitre, Sal ammoniac,
Tincture of Camphor – would be lost and vanish for ever.

This was the beginning and just around the corner a new
wonder was waiting – penicillin and the other antibiotics. At
last we had something to work with, at last we could use drugs
which we knew were going to do something.

All over the country, probably all over the world at that time,
vets were having these first spectacular results, going through
the same experience as myself; some with cows, some with
dogs and cats, others with valuable racehorses, sheep, pigs in
all kinds of environments. But for me it happened in that old
converted railway wagon among the jumble of rusting junk on
Willie Clark's farm.

Of course it didn't last – not the miraculous part of it anyway.

What I had seen at Willie Clark's was the impact of something new on an entirely unsophisticated bacterial population, but it didn't go on like that. In time the organisms developed a certain amount of resistance and new and stronger sulphonamides and antibiotics had to be produced. And so the battle has continued. We have good results now but no miracles, and I feel I was lucky to be one of the generation which was in at the beginning when the wonderful things did happen.

The arrival of new drugs to combat infection, first with the sulphonamides in the early 1940s, then sulpha drugs in the mid-1940s and a year or two later antibiotics, resulted in something of a golden age for veterinary practice which lasted into the early 1950s. Where once an animal might be sent to the knacker's yard, one injection in the rump might see a complete recovery overnight, much to its owner's delight. However, James has it drummed into him by Siegfried always to give a bleak prognosis for every case, so that if an animal dies, then they're proved right but if a patient recovers – which they did with more frequency with effective drugs – they would be hailed heroes.

By the time of *The Lord God Made Them All*, set in the years immediately after the Second World War, James is more often than not injecting animals with medication rather than pouring it down their throats.

I had had a disturbing morning. Everywhere I had gone I was reminded that I had come back to a world of change, and I did not like change. One old farmer saying 'It's all t'needle now, Mr Herriot' as I injected his cow, had made me look down almost with surprise at the syringe in my hand, realizing suddenly that this was what I was doing most of the time now.

I knew what he meant. Only a few years ago I would have been more likely to have 'drenched' his cow. Grabbed it by the nose and poured a pint of medicine down its throat.

We still carried a special drenching bottle around with us. An empty wine bottle because it had no shoulders and allowed the liquid to run more easily. Often we would mix the medicine with black treacle from the barrel which stood in the corner of most cow byres.

All this was disappearing and the farmer's remark about 'all t'needle' brought it home to me once more that things were never going to be the same again.

A revolution had begun in agriculture and in veterinary practice. Farming had become more scientific and concepts cherished for generations were being abandoned, while in the veterinary world the first trickles of the flood of new advances were being felt.

Previously undreamed-of surgical procedures were being carried out, the sulpha drugs were going full blast and, most exciting of all, the war, with its urgent need for better treatment of wounds, had given a tremendous impetus to the development of Sir Alexander Fleming's discovery of penicillin. This, the first of the antibiotics, was not yet in the hands of the profession except in the form of intra-mammary tubes for the treatment of mastitis, but it was the advance guard of the therapeutic army which was to sweep our old treatments into oblivion.

In the pre-war period, a highly contagious disease known as brucellosis ravaged cattle herds, causing pregnant cows to abort their foetuses or give birth to very weak calves. In *Vet in Harness* brucellosis breaks out at Frank Metcalfe's farm and his cows begin to abort their calves. The only drug James has at his disposal is to inject a mostly ineffective dead vaccine into the herd. A local farmer who reckons he knows better than James also advises that Frank try the quack remedy 'Professor Driscoll's Abortion Cure'. James wearily agrees that it probably wouldn't do any harm, knowing that his dead vaccine is likely to be just as ineffective.

Because this sort of thing was always happening in those days before the modern drugs appeared. Quack medicines abounded on the farms and the vets couldn't say a lot about them because their own range of pharmaceuticals was pitifully inadequate.

And in those diseases like abortion which had so far defeated all the efforts of the profession at control, the harvest for the quack men was particularly rich. The farming press and country newspapers were filled with confident advertisements for red drenches, black draughts, pink powders which were positively guaranteed to produce results. Professor Driscoll had plenty of competition.

After two cows calve normally, Frank is hopeful but it isn't long before three more cows abort their calves and then another two, and he knows there's nothing anyone can do to save the herd.

Driving home, I brooded on his words. Contagious Bovine Abortion has been recognized for centuries and I had read in old books of the filthy scourge which ravaged and ruined the ancient farmers just as it was doing to Frank Metcalfe today. The experts of those days said it was due to impure water, improper feeding, lack of exercise, sudden frights. They did note, however, that other cows which were allowed to sniff at the foetuses and afterbirths were likely to suffer the same fate themselves. But beyond that it was a black tunnel of ignorance.

We modern vets, on the other hand, knew all about it. We knew it was caused by a Gram-negative bacillus called *Brucella abortus* whose habits and attributes we had studied till we knew its every secret; but when it came to helping a farmer in Frank's situation we were about as much use as our colleagues of old who wrote those quaint books. True, dedicated researchers were working to find a strain of the bacillus which would form a safe and efficient vaccine to immunize cattle in calfhood and as far back as 1930 a certain strain 19 had been developed from which much was hoped. But even now it was still in the experimental stage. If Frank had had the luck to be born twenty years later the chances are that those cows he bought would have all been vaccinated and protected by that same strain 19. Nowadays we even have an efficient dead vaccine for the pregnant cows.

That autumn, Frank calls round to tell James he's had to sell up and move back to Middlesbrough. It's a disastrous and utterly underserved outcome for Frank, but like many Dales farmers, he's stoic about his misfortunes.

'Oh hell, Frank,' I said. 'I can't tell you how sorry I am. You haven't had a scrap of luck all the way through.' He looked at me and smiled with no trace of self-pity.

'Aye well,' he said. 'These things happen.'

I almost jumped at the words. 'These things happen!' That's what farmers always said after a disaster.

By the time Alf Wight wrote the final James Herriot book in the early 1990s, brucellosis had mostly been eradicated and herds were no longer being ravaged by it as they had in the 1940s and 1950s. Veterinary surgeons, however, had practically paddled in the bacteria when treating infected cattle and some would later suffer the effects, both physically and mentally. James thinks he has escaped without being affected, until he starts to experience what his family call 'funny turns'.

I was always apprehensive and ill at ease when I had Mrs Featherstone's problem dog on the table, but this time I felt relaxed and full of confidence. But then I was always like that when I was delirious.

Delirium was only one of the countless peculiar manifestations of brucellosis. This disease, which causes contagious abortion in cattle, ruined thousands of good farmers of my generation and was also a constant menace to the veterinary surgeons who had to deliver the premature calves and remove the afterbirths.

Thank heaven, the brucellosis scheme has now just about eradicated the disease but in the fifties such a thing hadn't been dreamed of and I and my contemporaries wallowed almost daily in the horrible infection.

I remember standing stripped to the waist in cow byres – parturition gowns were still uncommon and the long plastic protective gloves unknown in those days – working away inside infected cows for hours and looking with wry recognition at the leathery placenta and the light-coloured, necrotic cotyledons which told me that I was in contact with millions of the bacteria. And as I swilled myself with disinfectant afterwards, the place was filled with the distinctive acrid odour of abortion.

The effects on many of my fellow vets were wide and varied. One big fat chap faded away to a skeleton with undulant fever and was ill for years, others developed crippling arthritis and some went down with psychiatric conditions. One man wrote in the *Veterinary Record* that as part of his own syndrome he came home one night and decided it would be a good idea to murder his wife. He never got round actually to doing it, but recorded the impulse as an interesting example of what *Brucella abortus* could do to a man.

I used to pat myself on the back and thank God that I was immune. I had been bathing in the infection for years and had never experienced the slightest reaction and as I looked around at some of my suffering friends I was so thankful that I had been spared their ordeal. And after all this time I just knew that such a thing would never happen to me.

That was before I started my funny turns.

This was my family's term for a series of mysterious attacks which came unheralded and then passed off just as quickly. At first I diagnosed them as repeated chills — I was always stripping off in open fields, often in the middle of the night — then I thought I must have a type of flu of short duration. The symptoms were always the same — a feeling of depression, then an ice-cold shiveriness which drove me to my bed, where within an hour I shot up a temperature of 105 or 106. Once I had developed this massive fever I felt great: warm and happy, laughing heartily, chattering to myself and finally breaking into song. I couldn't help the singing — I felt so good.

This was a source of great amusement to my children. When I was at the singing stage I could always hear them giggling outside the bedroom door, but I didn't mind — I didn't mind anything.

However, I finally had to find out what was happening to me and a blood test by Dr Allinson dispelled all doubts by showing a nice positive titre to *Brucella abortus*. Reluctantly I had to admit that I had joined the club.

Alf suffered similar 'funny turns' that would eventually subside, but it has been suggested that these repeated attacks may have contributed to the depression he suffered in later life.

Alf was nonetheless aware, and thankful, that he had experienced rural life in Yorkshire as it once was, along with the introduction of effective modern drugs that would save the lives of the animals he treated.

'I consider that I am a very fortunate man,' Alf once said. 'I have lived through the golden years of vet practice – without doubt, the best years.' In *The Lord God Made Them All* Siegfried agrees as much although he also looks forward to great days ahead in veterinary practice.

'Do you know, James,' he said. 'I'm convinced that the same thing applies to our job. We're going through the best time there, too.'

'Do you think so?'

'Sure of it. Look at all the new advances since the war. Drugs and procedures we never dreamed of. We can look after our animals in a way that would have been impossible a few years ago and the farmers realize this. You've seen them crowding into the surgery on market day to ask advice — they've gained a new respect for the profession and they know it pays to call in the vet now.'

'That's true,' I said. 'We're certainly busier than we've ever been, with the Ministry work going full blast, too.'

'Yes, everything is buzzing. In fact, James, I'd like to bet that these present years are the high noon of country practice.'

I thought for a moment. 'You could be right. But if we are on the top now does it mean that our lives will decline later?'

'No, no, of course not. They'll be different, that's all. I sometimes think we've only touched the fringe of so many other things, like small animal work.' Siegfried brandished his gnawed piece of grass at me and his eyes shone with the enthusiasm which always uplifted me.

'I tell you this, James. There are great days ahead!'

Chapter 11

HURTLING AROUND
the HILLS

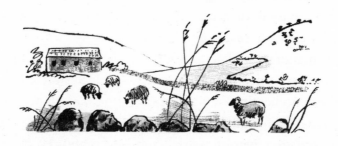

I hardly noticed the passage of the weeks as I rattled along the moorland roads on my daily rounds; but the district was beginning to take shape, the people to emerge as separate personalities. Most days I had a puncture. The tyres were through to the canvas on all wheels; it surprised me that they took me anywhere at all.

One of the few refinements on the car was a rusty 'sunshine roof'. It grated dismally when I slid it back, but most of the time I kept it open and the windows too, and I drove in my shirtsleeves with the delicious air swirling about me. On wet days it didn't help much to close the roof because the rain dripped through the joints and formed pools on my lap and the passenger seat.

I developed great skill in zig-zagging round puddles. To drive through was a mistake as the muddy water fountained up through the gaps in the floorboards.

On joining the Darrowby practice, James is given a tiny Austin 7 car 'of almost forgotten vintage' to do his rounds. Like all vets working in rural areas, James spends a great deal of time behind the wheel of a car, coaxing it up the hills of the Yorkshire Dales in all weathers. The car has seen better days: its tyres are worn and every morning it's touch and go whether it will start, the engine only coughing into life after several turns of the starting handle or a tow from Boardman.

These were still early days for cars – James's Austin was probably manufactured in the 1920s – and compared to modern cars, they were uncomfortable, noisy and bitterly cold in the winter with no heating. When working in Thirsk Alf also drove a rundown Austin 7 although by then he'd had some experience driving aged cars, getting by in a tiny, old-school Ford during his time in Sunderland. In a letter to his parents in January 1940, he described the experience of driving the Ford, his words infused with the humour he would later utilize to such great effect in his books: 'The car, using the word in its broadest sense, makes a colossal din and, in the country, the birds rise from the hedges in fright and the cows and horses in the fields look definitely startled. The vibration is terrific over thirty-five miles per hour and my liver will be in splendid condition after a month or two at it.'

Driving the Austin 7 across the rugged landscape of Yorkshire was also something of a challenge in a car that lacked the horsepower to make it up steep inclines. Around Thirsk, the approach to the Hambleton Hills via Sutton Bank was probably the worst – even in first gear the car struggled with its one-in-four gradient and Alf had no option but to reverse up it. In good weather, Alf could slide open the car's very primitive sunroof, but in wet weather, rain would leak through it even when closed, so that he had to put plastic sheeting on his knees.

The car's thin tyres were also prone to punctures and positively dangerous in snow or rain and, if the windscreen had iced up, Alf would often have to drive with his head out of the window. Out of desperation, he came up with an ingenious way to melt a few inches of the frost on his windscreen, referred to in *It Shouldn't Happen to a Vet*.

It was more than ten miles to the Clayton farm and it was one of those iron days when the frost piled thickly on the windscreen blotting out everything within minutes. But this morning I was triumphant. I had just bought a wonderful new invention – a couple of strands of wire mounted on a strip of Bakelite and fastened to the windscreen with rubber suckers. It worked from the car batteries and cleared a small space of vision.

No more did I have to climb out wearily and scrub and scratch at the frozen glass every half-mile or so. I sat peering delightedly through a flawlessly clear semicircle about eight inches wide at the countryside unwinding before me like a film show; the grey stone villages, silent and withdrawn under their smothering white cloak; the low, burdened branches of the roadside trees.

I was enjoying it so much that I hardly noticed the ache in my toes. Freezing feet were the rule in those days before car heaters, especially when you could see the road flashing past through the holes in the floorboards. On long journeys I really began to suffer towards the end. It was like that today when I got out of the car at the foot of the Pike Edge road; my fingers, too, throbbed painfully as I stamped around and swung my arms.

While driving up hills was a challenge for James's car, driving down them was even more alarming. The brakes on the Austin were always ineffective – as James found, violent pressure on the brake pedal would cause the car to stop, but only after a certain amount of veering across the road. But gradually, the brakes grow weaker until they become entirely absent, as one farmer discovers to his cost.

> I thought, not for the first time, that if you had to drive a car with no brakes one of the last places in England you'd want to be was the Yorkshire Dales. Even on the flat it was bad enough but I got used to it after a week or two and often forgot all about it. As when one day I was busy with a cow and the farmer jumped into my car to move it so that one of his men could get past with a tractor. I never said a word as the unsuspecting man backed round quickly and confidently and hit the wall of the barn with a sickening crash. With typical Yorkshire understatement, all he said was, 'Your brakes aren't ower savage, mister.'

Without brakes, Alf became adept at descending the many hill roads by putting his car into first gear, yet even this didn't stop it reaching terrifying speeds as it hurtled round bends, the engine screaming. In *It Shouldn't Happen to a Vet*, James is forced to run his brakeless car into a wall to avoid a flock of sheep, exactly as Alf did in the Witton Steeps in the Dales. Before launching himself down the hill, James sits for a long time looking down at Mr Robinson's farm, which lies a thousand feet below at the bottom of a steep track 'with two villainous S-bends. It was like a malevolent snake coiling almost headlong from where I sat'. With his heart thumping, he wrestles in his mind over which route he should take: to go back into Darrowby and take the low road into Worton, a safer detour of over ten miles, or to go straight down.

At last, I started the engine and did what I always did — took the quick way down.

But this hill really was a beauty, a notorious road even in this country, and as I nosed gingerly onto it, the whole world seemed to drop away from me. With the gear lever in bottom and my hand jammed against it I headed, dry-mouthed, down the strip of tarmac which now looked to be almost vertical.

It is surprising what speed you can attain in bottom gear if you have nothing else to hold you back and as the first bend rushed up at me the little engine started a rising scream of protest. When I hit the curve, I hauled the wheel round desperately to the right, the tyres spun for a second in the stones and loose soil of the verge, then we were off again.

This was a longer stretch and even steeper and it was like being on the big dipper with the same feeling of lack of control over one's fate. Hurtling into the bend, the idea of turning at this speed was preposterous but it was that or straight over the edge. Terror-stricken, I closed my eyes and dragged the wheel to the left. This time, one side of the car lifted and I was sure we were over, then it rocked back onto the other side and for a horrible second or two kept this up till it finally decided to stay upright and I was once more on my way.

Again a yawning gradient. But as the car sped downwards, engine howling, I was aware of a curious numbness. I seemed to have reached the ultimate limits of fear and hardly noticed as we shot round the third bend. One more to go and at last the road was levelling out; my speed dropped rapidly and at the last bend I couldn't have been doing more than twenty. I had made it.

It wasn't till I was right on to the final straight that I saw the sheep. Hundreds of them, filling the road. A river of woolly backs lapping from wall to wall. They were only yards from me and I was still going downhill. Without hesitation I turned and drove straight into the wall.

There didn't seem to be much damage. A few stones slithered down as the engine stalled and fell silent.

Slowly I sank back in my seat, relaxing my clenched jaws, releasing, finger by finger, the fierce grip on the wheel. The sheep continued to flow past and I took a sideways glance at the man who was shepherding them. He was a stranger to me and I prayed he didn't recognize me either because at that moment the role of unknown madman seemed to be the ideal one. Best not to say anything; appearing round a corner and driving deliberately into a wall is no basis for a rewarding conversation.

The sheep were still passing by and I could hear the man calling to his dogs. 'Get by, Jess. Come by, Nell.' But I kept up a steady stare at the layered stones in front of me, even though he passed within a few feet.

I suppose some people would have asked me what the hell I was playing at, but not a Dales shepherd. He went quietly by without invading my privacy, but when I looked in the mirror after a few moments I could see him in the middle of the road staring back at me, his sheep temporarily forgotten.

James had repeatedly spoken to Siegfried about the dangerous state of his Austin and the more senior vet had told him not to worry and to leave it with him. The problem was he never did anything about it and, as the car was Siegfried's property, there was little James could do but wait for him to take some action. It's only when Siegfried himself experiences the full terror of the car that he eventually does something about its sorry condition.

This occurs when the two vets head to a case together at a

farm just outside Darrowby. Siegfried decides to drive them in the Austin, with James 'huddled apprehensively next to him as he sets off at his usual brisk pace.'

Hinchcliffe's farm lies about a mile on the main road outside Darrowby. It is a massive place with a wide straight drive leading down to the house. We weren't going there, but as Siegfried spurted to full speed I could see Mr Hinchcliffe in his big Buick ahead of us proceeding in a leisurely way along the middle of the road. As Siegfried pulled out to overtake, the farmer suddenly stuck out his hand and began to turn right towards his farm directly across our path. Siegfried's foot went hard down on the brake pedal and his eyebrows shot right up as nothing happened. We were going straight for the side of the Buick and there was no room to go round on the left.

Siegfried didn't panic. At the last moment he turned right with the Buick and the two cars roared side by side down the drive, Mr Hinchcliffe staring at me with bulging eyes from close range. The farmer stopped in the yard, but we continued round the back of the house because we had to.

Fortunately, it was one of those places where you could drive right round and we rattled through the stackyard and back to the front of the house behind Mr Hinchcliffe who had got out and was looking round the corner to see where we had gone. The farmer whipped round in astonishment and, open-mouthed, watched us as we passed, but Siegfried, retaining his aplomb to the end, inclined his head and gave a little wave before we shot back up the drive.

Before we returned to the main road I had a look back at Mr Hinchcliffe. He was still watching us and there was a certain rigidity in his pose which reminded me of the shepherd.

Once on the road, Siegfried steered carefully into a layby and stopped. For a few moments he stared straight ahead without speaking and I realized he was having a little difficulty in getting his patient look properly adjusted; but when he finally turned to me his face was transfigured, almost saintly.

I dug my nails into my palms as he smiled at me with kindly eyes.

'Really, James,' he said, 'I can't understand why you keep things to yourself. Heaven knows how long your car has been in this condition, yet never a word from you.' He raised a forefinger and his patient look was replaced by one of sorrowing gravity. 'Don't you realize we might have been killed back there? You really ought to have told me.'

The experience of driving with Siegfried is just as hair-raising when he is at the wheel of his own car. His cars, in particular his battle-worn Hillman, bear testament to years of hard driving; sitting in the passenger seat requires nerves of steel and a strong stomach.

Outside the house, Farnon motioned me towards a battered Hillman and, as I moved round to the passenger's side, I shot a startled glance at the treadless tyres, the rusty bodywork, the almost opaque windscreen with its network of fine cracks. What I didn't notice was that the passenger seat was not fixed to the floor but stood freely on its sledge-like runners. I dropped into it and went over backwards, finishing with my head on the rear seat and my feet against the roof. Farnon helped me up, apologizing with great charm, and we set off.

Once clear of the market place, the road dipped quite suddenly and we could see all of the Dale stretching away from us in the evening sunshine. The outlines of the great hills were softened in the gentle light and a broken streak of silver showed where the Darrow wandered on the valley floor.

Farnon was an unorthodox driver. Apparently captivated by the scene, he drove slowly down the hill, elbows resting on the wheel, his chin cupped in his hands. At the bottom of the hill he came out of his reverie and spurted to seventy miles an hour. The old car rocked crazily along the narrow road and my movable seat slewed from side to side as I jammed my feet against the floorboards.

Then he slammed on the brakes, pointed out some pedigree shorthorns in a field and jolted away again. He never looked at the road in front; all his attention was on the countryside around and behind him. It was that last bit that worried me, because he spent a lot of time driving fast and looking over his shoulder at the same time.

Despite driving like a whirling dervish himself, Siegfried is disapproving of anyone else who does the same, particularly if they are driving a car he owns. When James's car returns from the garage, Siegfried advises him to take it easy when he drives it – no more 'belting along like a maniac' – although the elder partner does exactly this when he's next at its wheel.

Then there came the day when Siegfried decided to have my car rebored. It had been using a steady two pints of oil a day and he hadn't thought this excessive, but when it got to half a gallon a day he felt something ought to be done. What probably decided him was a farmer on market day saying he always knew when the young vet was coming because he could see the cloud of blue smoke miles away.

When the tiny Austin came back from the garage, Siegfried

fussed round it like an old hen. 'Come over here, James,' he called. 'I want to talk to you.'

I saw he was looking patient again and braced myself.

'James,' he said, pacing round the battered vehicle, whisking specks from the paintwork. 'You see this car?' I nodded.

'Well, it has been rebored, James, rebored at great expense, and that's what I want to talk to you about. You now have in your possession what amounts to a new car.' With an effort he unfastened the catch and the bonnet creaked open in a shower of rust and dirt. He pointed down at the engine, black and oily, with unrelated pieces of flex and rubber tubing hanging around it like garlands. 'You have a piece of fine mechanism here and I want you to treat it with respect. I've seen you belting along like a maniac and it won't do. You've got to nurse this machine for the next two or three thousand miles; thirty miles an hour is quite fast enough. I think it's a crime the way some people abuse a new engine — they should be locked up — so remember, lad, no flogging or I'll be down on you.'

He closed the bonnet with care, gave the cracked windscreen a polish with the cuff of his coat and left.

These strong words made such an impression on me that I crawled round the visits all day almost at walking pace.

The same night, I was getting ready for bed when Siegfried came in. He had two farm lads with him and they both wore silly grins. A powerful smell of beer filled the room.

Siegfried spoke with dignity, slurring his words only slightly. 'James, I met these gentlemen in the Black Bull this evening. We have had several excellent games of dominoes but unfortunately they have missed the last bus. Will you kindly bring the Austin round and I will run them home.'

I drove the car to the front of the house and the farm lads piled in, one in the front, the other in the back. I looked at

Siegfried lowering himself unsteadily into the driving seat and decided to go along. I got into the back.

The two young men lived in a farm up on the North Moors and, three miles out of the town, we left the main road and our headlights picked out a strip of track twisting along the dark hillside.

Siegfried was in a hurry. He kept his foot on the boards, the note of the engine rose to a tortured scream and the little car hurtled on into the blackness. Hanging on grimly, I leaned forward so that I could shout into my employer's ear. 'Remember this is the car which has just been rebored,' I bellowed above the din.

Siegfried looked round with an indulgent smile. 'Yes, yes, I remember, James. What are you fussing about?' As he spoke, the car shot off the road and bounded over the grass at sixty miles an hour. We all bounced around like corks till he found his way back. Unperturbed, he carried on at the same speed. The silly grins had left the lads' faces and they sat rigid in their seats. Nobody said anything.

The passengers were unloaded at a silent farmhouse and the return journey began. Since it was downhill all the way, Siegfried found he could go even faster. The car leaped and bumped over the uneven surface with its engine whining. We made several brief but tense visits to the surrounding moors, but we got home.

It was a month later that Siegfried had occasion to take his assistant to task once more. 'James, my boy,' he said sorrowfully, 'you are a grand chap, but by God, you're hard on cars. Look at this Austin. Newly rebored a short time ago, in tiptop condition, and look at it now – drinking oil. I don't know how you did it in the time. You're a real terror.'

When it comes to driving the practice cars, Siegfried is even more distrustful of his younger brother Tristan, and not without reason. In *It Shouldn't Happen to a Vet* Tristan must chauffeur for James, who has his arm in a sling after a bad calving, much to Siegfried's fury as it's only been a week since his brother had crashed and written off his Hillman. Their call-out involves taking the still-brakeless Austin across fields to Mr Prescott's farm, which, like some Dales farmsteads, has neither a road nor farm track leading to it. Now returning home, they have driven up the steep slope again, James has opened the last gate, where he joins Tristan, who has got out of the car and is sitting with his back against the gatepost. They take in the view of the farm far below and just as Tristan closes his eyes and takes in a long, deep gulp of moorland air and Woodbine smoke, there's suddenly a grinding noise coming from the car.

'Christ! She's off, Jim!' he shouted.

The little Austin was moving gently backwards down the slope – it must have slipped out of gear and it had no brakes to speak of. We both leaped after it. Tristan was nearest and he just managed to touch the bonnet with one finger; the speed was too much for him. We gave it up and watched.

The hillside was steep and the little car rapidly gathered momentum, bouncing crazily over the uneven ground. I glanced at Tristan; his mind invariably worked quickly and clearly in a crisis and I had a good idea what he was thinking. It was only a fortnight since he had turned the Hillman over, taking a girl home from a dance. It had been a complete write-off and the insurance people had been rather nasty about it; and of course Siegfried had gone nearly berserk and had finished by sacking him finally, once and for all – never wanted to see his face in the place again.

But he had been sacked so often, he knew he had only to keep out of his way for a bit and his brother would forget. And he had been lucky this time because Siegfried had talked his bank manager into letting him buy a beautiful new Rover and this blotted everything else from his mind.

It was distinctly unfortunate that this should happen when he, as driver, was technically in charge of the Austin. The car appeared now to be doing about 70 m.p.h. hurtling terrifyingly down the long, green hill. One by one the doors burst open till all four flapped wildly and the car swooped downwards looking like a huge, ungainly bird.

From the open doors, bottles, instruments, bandages, cotton wool cascaded out onto the turf, leaving a long, broken trail. Now and again a packet of nux vomica and bicarb stomach powder would fly out and burst like a bomb, splashing vivid white against the green.

Tristan threw up his arms. 'Look! The bloody thing's going straight for that hut.' He drew harder on his Woodbine.

There was indeed only one obstruction on the bare hillside – a small building near the foot where the land levelled out – and the Austin, as if drawn by a magnet, was thundering straight towards it.

I couldn't bear to watch. Just before the impact I turned away and focused my attention on the end of Tristan's cigarette, which was glowing bright red when the crash came. When I looked back down the hill the building was no longer there. It had been completely flattened and everything I had ever heard about houses of cards surged into my mind. On top of the shattered timbers the little car lay peacefully on its side, its wheels still turning lazily.

Fortunately, Mr Prescott has a horse that pulls the car upright again, although Tristan and James learn that the hut the runaway car had destroyed was in fact the clubhouse of the neighbouring Darrowby golf course. Thankfully, the sturdy little engine of the Austin starts up again and they are able to return to Skeldale House. Siegfried, however, who is coming down with a summer cold, is less than happy when he sees the car's broken rear light, raging at Tristan that he is a 'bloody young maniac . . . Go on, get to hell out of it. I'm finished with you.'

The following morning, Siegfried, now in bed with laryngitis, reads in the *Darrowby and Houlton Times* that the golf club-house has been mysteriously knocked down. It suddenly occurs to him that Tristan had been at Mr Prescott's but as soon as he mentions this, he slumps back and mutters, in a manner that is quite unlike Siegfried, that it's wrong of him always to blame Tristan for everything. He then gets a call about a cow with milk fever and tells Tristan to drive James straight to it. Tristan informs him the Austin is in the garage, and Siegfried has no choice but to let him take the Rover. In a menacing voice he hisses to Tristan: 'Right, so you'll have to take the Rover. I never thought I'd see the day when I'd let a wrecker like you drive it, but just let me tell you this. If you put a scratch on that car I'll kill you. I'll kill you with my own two hands.'

Undeterred, Tristan is thrilled to have the opportunity to drive Siegfried's Rover. He carefully backs it out of the yard, then on the Sorton road, nestling down into the car's rich leather upholstery, he puts his foot hard on the accelerator and brings it to an effortless eighty miles per hour. Ahead a large square-topped car is trying to overtake a milk lorry, and to James's horror they are thundering side by side towards the Rover. As they shoot past, the large car ends up crashing into one side of the Rover. When they stop, they discover that the entire left side of the Rover has lost its doors and is a 'desert of twisted metal where the old car, diving for the verge at the last split second, had ploughed its way.' They know they're in trouble and Tristan sets his agile mind on what to do next.

It seemed to me after a short appraisal of the situation that he had three possible courses of action. First, and most attractive, he could get out of Darrowby permanently — emigrate if necessary. Second, he could go straight to the railway station and board a train for Brawton where he could live quietly with his mother till this had blown over. Third, and it didn't bear thinking about, he could go back to Skeldale House and tell Siegfried he had smashed up his new Rover.

They bravely — or perhaps foolishly — take the third option and head back to the house. Siegfried is now very ill in bed, his face red with fever, barely able to whisper. Tristan tells him he has had 'a bit of a bump with the car' and that the 'front and rear wings pretty well mangled, I'm afraid — and both doors torn off the left side'.

As if operated by a powerful spring, Siegfried came bolt upright in the bed. It was startlingly like a corpse coming to life and the effect was heightened by the coils of Thermogene which had burst loose and trailed in shroud-like garlands from the haggard head. The mouth opened wide in a completely soundless scream.

'You bloody fool! You're sacked!'

He crashed back on to the pillow as though the mechanism had gone into reverse and lay very still. We watched him for a few moments in some anxiety, but when we heard the breathing restart we tiptoed from the room.

On the landing Tristan blew out his cheeks and drew a Woodbine from its packet. 'A tricky little situation, Jim, but you know what I always say.' He struck a match and pulled the smoke down blissfully. 'Things usually turn out better than you expect.'

Alf had in reality consulted with Brian Sinclair on many of the events related in *If Only They Could Talk*, including when he pranged his elder brother's Rover. 'You bloody fool! You're sacked!' is a faithful reproduction of the words used by Donald when he discovered what had happened to his beloved car. The demolishing of the hut was also based on a real incident and to this day Alf's son Jim still points out where that happened on the Leyburn road in North Yorkshire.

Brian wasn't the only culprit when it came to giving the practice cars a hard time. Many of the assistants who worked at 23 Kirkgate would drive them at maximum speed, careering across rough farm tracks and shooting around bends, only to end up in ditches. As a result, the cars were constantly in and out of the garage and a substantial drain on the finances of the practice. Cars suffered considerably in the hands of assistant Brian Nettleton, known in the books as Calum Buchanan, the 'vet wi' t'badger', as recounted in Chapter 4. Not only would he drive them at speed, returning one day with the front wing completely missing, but his pet badgers also caused havoc in the back seats.

When he wasn't crashing cars, Brian, who always delighted in pranks, couldn't resist having a bit of fun with them, much to the consternation of visitors to the practice. In *Vet in a Spin* Tristan enacts a well-worn stunt, while James and the local blacksmith Pat Jenner are in the practice yard seeing to a horse.

Some days Pat Jenner came in to check on the shoes and he and I were busy in the yard when I heard the familiar rattle of my little Austin in the back lane. The big double doors were open and I looked up as the car turned in and drew alongside us. Pat looked too, and his eyes popped.

'Bloody 'ell!' he exclaimed, and I couldn't blame him, because the car had no driver. At least it looked that way since there was nobody in the seat as it swung in from the lane.

A driverless car in motion is quite a sight, and Pat gaped open-mouthed for a few seconds. Then just as I was about to explain, Tristan shot up from the floor with a piercing cry.

'Hi there!' he shrieked.

Pat dropped his hammer and backed away. 'God 'elp us!' he breathed.

I was unaffected by the performance because it was old stuff to me. Whenever I was in the yard and a call came in, Tristan would drive my car round from the front street and this happened so many times that inevitably he grew bored and tried to find a less orthodox method.

After a bit of practice he mastered the driverless technique. He crouched on the floor with a foot on the accelerator and one hand on the wheel and nearly frightened the life out of me the first time he did it. But I was used to it now, and blasé.

When Siegfried knocks the exhaust off his car while bumping along a farm track, he realizes in *The Lord God Made Them All* that they need to acquire a spare car for the practice. Heading to Mr Hammond's garage, he decides to take a 1933 Morris Oxford for a quick spin and gives it a thorough testing before he makes up his mind.

'Hop in the back, James!' my partner cried. I opened the rear door and took my place behind Mr Hammond in the musty interior.

Siegfried took off abruptly with a roaring and creaking from the old vehicle and despite the garage man's outward calm I saw the back of his shirt collar rise a couple of inches above his blue serge jacket as we shot along Trengate.

The collar subsided a little when Siegfried slowed down at the church to make a left turn but reappeared spasmodically as we negotiated a series of sharp and narrow bends at top speed.

When we reached the long straight lane which runs parallel to Trengate Mr Hammond appeared to relax, but when Siegfried put his foot on the boards and sent the birds squawking from the overhanging branches as he thundered beneath them, I saw the collar again.

When we reached the end of the lane Siegfried came almost to a halt as he turned left.

'I think we'll test the brakes, Mr Hammond,' he said cheerfully, and hurled the car suddenly along the home straight for Trengate. He really meant to carry out a thorough test. The roar of the ancient engine rose to a scream and as the street approached with frightening rapidity the collar reappeared, then the shirt.

When Siegfried stood on the brakes the car slewed violently to the right and as we catapulted crabwise into Trengate, Mr Hammond's head was jammed against the roof and his entire shirt-back was exposed. When we came to a halt he slid slowly back into his seat and the jacket took over again. At no time had he spoken or, apart from his up-and-down movements, shown any emotion.

At the front door of the surgery we got out and my colleague rubbed his chin doubtfully. 'She does pull a little to the right on braking, Mr Hammond. I think we'd need to have that rectified. Or perhaps you have another vehicle available?'

The garage man did not answer for a few moments. His spectacles were askew and he was very pale. 'Aye . . . aye . . .' he said shakily. 'I 'ave another little job over there. It might suit you.'

Along with bumpy farm tracks, steep hills and the wild weather of the Dales, James and Siegfried often had to contend with packs of dogs chasing and barking at their cars as they drove out of farmyards. Alf frequently had large dogs escorting him as he made his way along tracks, some even dangerously darting close to the car and biting its wheels. This would then send Hector, the noisiest dog Alf owned, quite loopy if he was in the car, as he galloped around the inside defending his territory. If Alf's children were in the car, their job would be to load up syringes with water and squirt them at any chasing dogs, a tactic that proved remarkably effective.

In *Let Sleeping Vets Lie*, James meets a dog who is something of a professional when it comes to car chasing.

A lot of farm dogs are partial to a little light relief from their work. They like to play and one of their favourite games is chasing cars off the premises. Often I drove off with a hairy form galloping alongside and the dog would usually give a final defiant bark after a few hundred yards to speed me on my way. But Jock was different.

He was really dedicated. Car chasing to him was a deadly serious art which he practised daily without a trace of levity. Corner's farm was at the end of a long track, twisting for nearly a mile between its stone walls down through the gently sloping fields to the road below and Jock didn't consider he had done his job properly until he had escorted his chosen vehicle right to the very foot. So his hobby was an exacting one.

I watched him now as I finished stitching the foal's leg and began to tie on a bandage. He was slinking about the buildings, a skinny little creature who without his mass of black and white hair would have been an almost invisible mite, and he was playing out a transparent charade of pretending he was taking no notice of me – wasn't the least bit interested in my presence, in fact. But his furtive glances in the direction of the stable, his repeated criss-crossing of my line of vision gave him away. He was waiting for his big moment.

When I was putting on my shoes and throwing my Wellingtons into the boot I saw him again. Or rather part of him; just a long nose and one eye protruding from beneath a broken door. It wasn't till I had started the engine and begun to move off that he finally declared himself, stealing out from his hiding place, body low, tail trailing, eyes fixed intently on the car's front wheels, and as I gathered speed and headed down the track he broke into an effortless lope.

I had been through this before and was always afraid he might run in front of me so I put my foot down and began to hurtle downhill. This was where Jock came into his own. I often wondered how he'd fare against a racing greyhound because by golly he could run. That sparse frame housed a perfect physical machine and the slender limbs reached and flew again and again, devouring the stony ground beneath, keeping up with the speeding car with joyful ease.

There was a sharp bend about halfway down and here Jock invariably sailed over the wall and streaked across the turf, a little dark blur against the green, and having craftily cut off the corner he reappeared like a missile zooming over the grey

351

stones lower down. This put him into a nice position for the run to the road and when he finally saw me onto the tarmac my last view of him was of a happy, panting face looking after me. Clearly he considered it was a job well done and he would wander contentedly back up to the farm to await the next session, perhaps with the postman or the baker's van.

In the final book, James is finally able to upgrade to an Austin 10, which is still second-hand but has been well maintained and looked like new with black, sparkling bodywork. When he turns up at farms in a new-looking car, he is invariably met with a certain amount of leg-pulling from the farmers, who joke they are paying too much for his services. Alf similarly used to get a lot of usually good-natured ribbing from farmers if he turned up in a brand-new car and it was almost a relief when he reverted to buying a second-hand one in the 1960s.

As James muses in *Every Living Thing*, veterinary work is not a path to riches – he works hard seven days a week, in the evenings and often during the night 'rolling about on cobbled floors fighting with tough calvings to the point of exhaustion, getting kicked, crushed, trodden on and sprayed with muck'. Despite all of this, he still has a hefty overdraft, compensated by the fact he spends much of his time driving around the glorious countryside of the Dales. And for this, he counts himself lucky in whatever car he drives.

Chapter 12

HORSES

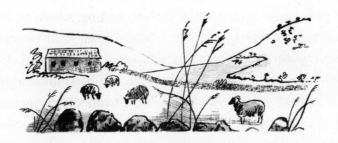

Probably the most dramatic occurrence in the history of veterinary practice was the disappearance of the draught horse. It is an almost incredible fact that this glory and mainstay of the profession just melted quietly away within a few years. And I was one of those who were there to see it happen.

When I first came to Darrowby the tractor had already begun to take over, but tradition dies hard in the agricultural world and there were still a lot of horses around. Which was just as well because my veterinary education had been geared to things equine with everything else a poor second. It had been a good scientific education in many respects but at times I wondered if the people who designed it still had a mental picture of the horse doctor with his top hat and frock coat busying himself in a world of horse-drawn trams and brewers' drays.

We learned the anatomy of the horse in great detail, then that of the other animals much more superficially. It was the same with the other subjects; from animal husbandry with such insistence on a thorough knowledge of shoeing that we developed into amateur blacksmiths — right up to medicine and surgery where it was much more important to know about glanders and strangles than canine distemper. Even as we were learning, we youngsters knew it was ridiculous, with the draught horse already cast as a museum piece and the obvious potential of cattle and small animal work.

Still, as I say, after we had absorbed a vast store of equine lore it was a certain comfort that there were still a lot of patients on which we could try it out. I should think in my first two years I treated farm horses nearly every day and though I never was and never will be an equine expert there was a strange thrill in meeting with the age-old conditions whose names rang down almost from medieval times. Quittor, fistulous withers, poll evil, thrush, shoulder slip — vets had been wrestling with them for hundreds of years using very much the same drugs and procedures as myself. Armed with my firing iron and box of blister I plunged determinedly into what had always been the surging mainstream of veterinary life.

Alfred Wight had similarly undertaken a programme of education that placed much of its attention on the horse. In his final year at the Glasgow Veterinary College he gained some practical experience working at the busy Glasgow practice of Professor Willie Robb. A renowned horse specialist, Robb, like his fellow professors, had lived through the days when heavy draught horses were a familiar sight in both the city streets of Glasgow and the rural pastures of Yorkshire.

Alf, however, had had little experience of horses prior to his studies and was all too aware he still had a huge amount to learn when he finally graduated as a veterinary surgeon in 1939. After five years of 'a slow and painful assimilation of thousands of facts', as James Herriot puts it in *If Only They*

Could Talk, he feels as if he knows nothing, like an 'astronomer looking through a telescope at an unknown galaxy'. He wasn't always plagued with such doubt and in the same book he reminisces about his seventeen-year-old self, when after just one lecture in animal husbandry, he felt he 'really knew about horses' and was thus keen to try out his new-found expertise.

I could hardly believe my luck when I saw the horse. It was standing outside the library below Queen's Cross like something left over from another age. It drooped dispiritedly between the shafts of a coal cart which stood like an island in an eddying stream of cars and buses. Pedestrians hurried by, uncaring, but I had the feeling that fortune was smiling on me.

A horse. Not just a picture but a real, genuine horse. Stray words from the lecture floated up into my mind; the pastern, cannon bone, coronet and all those markings — snip, blaze, white sock near hind. I stood on the pavement and examined the animal critically.

I thought it must be obvious to every passer-by that here was a true expert. Not just an inquisitive onlooker but a man who knew and understood all. I felt clothed in a visible aura of horsiness.

I took a few steps up and down, hands deep in the pockets of the new riding mac, eyes probing for possible shoeing faults or curbs or bog spavins. So thorough was my inspection that I worked round to the off side of the horse and stood perilously among the racing traffic.

I glanced around at the people hurrying past. Nobody seemed to care, not even the horse. He was a large one, at least seventeen hands, and he gazed apathetically down the street, easing his hind legs alternately in a bored manner. I hated to leave him but I had completed my examination and it was time I was on my way. But I felt that I ought to make a gesture before I left; something to communicate to the horse that I understood his problems and that we belonged to the same brotherhood. I stepped briskly forward and patted him on the neck.

Quick as a striking snake, the horse whipped downwards and seized my shoulder in his great strong teeth. He laid back his ears, rolled his eyes wickedly and hoisted me up, almost off my feet. I hung there helplessly, suspended like a lopsided puppet. I wriggled and kicked but the teeth were clamped immovably in the material of my coat.

There was no doubt about the interest of the passers-by now. The grotesque sight of a man hanging from a horse's mouth brought them to a sudden halt and a crowd formed with people looking over each other's shoulders and others fighting at the back to see what was going on.

A horrified old lady was crying: 'Oh, poor boy! Help him, somebody!' Some of the braver characters tried pulling at me but the horse whickered ominously and hung on tighter. Conflicting advice was shouted from all sides. With deep shame I saw two attractive girls in the front row giggling helplessly.

Appalled at the absurdity of my position, I began to thrash about wildly; my shirt collar tightened round my throat; a stream of the horse's saliva trickled down the front of my mac. I could feel myself choking and was giving up hope when a man pushed his way through the crowd.

He was very small. Angry eyes glared from a face blackened by coal dust. Two empty sacks were draped over an arm.

'Whit the hell's this?' he shouted. A dozen replies babbled in the air.

'Can ye no leave the bloody hoarse alone?' he yelled into my face. I made no reply, being pop-eyed, half throttled and in no mood for conversation. The coalman turned his fury on the horse. 'Drop him, ya big bastard! Go on, let go, drop him!'

Getting no response he dug the animal viciously in the belly with his thumb. The horse took the point at once and released me like an obedient dog dropping a bone. I fell on my knees and ruminated in the gutter for a while till I could breathe more easily. As from a great distance I could still hear the little man shouting at me.

After some time I stood up. The coalman was still shouting and the crowd was listening appreciatively. 'Whit d'ye think you're playing at – keep yer hands off ma bloody hoarse – get the poliss tae ye.'

I looked down at my new mac. The shoulder was chewed to a sodden mass. I felt I must escape and began to edge my way through the crowd. Some of the faces were concerned but most were grinning. Once clear I started to walk away rapidly and as I turned the corner the last faint cry from the coalman reached me.

'Dinna meddle wi' things ye ken nuthin' aboot!'

Five years later and a newly qualified James Herriot has recently arrived in Darrowby and is eagerly awaiting his first call-out without Siegfried. The phone rings and it's Lord Hulton's farm manager, Mr Soames, who explains he has a valuable hunting horse with colic. James's hopes for a straightforward case are dashed: not only is colic in horses notoriously tricky, but he must also deal with Soames, who is a prickly character.

James, nonetheless, has no choice but to steel himself for the visit, the well-thumbed pages of *Common Colics of the Horse* hovering in front of him 'phantom-like' as he drives to the farm.

I opened the door and went inside. And I stopped as though I had walked into a wall. It was a very large box, deeply bedded with peat moss. A bay horse was staggering round and round the perimeter where he had worn a deep path in the peat. He was lathered in sweat from nose to tail, his nostrils were dilated and his eyes stared blankly in front of him. His head rolled about at every step and, through his clenched teeth, gobbets of foam dripped to the floor. A rank steam rose from his body as though he had been galloping.

My mouth had gone dry. I found it difficult to speak and when I did, it was almost in a whisper. 'How long has he been like this?'

'Oh, he started with a bit of belly ache this morning. I've been giving him black draughts all day, or at least this fellow has. I wouldn't be surprised if he's made a bloody mess of it like he does everything.'

I saw that there was somebody standing in the shadows in the corner; a large, fat man with a head collar in his hand.

'Oh, I got the draught down him, right enough, Mr Soames, but they haven't done 'im no good.' The big man looked scared.

'You call yourself a horseman,' Soames said, 'but I should have done the damn job myself. I reckon he'd have been better by now.'

'It would take more than a black draught to help him,' I said. 'This is no ordinary colic.'

'What the hell is it, then?'

'Well, I can't say till I've examined him, but severe, continuous pain like that could mean a torsion – a twisted bowel.'

'Twisted bowel, my foot! He's got a bit of belly ache, that's all. He hasn't passed anything all day and he wants something to shift him. Have you got the arecoline with you?'

'If this is torsion, arecoline would be the worst thing you could give him. He's in agony now, but that would drive him mad. It acts by contracting the muscles of the intestines.'

'God dammit,' snarled Soames, 'don't start giving me a bloody lecture. Are you going to start doing something for the horse or aren't you?'

I turned to the big man in the corner. 'Slip on that head collar and I'll examine him.'

With the collar on, the horse was brought to a halt. He stood there, trembling and groaning as I passed a hand between ribs and elbows, feeling for the pulse. It was as bad as it could be — a racing, thready beat. I everted an eyelid with my fingers; the mucous membrane was a dark, brick red. The thermometer showed a temperature of a hundred and three.

I looked across the box at Soames. 'Could I have a bucket of hot water, soap and a towel, please?'

'What the devil for? You've done nothing yet and you want to have a wash?'

'I want to make a rectal examination. Will you please bring me the water?'

'God help us, I've never seen anything like this.' Soames passed a hand wearily over his eyes then swung round on the big man. 'Well, come on, don't stand around there. Get him hot water and we'll maybe get something done.'

When the water came, I soaped my arm and gently inserted it into the animal's rectum. I could feel plainly the displacement of the small intestine on the left side and a tense, tympanitic mass which should not have been there. As I touched it, the horse shuddered and groaned again.

As I washed and dried my arms, my heart pounded. What was I to do? What could I say?

Soames was stamping in and out of the box, muttering to himself as the pain-maddened animal writhed and twisted. 'Hold the bloody thing,' he bellowed at the horseman who was gripping the head collar. 'What the bloody hell are you playing at?'

The big man said nothing. He was in no way to blame but he just stared back stolidly at Soames.

I took a deep breath. 'Everything points to the one thing. I'm convinced this horse has a torsion.'

'All right then, have it your own way. He's got a torsion. Only for God's sake do something, will you? Are we going to stand in here all night?'

'There's nothing anybody can do. There is no cure for this. The important thing is to put him out of his pain as quickly as possible.'

Soames screwed up his face. 'No cure? Put him out of his pain? What rubbish is this you're talking? Just what are you getting at?'

I took a hold of myself. 'I suggest you let me put him down immediately.'

'What do you mean?' Soames' mouth fell open.

'I mean that I should shoot him now, straight away. I have a humane killer in the car.'

Soames looked as if he was going to explode. 'Shoot him! Are you stark raving mad? Do you know how much that horse is worth?'

'It makes no difference what he's worth, Mr Soames. He has been going through hell all day and he's dying now. You should have called me out long ago. He might live a few hours more but the end would be the same. And he's in dreadful pain, continuous pain.'

Soames sank his head in his hands. 'Oh God, why did this have to happen to me? His lordship is on holiday or I'd call him out to try to make you see some sense. I tell you, if your boss had been here he'd have given that horse an injection and put him right in half an hour. Look here, can't we wait till Mr Farnon gets back tonight and let him have a look at him?'

Something in me leaped gladly at the idea. Give a shot of morphine and get away out of it. Leave the responsibility to somebody else. It would be easy. I looked again at the horse. He had recommenced his blind circling of the box, stumbling round and round in a despairing attempt to leave his agony behind. As I watched, he raised his lolling head and gave a little whinny. It was a desolate, uncomprehending, frantic sound and it was enough for me.

I strode quickly out and got the killer from the car. 'Steady his head,' I said to the big man and placed the muzzle between the glazing eyes. There was a sharp crack and the horse's legs buckled. He thudded down on the peat and lay still.

While Soames stares at the body of the horse in disbelief, James explains that Siegfried will carry out a post-mortem in the morning to confirm his diagnosis. Soames is now furious and threatens to sue James over the whole affair, convinced that the young vet has made a grave error. James heads back to the surgery, worried that he may have scuppered his career before it had even started, although he still feels that he had no option but to put the horse out of its misery. The next morning, however, Siegfried informs him that the post-mortem had indeed shown torsion of the bowel, meaning James had taken exactly the right course of action and that, if anything, Soames had taken too long in sending for a vet.

Despite the advent of tractors, there were still plenty of young and healthy horses in the Yorkshire Dales who needed the services of vets like James. The area even had its own breed, the strong and hardy Dales pony. Spring was a busy time for foaling, followed by docking and castration in May and June.

Docking removed part of the tail, a procedure usually carried out on heavy draught horses to prevent it getting caught in harnesses or carriage equipment. The castration of year-old colts was a job Alf never enjoyed, principally because in the 1940s castrations were often performed on a conscious, standing horse, with the aid of just local anaesthesia. The actual procedure is fairly simple but vets were obviously vulnerable to injury should a horse prove non-compliant. 'It's dead easy to remove the testicles from a horse,' Alf frequently said. 'The real skill lies in persuading him to part with them!'

The real-life experiences of Alf and partner Donald Sinclair bore testament to the dangers and occasional mayhem that ensued when treating horses. While performing a castration, Donald narrowly escaped a nasty injury when the horse kicked the knife he was holding out of his hand, so that it sailed through the air, missing his head by inches. Alf applied a chloroform muzzle to anaesthetize the horse which promptly bolted into a field. Alf was 'hanging on grimly to the head rope' as it crashed through a fence into a garden.

Not unsurprisingly, in *If Only They Could Talk* the young James Herriot is apprehensive whenever he is sent to perform a castration or delicate equine surgery, knowing that, while he is competent in his work, he perhaps lacks the innate skills to tame an unruly horse.

Out of ten jobs nine would be easy and the tenth would be a rodeo. I don't know how much apprehension this state of affairs built up in other vets but I was undeniably tense on castration mornings.

Of course, one of the reasons was that I was not, am not and never will be a horseman. It is difficult to define the term but I am convinced that horsemen are either born or acquire the talent in early childhood. I knew it was no good my trying to start in my mid-twenties. I had the knowledge of equine diseases, I believed I had the ability to treat sick horses efficiently but that power the real horseman had to soothe and quieten and mentally dominate an animal was beyond my reach. I didn't even try to kid myself.

It was unfortunate because there is no doubt horses know. It is quite different with cows; they don't care either way; if a cow feels like kicking you she will kick you; she doesn't give a damn whether you are an expert or not. But horses know.

So on those mornings my morale was never very high as I drove out with my instruments rattling and rolling about on an enamel tray on the back seat. Would he be wild or quiet? How big would he be? I had heard my colleagues airily stating their preference for big horses — the two-year-olds were far easier, they said, you could get a better grip on the testicles. But there was never any doubt in my own mind. I liked them small; the smaller the better.

One morning when the season was at its height and I had had about enough of the equine race, Siegfried called to me as he was going out. 'James, there's a horse with a tumour on its belly at Wilkinson's of White Cross. Get along and take it off — today if possible but otherwise fix your own time; I'll leave it with you.'

Feeling a little disgruntled at fate having handed me something on top of the seasonal tasks, I boiled up a scalpel, tumour spoons and syringe and put them on my tray with local anaesthetic, iodine and tetanus antitoxin.

I drove to the farm with the tray rattling ominously behind me. That sound always had a connotation of doom for me. I wondered about the horse — maybe it was just a yearling; they did get those little dangling growths sometimes — nanberries, the farmers called them. Over the six miles I managed to build up a comfortable picture of a soft-eyed little colt with pendulous abdomen and overlong hair; it hadn't done well over the winter and was probably full of worms — shaky on its legs with weakness, in fact.

At Wilkinson's all was quiet. The yard was empty except for a lad of about ten who didn't know where the boss was.

'Well, where is the horse?' I asked.

The lad pointed to the stable. 'He's in there.'

I went inside. At one end stood a high, open-topped loose box with a metal grille topping the wooden walls and from within I heard a deep-throated whinnying and snorting followed by a series of tremendous thuds against the sides of the box. A chill crept through me. That was no little colt in there.

I opened the top half door and there, looking down at me, was an enormous animal; I hadn't realized horses ever came quite as big as this; a chestnut stallion with a proud arch to his neck and feet like manhole covers. Surging swathes of muscle shone on his shoulders and quarters and when he saw me he laid back his ears, showed the whites of his eyes and lashed out viciously against the wall. A foot-long splinter flew high in the air as the great hoof crashed against the boards.

'God almighty,' I breathed and closed the half door hurriedly. I leaned my back against the door and listened to my heart thumping.

I turned to the lad. 'How old is that horse?'

'Over six years, sir.'

I tried a little calm thinking. How did you go about tackling a man-eater like this? I had never seen such a horse — he must weigh over a ton. I shook myself; I hadn't even had a look at the tumour I was supposed to remove. I lifted the latch, opened the door about two inches and peeped inside. I could see it plainly dangling from the belly; probably a papilloma, about the size of a cricket ball, with a lobulated surface which made it look like a little cauliflower. It swung gently from side to side as the horse moved about.

On walking back to the house to ask for soap and water, he discovers no one is in so is forced to return – in something of a gleeful gallop – to his car. A few weeks later, however, he is called back in to perform the dreaded procedure.

Stepping out of the car, I felt almost disembodied. It was like walking a few inches above the ground. I was greeted by a reverberating din from the loose box; the same angry whinnies and splintering crashes I had heard before. I tried to twist my stiff face into a smile as the farmer came over.

'My chaps are getting a halter on him,' he said, but his words were cut short by an enraged squealing from the box and two tremendous blows against the wooden sides. I felt my mouth going dry.

The noise was coming nearer; then the stable doors flew open and the great horse catapulted out into the yard, dragging two big fellows along on the end of the halter shank. The cobbles struck sparks from the men's boots as they slithered about but they were unable to stop the stallion backing and plunging. I imagined I could feel the ground shudder under my feet as the hooves crashed down.

At length, after much manoeuvring, the men got the horse standing with his off side against the wall of the barn. One of them looped the twitch onto the upper lip and tightened it expertly, the other took a firm grip on the halter and turned towards me. 'Ready for you now, sir.'

I pierced the rubber cap on the bottle of cocaine, withdrew the plunger of the syringe and watched the clear fluid flow into the glass barrel. Seven, eight, ten cc's. If I could get that in, the rest would be easy; but my hands were trembling.

Walking up to the horse was like watching an action from a film. It wasn't really me doing this — the whole thing was unreal. The near-side eye flickered dangerously at me as I raised my left hand and passed it over the muscles of the neck, down the smooth, quivering flank and along the abdomen till I was able to grasp the tumour. I had the thing in my hand now, the lobulations firm and lumpy under my fingers. I pulled gently downwards, stretching the brown skin joining the growth to the body. I would put the local in there — a few good weals. It wasn't going to be so bad. The stallion laid back his ears and gave a warning whicker.

I took a long, careful breath, brought up the syringe with my right hand, placed the needle against the skin then thrust it in.

The kick was so explosively quick that at first I felt only surprise that such a huge animal could move so swiftly. It was a lightning outward slash that I never even saw and the hoof struck the inside of my right thigh, spinning me round helplessly. When I hit the ground I lay still, feeling only a curious numbness. Then I tried to move and a stab of pain went through my leg.

When I opened my eyes Mr Wilkinson was bending over me. 'Are you all right, Mr Herriot?' The voice was anxious.

'I don't think so,' I was astonished at the matter-of-fact sound of my own words; but stranger still was the feeling of being at peace with myself for the first time for weeks. I was calm and completely in charge of the situation.

'I'm afraid not, Mr Wilkinson. You'd better put the horse back in his box for now — we'll have a go at him another day

— and I wonder if you'd ring Mr Farnon to come and pick me up. I don't think I'll be able to drive.'

My leg wasn't broken but it developed a massive haematoma at the point of impact and then the whole limb blossomed into an unbelievable range of colours from delicate orange to deepest black. I was still hobbling like a Crimean veteran when, a fortnight later, Siegfried and I with a small army of helpers went back and roped the stallion, chloroformed him and removed that little growth.

I have a cavity in the muscle of my thigh to remind me of that day, but some good came out of the incident. I found that the fear is worse than the reality and horse work has never worried me as much since then.

Horse work also involved a considerable amount of dentistry. A horse that cannot chew properly rapidly loses condition so any problems with teeth require prompt attention. Years of grinding could leave sharp spikes on teeth which needed to be rasped (filed down) or clipped off to prevent them catching on the tongue or cheek. It was also commonly thought that 'wolf teeth' – small teeth in front of the first molars – hindered chewing and required knocking out, although James is less convinced of the benefits of this procedure.

As a result, veterinary practices had an array of medieval-like instruments to grind, shear off and knock out the teeth of their equine patients, including, as James Herriot writes, 'vicious forceps with two-feet-long arms, sharp-jawed shears, mouth gags, hammers and chisels, files and rasps; it was rather like a quiet corner in the Spanish Inquisition'.

In *If Only They Could Talk*, James is called in to look at a couple of aged horses belonging to John Skipton at Dennaby Close. He, like many Dalesmen, has grown attached to the majestic beasts that once toiled by his side and he has cared for them well beyond their working years. The character of John Skipton was based on a client of the Thirsk practice, John Sowerby, who typified the type of hard-working, decent farmer who had lived a life of hard graft labouring alongside men and horses rather than machines.

As James arrives, old Mr Skipton effortlessly hoists a pitchfork of hay over his shoulder and sets off at a brisk pace. James, lugging his wooden box of instruments, staggers across the large estate, far down to the river where two horses stand in the autumn sunshine.

'They're in a nice spot, Mr Skipton,' I said.

'Aye, they can keep cool in the hot weather and they've got the barn when winter comes.' John pointed to a low, thick-walled building with a single door. 'They can come and go as they please.'

The sound of his voice brought the horses out of the river at a stiff trot and as they came near you could see they really were old. The mare was a chestnut and the gelding was a light bay but their coats were so flecked with grey that they almost looked like roans. This was most pronounced on their faces where the sprinkling of white hairs, the sunken eyes and the deep cavity above the eyes gave them a truly venerable appearance.

For all that, they capered around John with a fair attempt at skittishness, stamping their feet, throwing their heads about, pushing his cap over his eyes with their muzzles.

'Get by, leave off!' he shouted. 'Daft awd beggars.' But he tugged absently at the mare's forelock and ran his hand briefly along the neck of the gelding.

'When did they last do any work?' I asked.

'Oh, about twelve years ago, I reckon.'

I stared at John. 'Twelve years! And have they been down here all that time?'

'Aye, just lakin' about down here, retired like. They've earned it an' all.' For a few moments he stood silent, shoulders hunched, hands deep in the pockets of his coat, then he spoke quietly as if to himself. 'They were two slaves when I was a slave.' He turned and looked at me and for a revealing moment I read in the pale blue eyes something of the agony and struggle he had shared with the animals.

'But twelve years! How old are they, anyway?'

John's mouth twisted up at one corner. 'Well, you're t'vet. You tell me.'

I stepped forward confidently, my mind buzzing with Galvayne's groove, shape of marks, degree of slope and the rest; I grasped the unprotesting upper lip of the mare and looked at her teeth.

'Good God!' I gasped. 'I've never seen anything like this.' The incisors were immensely long and projecting forward till they met at an angle of about forty-five degrees. There were no marks at all — they had long since gone.

I laughed and turned back to the old man. 'It's no good, I'd only be guessing. You'll have to tell me.'

'Well, she's about thirty and gelding's a year or two younger. She's had fifteen grand foals and never ailed owt except a bit of teeth trouble. We've had them rasped a time or two and it's time they were done again, I reckon. They're both losing ground and dropping bits of half-chewed hay from their mouths. Gelding's the worst — has a right job champin' his grub.'

I put my hand into the mare's mouth, grasped her tongue and pulled it out to one side. A quick exploration of the molars with my other hand revealed what I suspected: the outside edges of the upper teeth were overgrown and jagged and were irritating the cheeks while the inside edges of the lower molars were in a similar state and were slightly excoriating the tongue.

'I'll soon make her more comfortable, Mr Skipton. With those sharp edges rubbed off she'll be as good as new.' I got the rasp out of my vast box, held the tongue in one hand and worked the rough surface along the teeth, checking occasionally with my fingers till the points had been sufficiently reduced.

'That's about right,' I said after a few minutes. 'I don't want to make them too smooth or she won't be able to grind her food.'

John grunted. 'Good enough. Now have a look at t'other. There's summat far wrong with him.'

I had a feel at the gelding's teeth. 'Just the same as the mare. Soon put him right, too.'

But pushing at the rasp, I had an uncomfortable feeling that something was not quite right. The thing wouldn't go fully to the back of the mouth; something was stopping it. I stopped rasping and explored again, reaching with my fingers as far as I could. And I came upon something very strange, something which shouldn't have been there at all. It was like a great chunk of bone projecting down from the roof of the mouth.

It was time I had a proper look. I got out my pocket torch and shone it over the back of the tongue. It was easy to see the trouble now; the last upper molar was overlapping the lower one resulting in a gross overgrowth of the posterior border. The result was a sabre-like barb about three inches long stabbing down into the tender tissue of the gum.

That would have to come off — right now. My jauntiness vanished and I suppressed a shudder; it meant using the horrible shears — those great long-handled things with the screw operated by a crossbar. They gave me the willies because I am one of those people who can't bear to watch anybody blowing up a balloon and this was the same sort of thing only worse. You fastened the sharp blades of the shears on to the tooth and began to turn the bar slowly, slowly. Soon the tooth began to groan and creak under the tremendous leverage and you knew that any second it would break off and when it did it was like somebody letting off a rifle in your ear. That was when all hell usually broke loose but mercifully this was a quiet old horse and I wouldn't expect him to start dancing around on his hind legs. There was no pain for the horse because the overgrown part had no nerve supply — it was the noise that caused the trouble.

Returning to my crate I produced the dreadful instrument and with it a Haussman's gag which I inserted on the incisors and opened on its ratchet till the mouth gaped wide. Everything was easy to see then and, of course, there it was — a great prong at the other side of the mouth exactly like the first. Great, great, now I had two to chop off.

The old horse stood patiently, eyes almost closed, as though he had seen it all and nothing in the world was going to bother him. I went through the motions with my toes curling and when the sharp crack came, the white-bordered eyes opened wide, but only in mild surprise. He never even moved. When I did the other side he paid no attention at all; in fact, with the gag prising his jaws apart he looked exactly as though he was yawning with boredom.

As I bundled the tools away, John picked up the bony spicules from the grass and studied them with interest. 'Well, poor awd beggar. Good job I got you along, young man. Reckon he'll feel a lot better now.'

Alongside looking after heavy draught horses, many of which have seen years of farm labour, James and Siegfried also treat a variety of ponies, riding horses and thoroughbreds. Their real-life counterparts, Donald and Alf, were also frequently asked to judge at local horse shows, an unenviable task, often causing resentment among those without rosettes. On attending such events, Donald advised: 'Be friendly but firm. Thoroughly examine every animal . . . and keep the car engine running!'

Call-outs to racing stables were also part of the job: Yorkshire has had a long association with horse racing and there are still nine racecourses in the county, including in Thirsk itself. Of the two vets, Siegfried is the horse specialist just like Donald Sinclair who was the Thirsk Racecourse Veterinary Surgeon for over forty years.

Like Alf, James proves himself a very capable equine vet but visits to racing stables often prove challenging. The patients are valuable animals and James is always compared unfavourably with his senior partner Siegfried who is a well-known figure in the racing fraternity and very comfortable in that world. In *Vets Might Fly*, James must visit a racing stable where he is given a distinctly hostile reception.

Even now I can recall the glowering face of Ralph Beamish the racehorse trainer, as he watched me getting out of my car.

'Where's Mr Farnon?' he grunted.

My toes curled. I had heard that often enough, especially among the horse fraternity around Darrowby.

'I'm sorry, Mr Beamish, but he'll be away all day and I thought I'd better come along rather than leave it till tomorrow.'

He made no attempt to hide his disgust. He blew out his fat, purpled cheeks, dug his hands deep in his breeches pockets and looked at the sky with a martyred air.

'Well, come on, then.' He turned and stumped away on his short, thick legs towards one of the boxes which bordered the yard. I sighed inwardly as I followed him. Being an unhorsey vet in Yorkshire was a penance at times, especially in a racing stable like this which was an equine shrine. Siegfried, apart altogether from his intuitive skill, was able to talk the horse language. He could discuss effortlessly and at length the breeding and points of his patients; he rode, he hunted, he even looked the part with his long aristocratic face, clipped moustache and lean frame.

The trainers loved him and some, like Beamish, took it as a mortal insult when he failed to come in person to minister to their valuable charges.

James goes on to examine three horses, Mr Beamish dismissing all of his diagnoses. When James attempts to take the third horse's temperature, Mr Beamish stops Harry the stable lad lifting one of the horse's fore legs, enabling it to raise its two hind feet and thrust them into James, who sails backwards through the door. Stretched out on the concrete, he struggles for breath.

There was a moment when I was convinced I was going to die but at last a long wailing respiration came to my aid . . . Mr Beamish, on the other hand, showed no interest in my plight; he was anxiously examining the horse's hind feet one after the other. Obviously he was worried lest they have sustained some damage by coming in to contact with my nasty hard ribs.

Having recovered from the unfortunate incident, James is then alerted to another horse that has started to choke and wheeze alarmingly, as if on the verge of death. After a hasty examination, James diagnoses oedema of the larynx, caused by the allergic condition urticaria. He injects adrenaline into the jugular furrow and within fifteen minutes the filly is almost back to normal in what appears to be a miraculous recovery. Beamish looks on with amazement, while James walks back to his car 'riding on a pink cloud with all the tension and misery flowing from me in a joyful torrent'. It's an event that typifies how veterinary work can in a moment transition from despair to triumph, prompting Mr Beamish to put his face to the car window and utter: 'Mr Herriot, I've been thinking . . . you don't have to be a horsey man to cure horses, do you?'

The Darrowby practice also has a long line of assistants who share the load when it comes to horse work. In *Every Living Thing*, Siegfried, who has always embraced new ideas and contraptions, sends the latest assistant John Crooks out to test a new electrical treatment on a horse belonging to Darrowby's lord of the manor.

John had his own ideas about treatment and wasn't afraid to express them. One day Siegfried found the two of us in the operating room.

'I've been reading about this Inductotherm. Revolutionary new treatment for strained tendons in horses. You just wrap this electric cable round the leg for a certain time every day and the heat clears up the strain.'

I gave a non-committal grunt. I seldom had any ideas and, in fact, was constitutionally opposed to any change, any innovation. This trait, I knew, irritated my partner intensely so I remained silent.

John, however, spoke up. 'I've read about it, too, but I don't fancy it.'

'Why not?' Siegfried's eyebrows went up.

'Smacks of witchcraft to me,' John said.

'Oh, rubbish!' Siegfried frowned at him. 'I think it sounds perfectly rational. Anyway, I've ordered one of the things and I'd like to bet it'll be a big help to us.'

Siegfried was the horse specialist so I didn't argue, but I was very interested to see how the thing worked and we soon had the opportunity to find out. The Lord of the Manor of Darrowby, usually called the Squire, kept his horses in some stables at the foot of our street, a mere hundred yards away, and it seemed like fate when he reported a case of strained tendons.

Siegfried rubbed his hands. 'Just what we wanted. I've got to go over to Whitby to inspect a stallion, so I'll leave it to you to handle this case, John. I've got a feeling you'll think the treatment is a great advance.'

I know my partner was looking forward to saying 'I told you so' to the young man, but after a week of the treatment, John still wasn't impressed.

'I've been winding this thing round the horse's leg every day and hanging about for the required time, but I can't see any difference. I'm having another session this afternoon, but if it still isn't any better I'm going to suggest a return to the old treatment.'

Around five o'clock that afternoon, with heavy rain sweeping along on the wind, I was drawing up outside the surgery when I froze in my seat. I was looking out at something terrible. Several of the Squire's men were carrying a body down the street. It was John. As I got out of the car they bore him into the house and deposited him at the foot of the stairs. He seemed to be unconscious.

'What on earth's happened?' I gasped, looking down in horror at the form of my colleague draped over the lower steps.

'T'yoong man's electrocuted 'isself,' one of the men said.

'What!'

'Aye, it's right. He were soaked wi' rain and when 'e went to connect up the machine to the plug, 'e must have got his fingers on the live metal. He started to yell, but 'e couldn't let go. He went on yellin', but I were hangin' on to the horse's head and I couldn't help 'im. He sort of staggered about, like, and at t'finish he fell over the horse's hind leg and that broke 'is grip on the thing or I think he'd have been a goner!'

'My God! What can we do?' I turned to Helen who had appeared from the kitchen. 'Could you phone the doctor,' I cried. 'But wait a minute, I think he's coming round.'

John, stretched out on the stairs, had begun to stir, and as he peered up at us through half-closed eyes, an amazing flow of colourful language began to pour from him. He went on and on and on.

Helen stared at me, open-mouthed. 'Just listen to that! And he's such a nice young man, too!'

I could understand her astonishment, because John was an upright, very correct lad who, unlike most vets, did not swear. However, he had a wonderful store within him because some of the words were new even to me, which was surprising considering that I grew up in Glasgow.

After a while the torrent slowed down to an unintelligible mumble, and Siegfried, who had just come in from his round, began to ply him with neat gin which, I believe, is contraindicated in these cases.

There is no doubt that John could have lost his life but, mercifully, as the minutes passed he recovered steadily until he was able to sit up on the stairs. At last, as we adjured him to take it easy and stay where he was, he shook himself, got up, drew himself up to his considerable height and faced Siegfried.

'Mr Farnon,' he said with great dignity, 'if you ask me to operate that bloody apparatus again I shall tender my resignation.'

And so that was the end of the short career of the Inductotherm.

When horses provided the power on farms, veterinary surgeons were often required to investigate lameness, which nine times out of ten was caused by problems with the feet. They had the tools and training required to remove horseshoes, which they frequently did, although occasionally they had to call in the experts if a large horse was proving particularly troublesome.

In *Every Living Thing*, James calls in the local expert in the form of blacksmith Denny Boynton to help with Farmer Dickson's big Clydesdale who has 'gravel', a local term for infection of the foot.

'Right,' I said, 'let's have a look at it.' I ran my hand down the leg and was reaching for the foot when the horse whickered with anger, turned quickly and lashed out at me, catching me a glancing blow on the thigh.

'He can still kick with that bad foot, anyway,' I murmured.

The farmer took a firmer grip on the halter and braced his feet. 'Aye, he's a cheeky sod. Watch yourself. He's given me a clout or two.'

I tried again with the same result and, at the third attempt, after the flailing foot had narrowly missed me, the horse swung round and sent me crashing against the side of the box. As I got up and, grimly determined, had another go at reaching the foot, he reared round at me, brought a fore foot crashing on my shoulder, then tried to bite me.

The farmer was an elderly man, slightly built and he didn't look happy as he was dragged around by the plunging animal.

'Look,' I said, panting and rubbing my shoulder, 'we've got a bit of a problem. I have to bring Denny Boynton out to another gravelled horse near here this afternoon. We'll call in about two o'clock and treat this chap. He's got a shoe on, anyway, and it's a lot easier to do the job with a blacksmith.'

Farmer Hickson looked relieved. 'Aye, that'll be best. I could see we were goin' to have a bit of a rodeo!'

As I drove away, I mused on my relationship with Denny. He and I were old friends. He was a bit younger than I and accompanied me regularly on horse visits. In the fifties, the tractor had more or less taken over on the farms but some farmers still liked to keep a carthorse and took a pride in them. Most of them were big, docile animals and I had always had a strong empathy with them as they plodded patiently through their daily tasks, but that one back there was an exception.

Normally I would have taken the shoe off without much trouble before exploring the foot. All vets did courses in shoeing early in their education and I carried the tools with me, but I would have had some fun trying to do that with Hickson's animal. It was a job for Denny.

Denny Boynton is one of the few blacksmiths to have survived in the area. At one point nearly every village had a forge and a town like Darrowby would have had several. 'But with the disappearance of the draught horse,' as James Herriot puts it, 'they had just melted away. The men who had spent their lives in them for generations had gone and their work places which had echoed to the clatter of horses' feet and the clang of iron were deserted and silent.' Alf Wight based Denny on the Thirsk blacksmith Billy Keel, who was entirely fearless when it came to horses, even fierce stallions, but was bizarrely anxious around little dogs.

James heads to the Boynton smithy in Rolford village, where
Denny is found bent over the foot of a strapping hunter, his
father hammering the glowing metal on the anvil. James
explains he needs help with Hickson's horse, warning him of
his wildness, although knowing that Denny had dealt with
dangerous horses since childhood – 'I had seen him again and
again pushing big, explosive animals around effortlessly as
though they were kittens.' Denny is happy to help, untroubled
by what James has in store for him.

The farmer gripped the halter tightly and smiled uncertainly at
Denny as he came in. 'Watch 'im, lad. He's a funny sod.'

'Funny, is he?' The young man, hammer dangling from his
hand, grinned and stepped close to the horse, and the animal,
as though determined to prove the words, laid back his ears
and lashed out.

Denny avoided the flying foot with practised ease and gave
a demon king's laugh, throwing back his head. 'Aha! You're
like that, are ye? Right, ya bugger, we'll see!' Then he moved
in again. I don't know how he kept clear of the horse's repeated
attempts to injure him, but within a minute he caught the claw
of his hammer in the iron shoe in full flight and pulled it towards
him. 'OK, ya big bugger, I've got ye now, haven't I, eh?'

The horse, on three legs, made a few half-hearted attempts
to pull his foot away as Denny hung on and chattered at him
but it was clear that he realized that this new man was an
entirely different proposition. Denny, with the foot on his knee,
reached for his tools, muttering threats all the time and as I
watched unbelievingly, he knocked up the clenches, drew out
the nails with his pincers and removed the shoe. The horse,
motionless except for a quivering of the flanks, was totally
subjugated.

Denny displayed the sole for my inspection. 'Now, where d'you want me, Mr Herriot?' he asked.

I tapped along the sole until I found a place which seemed tender. To make sure, I squeezed at the place with the pincers and the animal flinched.

'That's the spot, Denny,' I said. 'There's a crack there.'

The young farrier began to cut away the horn with expert sweeps of his sharp knife. This was a job I had done so often by myself, but it was a joy to see an expert doing it. In no time at all he had followed the crack down and there was a hiss then a trickle of pus as he reached the site of the infection. It was one of the most satisfactory things in veterinary practice because, if the abscess is not evacuated, it causes the most acute agony for the animal. Sometimes the pus can work up under the wall of the hoof until it bursts out at the coronet after a long period of pain, and in other cases I have seen horses having to be put down when all attempts to relieve the infection have failed and the poor animal was laid groaning with a hugely swollen foot. Such memories from the old carthorse days always haunted me.

Nothing of that was going to happen this time and my relief was as strong as always. 'Thanks, Denny, that's great.' I administered antibiotic and anti-tetanus injections and said to the farmer, 'He'll soon be sound now, Mr Hickson.'

Then Denny and I set off for our next appointment. As we drove out of the yard I looked at the young blacksmith. 'Well, you certainly dealt with that wild horse. It was amazing how you quietened him.'

He leaned back in his seat, lit another cigarette and spoke lazily. 'Nobbut a bit daft, 'e was. It was nowt. There's lots like 'im — silly big bugger.'

EPILOGUE

The James Herriot books firmly established Alfred Wight as the world's most famous vet. It is in many ways an incongruous epithet for such a private man, who loved his family, profession and the peace of the Yorkshire countryside but nonetheless achieved worldwide success and fame by dint of writing such wonderful stories.

As with everything Alf Wight did in life, he put his heart and soul into every book he wrote, including the final volume in the series, *Every Living Thing*, which like all its predecessors shot into the bestseller lists when it was published in 1992. Sadly, there were two people central to the stories who didn't see its publication. Brian Nettleton, the inimitable 'vet with t' badger' who features so much in the final book as Calum Buchanan, was killed in a road accident in Chicago in the late seventies, twenty years after he left the Thirsk practice bound for Canada.

Brian Sinclair, who always rejoiced in his portrayal as the exuberant Tristan, had also died, of a heart attack in 1988. He continued to work for the Ministry of Agriculture in Leeds until his retirement in 1977. Thereafter, he and Alf would meet in Harrogate every Thursday afternoon. Sitting in a tea shop by the railway station, Brian would regale Alf with his latest stock of jokes and stories, the two roaring with laughter just as they had done all those years before in the sitting room of 23 Kirkgate. An extraordinary character in life and on the page, Brian was pivotal to the James Herriot stories. Donald was similarly deeply affected by the death of his younger brother, and Alf felt keenly the death of his much-treasured friend.

Alf and Donald remained practice partners and good friends, and Alf, Joan, Rosie and Jim were frequent guests at Donald and Audrey's nearby estate, Southwoods Hall. In his later years, Donald showed no signs of mellowing or slowing down. He continued to come up with various schemes to generate money for the Thirsk practice, including in 1975 setting up a dog trimming parlour, which lasted a matter of days after Donald attempted to trim a Pekinese with some horse clippers – the dog was fine but the owner promptly burst into tears when she saw the results. In 1981, at the age of sixty-six, Donald suffered a bad fracture of his leg after stepping in front of a speeding motorbike in the Thirsk market place. Impatient as ever, he discharged himself from hospital – no doubt to the relief of the sister there, who considered him the worst patient she'd ever had – and he carried on working at the practice, despite wearing a plaster cast for almost a year. It was only after he suffered a stroke in 1991, at the age of eighty, that Donald finally retired.

By the time *Every Living Thing* was published, Alf was also not in the best of health, having been diagnosed with prostate cancer at the end of 1991. The disease kept a low profile for two years, but from late 1993 his condition worsened, compounded by a bout of depression, which was thankfully short-lived. He bore his illness stoically and remained determinedly mobile until just before his death on 23 February 1995. Donald, already distressed by Alf's death, lost his wife Audrey three months later and not long after he was found in a coma having taken an overdose of barbiturate. Donald had always been a proponent of voluntary euthanasia so the manner of his death, although tragic, was perhaps not entirely surprising to those who knew him well.

Throughout Alf's illness, and brief episode of melancholy, he nonetheless gleaned satisfaction from the success of *Every Living Thing* and his days were undoubtedly lightened by the piles of fan mail that arrived at the house every day. Always a modest man, he never considered himself a great writer, just an average one who had got lucky, but his fans thought differently and when he died, tributes poured in from across the world – all of which illustrated the great respect there was for his books and the huge affection there was for him. One particular tribute written by Mary Ann Grossman for *The Chicago Tribune* seemed to capture the magic of his writing: his empathy for animals and humans, his respect for hard-working people and love of the land, as well as 'a glow of decency that makes people want to be better humans. I guess we'd call it spirituality these days, this proud belief of Herriot's that humans are linked to all animals whether they be the cows he helped birth or pampered pets like Tricki Woo, a lovable but overfed Pekinese.'

Alf's wife Joan supported her husband through his illness, as she had throughout their married lives together. He always thought the world of her and could never have achieved such success without her love and gentle encouragement, and she of course bore the brunt of his worsening illness and eventual death. After he died, her health slowly declined and four years later on 14 July 1999 she too passed away.

Like so many others, Joan is now immortalized in the James Herriot books, as the endearing and capable Helen, just as Donald, Brian and the array of Alf's friends, farming clients and the animals of North Yorkshire live on for ever in his writing. The people he met, the world in which he lived and the stories he crafted are still read by millions across the world. His legacy lives on, both in his books and screen adaptations, and in the Herriot name which remains a force for good. Alf's daughter Rosie has worked for many years with a local charity called Herriot Hospice Homecare. The James Herriot estate has also supported the Yorkshire Dales Millennium Trust, which looks after and preserves the Dales, including its barns, walls and hay meadows, and in Swaledale there is to be a newly planted woodland, bearing the plaque 'James Herriot Plantation'. Both of these charities have benefited enormously from the use of the James Herriot name and will make lasting contributions to the landscape and community that he loved.

In the days and weeks after Alf's death, Joan and the family also received thousands of letters of condolences from close friends, clients, former assistants, and fans across the world. Decades later, the family still receive letters from Herriot enthusiasts, and there is a common thread running through all of them. Many fans are keen to express the gratitude they feel to James Herriot, emphasizing how much they have been comforted by reading his books, which have, in their words, saved their lives. The warmth and decency in the stories, the humour, the depiction of a gentler time, and the affection and respect James Herriot has for humans and animals alike, act as a kind of balm for many readers and to all of us grappling with the complexities of life.

We welcome the change of pace his books bring and are

happy to be immersed in its world. Many years ago Phoebe Adams in an *Atlantic Monthly* review of the omnibus edition of the first two books described the James Herriot world as 'full of recalcitrant cows, sinister pigs, neurotic dogs, Yorkshire weather and pleasantly demented colleagues. It continues to be one of the funniest and most likeable books around' – a review that would have undoubtedly pleased Alf Wight and could summarize all eight books in the series. While many of the small farms and cobbled byres have gone, as have the hard-working farmers and animals depicted in the books, North Yorkshire and the Dales still retain their beauty – we too can breathe in that pure air, the scent of wildflowers carried on the breeze and enjoy the landscape that so enchanted the much-loved veterinary surgeon and author James Herriot.

Bibliography

Herriot, James, *If Only They Could Talk* (1970)

Herriot, James, *It Shouldn't Happen to a Vet* (1972)

Herriot, James, *Let Sleeping Vets Lie* (1973)

Herriot, James, *Vet in Harness* (1974)

Herriot, James, *Vets Might Fly* (1976)

Herriot, James, *Vet in a Spin* (1977)

Herriot, James, *The Lord God Made Them All* (1981)

Herriot, James, *Every Living Thing* (1992)

Herriot, James, *James Herriot's Yorkshire* (1993)

Herriot, James, *James Herriot's Dog Stories* (2020)

Reader's Digest Association, The, *The Best of James Herriot* (1982)

Wight, Jim, *The Real James Herriot: The Authorized Biography* (1999)

Acknowledgements

Our heartfelt thanks go to Emma Marriott for her invaluable contribution to this book. Emma immersed herself in the works of James Herriot; we believe that she came to love and appreciate our father's writings almost as much as we do.

We would also like to thank our agent, Georgia Glover. She has overseen this project with her customary calm and efficiency, safeguarding our best interests as she has done for many years.